CANCER FACTS

CANCER FACTS

A Concise Oncology Text

Edited by

James F. Bishop

Professor of Cancer Medicine
University of Sydney

and

Director
Sydney Cancer Centre
Australia

harwood academic publishers
Australia • Canada • China • France • Germany • India • Japan
Luxembourg • Malaysia • The Netherlands • Russia • Singapore • Switzerland

Amsteldijk 166
1st Floor
1079 LH Amsterdam
The Netherlands

British Library Cataloguing in Publication Data

A catalogue record for this book is available from the British Library.

ISBN 90-5702-470-5

Cover design by Kerry Klinner.

CONTENTS

PLATES

PREFACE

Cancer represents a series of diseases resulting from multiple genetic changes, often over years, leading to cell proliferation or immortalisation. The clinical consequence of this is a complex and dazzling array of clinical presentations which will result in the untimely death of 25–30% of the population.

As clinicians, we are obliged to suspect the cancer, quickly and accurately make a histological diagnosis, stage and understand the prognosis and have an optimal management plan. Most importantly, we should support the patient as a genuine friend and adviser, while they adjust to the diagnosis and prognosis, make decisions about treatment, goals and how to re-adjust their lives.

Oncology is a rapidly evolving field of medicine which has attracted a wealth of talent in epidemiology, molecular biology, statistics, clinical trial methodology, surgery, medical oncology, radiation oncology, palliative care and allied health areas. Clinically, most cancers need such a multi-disciplinary approach, involving all the treating medical specialties, allied health workers, psychologists and educators working together to do the best for the patient.

There have been important advances in molecular biology, new anti-cancer drugs, imaging and adjuvant therapy in recent years as a result of this large effort. The daily needs and poor outcome of many of our patients are a powerful motivation to provide the world's best, evidence-based treatment, and to discover new approaches as quickly as possible.

The objective of this text is to concisely document the most essential, highest priority information in cancer. Authors were chosen for their particular expertise in their field. Each author was given the challenge of only preparing the most important information in their field. The reading lists at the end of each chapter are not references for the text, but are designed to allow wider, more detailed reading on the essential elements of each chapter.

This text is designed to be read quickly and to be assimilated completely. Having read the text, you will have a comprehensive knowledge of cancer and its management. It should provide a solid framework on which to build additional knowledge. Since 20–30% of all patients have cancer and its various complications, an understanding of the essentials of oncology is obviously of utmost importance in medicine.

This text is dedicated, firstly, to my patients, who have taught me most of the essential elements of cancer management. Secondly, to my colleagues, peers and friends who taught me about a systematic, evidence-based approach to cancer. Finally, this text is dedicated to my wife Ruby, for enduring me while developing the text.

To the readers, I wish you well in your pursuit of knowledge in this most exciting but demanding field of medicine.

FOREWORD

Some areas of medicine seem to outstrip others in their rate of growth and complexity. Oncology fits into this category but it also has an impact on almost every other discipline in medicine. Thus not only the active oncologist but also almost every health practitioner needs access to up to date information in this rapidly advancing field. To further complicate the learning problem, oncology has emerged as a truly multi-disciplinary and teamwork-based field of medical practice incorporating many other disciplines and professionals ranging through surgery, basic science, social work, epidemiology, radiotherapy, nursing, etc.

The specialist oncologist will benefit from the perspective generated by this concise text written by 55 experts collated, integrated and edited by an outstanding authority with a broad view of the whole field. For the non-oncologist seeing patients with malignant disease the book provides an outstanding distilled overview of conventional contemporary wisdom and indicates where to find more in-depth discussion and analysis of debatable areas.

Evidence based medicine is correctly hailed as the essential basis of modern practice and is embraced by the authors contributing to this text. However there is an unarguable role for a concise statement of contemporary consensus views which also indicates extra sources of more detailed information. Another key element of modern practice is the fundamental role of patient education. Informed understanding can be easily distorted by inaccurate and misleading misinformation which again is less likely to occur if the health professional has access to a text such as this one. Inevitably any comprehensive book will not be totally 'cutting edge' at the time of publication but it can indicate the present trends, accepted consensus and point to expected innovations.

It has been an ambitious project requiring immense breadth and insight as well as very considerable energy. Inevitably there will be some disparities in quality and opinion but the overall structure appears to me to be admirable and it should rapidly find a valued place on the bookshelves and desks of trainees and practising health professionals.

JAMES R. LAWRENCE

CONTRIBUTORS

Stephen P. Ackland
Staff Specialist Medical Oncology
Department of Medical Oncology
Newcastle Mater Misericordiae Hospital
Newcastle, NSW, Australia

Michael Barton
Division of Radiation Oncology
Westmead Hospital, Sydney
NSW, Australia

Jane Beith
Staff Specialist Medical Oncology
Royal Prince Alfred Hospital, Sydney
NSW, Australia

James F. Bishop
Professor of Cancer Medicine
University of Sydney
Director, Sydney Cancer Centre
Royal Prince Alfred Hospital, Sydney
NSW, Australia

E. L. Bokey
Professor of Colon and Rectal Surgery
Head, Department of Surgery
University of Sydney
NSW, Australia

Michael Boyer
Staff Specialist and Head
Department of Medical Oncology
Royal Prince Alfred Hospital, Sydney
Senior Lecturer, University of Sydney
NSW, Australia

Ken F. Bradstock
Clinical Associate Professor, Senior Staff Specialist
Head, Bone Marrow Transplantation Service
Westmead Hospital, Sydney
NSW, Australia

Rhonda F. Brown
Senior Research Officer
Medical Psychology Unit
Royal Prince Alfred Hospital, Sydney
NSW, Australia

Robert C. Burton
Director, Anti-Cancer Council of Victoria,
Melbourne, VIC, Australia

Jonathan Carter
Head, Gynaecologic Oncology
King George V and Royal Prince Alfred Hospitals,
  Sydney
Senior Lecturer, Department of Obstetrics and
  Gynaecology
University of Sydney
NSW, Australia

Elizabeth Chua
Department of Endocrinology
University of Sydney
NSW, Australia

Stephen J Clarke
Senior Lecturer, University of Sydney
Staff Specialist Medical Oncology, Royal Prince
  Alfred Hospital, Sydney
Head, Medical Oncology, Concord Hospital
NSW, Australia

Alan Coates
Australian New Zealand Breast Cancer Trials
  Group
Staff Specialist Medical Oncology
Royal Prince Alfred Hospital, Sydney
Associate Professor, Department of Medicine,
  University of Sydney
NSW, Australia

Alison Davis
Senior Registrar in Oncology
Prince of Wales Hospital, Sydney
NSW, Australia

Brian D. Draganic
Senior Registrar
Colon and Rectal Surgery
Concord Hospital, Sydney
NSW, Australia

Stewart M. Dunn
Professor of Psychological Medicine
University of Sydney and Royal North Shore
  Hospital, Sydney
NSW, Australia

Michael P. N. Findlay
Staff Specialist Medical Oncology
Royal Prince Alfred Hospital, Sydney
Senior Lecturer, University of Sydney
NSW, Australia

Michael Friedlander
Director of Medical Oncology
Institute of Oncology, Prince of Wales Hospital,
  Sydney
Associate Professor of Medicine, University of
  NSW
NSW, Australia

Graham G. Giles
Director, Cancer Epidemiology
Anti-Cancer Council of Victoria
Melbourne, VIC, Australia

David Gillett
Associate Professor, University of Sydney
The Strathfield Breast Centre
Strathfield Private Hospital, Sydney
NSW, Australia

Afaf Girgis
Deputy Director, Cancer Education Research
  Program
New South Wales Cancer Council, Westmead
NSW, Australia

Paul Glare
Staff Specialist Physician in Palliative Medicine
Westmead Hospital, Sydney
NSW, Australia

Paul R. Harnett
Director, Department of Medical Oncology and
  Palliative Care
Division of Medicine
Westmead Hospital, Sydney
Clinical Associate Professor, University of Sydney
NSW, Australia

Harry J. Iland
Senior Staff Specialist, The Kanematsu
  Laboratories
Royal Prince Alfred Hospital, Sydney
Clinical Associate Professor
Department of Medicine
University of Sydney
NSW, Australia

Michael Jackson
Staff Specialist Radiation Oncology
Royal Prince Alfred Hospital, Sydney
NSW, Australia

Jeremy R. Jass
Professor of Anatomical Pathology
Head, Department of Pathology
Medical School
University of Queensland, Brisbane
Qld, Australia

Douglas E. Joshua
Clinical Professor in Medicine, University of
  Sydney
Director, Institute of Haematology
Royal Prince Alfred Hospital, Sydney
NSW, Australia

John H. Kearsley
Professor, Director, Division of Cancer Services
Cancer Care Centre
St George Hospital, Sydney
NSW, Australia

Richard F. Kefford
Professor of Medicine
Director, Westmead Institute for Cancer Research
Department of Medicine
Westmead Hospital, Sydney
University of Sydney at Westmead Hospital,
  Sydney
NSW, Australia

Mohamed H. Khadra
Senior Lecturer, The University of Sydney
Urological Surgeon, Royal Prince Alfred Hospital,
  Sydney
NSW, Australia

James R. Lawrence
Professor of Medicine, University of Sydney
Concord Repatriation General Hospital, Sydney
NSW, Australia

John A. Levi
Head, Department of Clinical Oncology
Royal North Shore Hospital, Sydney
Clinical Professor of Medicine, University of
  Sydney
NSW, Australia

J. Norelle Lickiss
Director of Palliative Care
Royal Prince Alfred Hospital, Sydney
Clinical Associate Professor, University of Sydney
Associate Professor, University of New South
  Wales
NSW, Australia

William H. McCarthy
Professor of Surgery (Melanoma and Skin
  Oncology), University of Sydney
Director, Sydney Melanoma Unit
Royal Prince Alfred Hospital, Sydney
NSW, Australia

Brian C. McCaughan
Department of Surgery
Royal Prince Alfred Hospital, Sydney
Clinical Associate Professor, University of Sydney
NSW, Australia

Jane P. Matthews
Director, Statistical Centre
Peter MacCallum Cancer Institute, Melbourne
Victoria, Australia

Andrew A. Miller
Senior Registrar, Cancer Care Centre
St George Hospital, Sydney
NSW, Australia

Sam Milliken
Senior Staff Specialist in Haematology and HIV
  Medicine
St Vincents Hospital and University of New South
  Wales, Sydney
NSW, Australia

Michael Millward
Consultant Medical Oncologist
Division of Haematology and Medical Oncology
Peter MacCallum Cancer Institute, Melbourne
VIC, Australia

David Mitchell
Staff Specialist, Centre for Infectious Diseases and
  Microbiology
Institute of Clinical Pathology and Medical
  Research
Westmead Hospital, Sydney
NSW, Australia

Peter Mollee
Haematology Registrar
Mater Hospital, Brisbane
Qld, Australia

Robin Murray
Consultant Endocrinologist and Head, Endocrine
  Department
Peter MacCallum Cancer Institute, Melbourne
VIC, Australia

Christopher J. O'Brien
Attending Surgeon Department of Head and Neck
  Surgery
Royal Prince Alfred Hospital, Sydney
Clinical Associate Professor of Surgery
Department of Surgery
University of Sydney
NSW, Australia

Ian N. Olver
Clinical Director
Royal Adelaide Hospital Cancer Centre, Adelaide
Director Medical Oncology
Clinical Associate Professor
University of Adelaide
SA, Australia

Susan C. Pendlebury
Staff Specialist
Radiation Oncology
Royal Prince Alfred Hospital, Sydney
NSW, Australia

Ronald Penny
Professor of Clinical Immunology
Directory, of the Centre of Immunology
St Vincents Hospital and University of New South
  Wales, Sydney
NSW, Australia

Kelly-Anne Phillips
Research Fellow in Cancer
Princess Margaret Hospital
Toronto, Canada

Danny Rischin
Consultant Medical Oncology
Division of Haematology and Medical Oncology
Peter MacCallum Cancer Institute, Melbourne
VIC, Australia

Laurent P. Rivory
Senior Scientist
Sydney Cancer Centre Pharmacology Laboratory
Royal Prince Alfred Hospital
Sydney, Australia

Robert W. Sanson-Fisher
Professor, Director National Cancer Control
  Initiative,
Melbourne, VIC, Australia

Paul D. Stalley
Department of Orthopaedic Surgery
Bone and Soft Tissue Sarcoma Unit
Royal Prince Alfred Hospital, Sydney
NSW, Australia

Graham Stevens
Department of Radiation Oncology
Royal Prince Alfred Hospital, Sydney
NSW, Australia

John F. Stewart
Director, Medical Oncology
Newcastle Mater Misericordiae Hospital,
  Newcastle
NSW, Australia

Martin Stockler
Senior Lecturer, Department of Medicine,
  University of Sydney
Coordinator of Medical Education, Royal Prince
  Alfred Hospital, Sydney
NSW, Australia

David W. Storey
Visiting Surgeon
Royal Prince Alfred Hospital, Sydney
NSW, Australia

Robert L. Sutherland
Professor, Director, Cancer Research Program
Garvan Institute of Medical Research, Sydney
St Vincent's Hospital,
University of New South Wales, Sydney
NSW, Australia

Andrea Szendroe
Senior Social Worker/Counsellor
Sydney Cancer Centre
Royal Prince Alfred Hospital, Sydney
NSW, Australia

Martin H. N. Tattersall
Professor of Cancer Medicine
University of Sydney
NSW, Australia

Kerry Taylor
Associate Professor of Medicine
Director of Haematology
Director, Division of Cancer Services
Mater Hospital, Brisbane
Qld, Australia

John F. Thompson
Associate Professor, Department of Surgery,
  University of Sydney
Deputy Director, The Sydney Melanoma Unit
Head, Department of Surgical Oncology
Royal Prince Alfred Hospital, Sydney
NSW, Australia

Guy C. Toner
Head, Medical Oncology Unit
Peter MacCallum Cancer Institute, Melbourne
Victoria, Australia

Ronald J. Trent
Head, Department of Molecular and Clinical
  Genetics
Royal Prince Alfred Hospital, Sydney
Professor of Molecular Genetics
University of Sydney
NSW, Australia

John R. Turtle
Professor of Medicine
Head, Department of Endocrinology
Royal Prince Alfred Hospital, Sydney
NSW, Australia

Keith Waters
Consultant Haematologist/Oncologist
Department of Haematology and Oncology
Royal Children's Hospital, Melbourne
Victoria, Australia

John E. L. Wong
Diplomate, American Board of Internal Medicine
Medical Oncology, Haematology
Associate Professor of Medicine
Chief, Department of Medical Oncology
National University Hospital, Singapore

Graham A. R. Young
Clinical Assoc Professor
Department of Medicine, University of Sydney
Deputy Director, The Kanematsu Laboratories
Royal Prince Alfred Hospital, Sydney
NSW, Australia

PART I

THE INCIDENCE AND AETIOLOGY OF CANCER

CHAPTER 1

CANCER INCIDENCE, MORTALITY AND TRENDS

Bruce K. Armstrong

WORLD BURDEN OF CANCER

It has been estimated that, in 1985, some 7.6 million cancers were diagnosed worldwide and about 5 million people died from cancer (Table 1.1)[1,2]. These estimates excluded non-melanocytic skin cancers, which added about an additional 2.75 million cases in that year[3]. The numbers of new cancers and deaths from cancer undoubtedly rose over the succeeding decade, because of population growth, increasing average age, and increasing incidence of some cancers. Deaths were projected to increase to about 5.7 million by 1990 and 7.1 million by the year 2000. If we assume constant incidence to mortality ratios, the number of new cases in the year 2000 (excluding nonmelanocytic skin cancers) will be about 10.6 million.

The major cancers divide, roughly, into two broad groups. Cancers that occur most frequently in wealthy countries (cancers of the colon and rectum, lung, melanoma of the skin, breast, corpus uteri, ovary, prostate, bladder, kidney and lymphoma and leukaemia) and those that occur most frequently in poor countries (cancers of the mouth and pharynx, oesophagus, stomach, liver and cervix). Some follow rather different geographical patterns, such as cancers of the pancreas (highest in Eastern Europe and East Asia, but high also in many wealthier parts of the world) and cancer of the larynx (high in Western Asia, the Middle East, and around the Mediterranean more generally, perhaps because of a local predilection for dark tobaccos). North America is distinguished by having the highest estimated, age standardised rates of most of the cancers associated with affluence. The low rates in Western Africa for many cancers are probably due to underestimation.

Australia and New Zealand together are in the top third of countries for 14 of the 18 cancers listed in Table 1.1, and in third place, to North America and Western Europe, for all cancers. They are second only to North America in their age-standardised incidence rates of cancers of the colon and rectum (may now be in first place[4]), prostate, lymphoma and leukaemia; and, of course, they are first in melanoma of the skin.

Table 1.1 Estimated world burden of cancer in 1985 with the rank position of Australia and New Zealand, among 24 regions of the world, with respect to estimated number of new cases of the major cancers in that year[1,2].

Site or type of cancer	Number of new cases	Number of deaths	Region of highest incidence	Region of lowest incidence	Rank position of Australia and New Zealand
Mouth and pharynx	412,400	262,400	Melanesia	Western Africa	8
Oesophagus	303,500	287,000	Southern Africa	Western Africa	15
Stomach	754,800	620,100	Eastern Asia	Northern Africa	16
Colon and rectum	677,500	394,100	North America	Western Africa	2
Liver	314,900	312,200	Eastern Asia	Central America	23
Pancreas	185,100	181,100	Eastern Europe	Melanesia	5
Larynx	141,200	72,600	Western Asia	Western Africa	14
Lung	895,800	785,400	North America	Western Africa	5
Melanoma of skin	91,700	31,100	Australia and New Zealand	Southern Asia	1
Breast	719,100	308,100	North America	Western Africa	3
Cervix	437,300	202,900	Southern Africa	Western Asia	20
Corpus uteri	140,000	54,900	North America	Southern Asia	6
Ovary	161,500	105,500	Northern Europe	Northern Africa	5
Prostate	291,200	148,600	North America	Eastern Asia	2
Bladder	243,100	112,700	North America	Melanesia	5
Kidney	126,500	73,900	North America	Middle Africa	4
Lymphoma	316,000	188,400	North America	Southern Asia	2
Leukaemia	216,000	177,900	North America	Middle Africa	2
All (except nonmelanocytic skin cancer)	7,623,600	5,100,200	North America	Western Africa	3

INCIDENCE OF AND MORTALITY FROM CANCER IN AUSTRALIA

The eighteen most prevalent types of cancer in Australia (excluding non-melanocytic skin cancers) are listed in Table 1.2. These cancers comprise about 86% of all internal cancers diagnosed in Australia. In 1989–90, colorectal cancer was the most numerous internal cancer. However, it has since been overtaken by prostate cancer[5]. Breast cancer is the most numerous cancer in Australian women. Some may find the numbers of non-Hodgkin's lymphomas unexpectedly large, now over 2 200 a year. They are, however, rising in incidence more rapidly than most other cancers, and for unknown reasons, thus their prominence will increase.

Non-melanocytic skin cancers are, of course, the most numerous cancers in Australia. They are not listed in Table 1.2 because cancer registries do not usually record them. It can be estimated, however, on the basis of a population survey of diagnosed skin cancer confirmed histopathologically, that there were about 126 000 basal cell and 49 000 squamous cell carcinomas of the skin diagnosed in 1990 in Australia[6]. This is about three times the number of all other cancers combined.

It may be estimated from the data in Table 1.2, that 1 in 2.8 men and 1 in 3.8 women will have been diagnosed with cancer (except non-melanocytic skin cancer) by 75 years of age, assuming survival to that age. Individually, the highest cumulative probabilities to age 75 are 1 in 13.6 for breast cancer in women (now probably about 1 in 11), 1 in 16.7 for lung cancer in men (now probably about 1 in 19), and 1 in 18.5 for cancers of the colon and rectum, and prostate in men (prostate is now probably about 1 in 8 due to the extremely high rate of increase since 1990).

TRENDS IN CANCER INCIDENCE

Age-standardised cancer incidence is currently rising in both sexes (Table 1.3), principally because of increasing rates of breast cancer in women and prostate cancer in men caused by screening. These screening-induced rises in incidence probably came to an end in about 1995 for breast cancer and 1994 for prostate cancer[7] and succeeding falls will bring them back towards, but probably never right down to, their pre-screening levels.

In addition to the rising incidence rates of non-Hodgkin's lymphomas and cancer of the kidney shown in Table 1.3, there are also important upward trends in cancers of the testis and thyroid that are currently unexplained[5]. Other trends can usually be explained in terms of trends in known risk factors (e.g. increased tobacco smoking by women in relation to cancer of the lung).

As shown in Table 1.3, the trends in cancer incidence in Australia are generally similar to those occurring in the United Kingdom and the United States[8]. There are, however, some notable differences. Incidence of cancer of the lip appears to be increasing in Australia, perhaps quite rapidly in women (although the numbers are small and the trend quite unstable), whereas it is falling in males in England, Scotland and the USA. Melanoma mortality, and possibly incidence, appears to have stopped rising in Australia whereas it is still going up in most other populations of European origin[5,9]. Bladder cancer incidence is clearly falling in Australia but it was not falling in the United Kingdom and the United States in the mid 1980s. However, the downturn in Australia only began in the mid 1980s[5].

SURVIVAL AFTER DIAGNOSIS OF CANCER

The only comprehensive, whole-population data available on survival after diagnosis of cancer in Australia are those published by the South Australian Cancer Registry[10]. Average five-year relative survival proportions (i.e. survival relative to that of the whole population of the same age and sex) for

Table 1.2 Average numbers of new cases of cancer (excluding nonmelanocytic skin cancer) diagnosed each year in Australia 1989–90 with average, age-standardised incidence and mortality rates[a] and cumulative incidence to 75 years of age[b].

Cancer site or type	New cases per year	Incidence[a] per 100,000		Cumulative incidence %[b]		Mortality[a] per 100,000	
		Males	Females	Males	Females	Males	Females
Lip	868	6.4	1.6	0.8	0.2	0.1	0.05
Head and neck	1,464	10.6	3.6	1.3	0.4	4.6	1.3
Oesophagus	760	4.7	1.9	0.6	0.2	4.8	1.6
Stomach	1,738	10.6	4.4	1.2	0.5	7.3	3.4
Colon and rectum	8,732	45.1	31.6	5.4	3.8	20.6	14.2
Pancreas	1,288	6.5	4.3	0.8	0.5	6.8	4.7
Lung	6,732	46.7	15.2	6.0	2.0	42.9	12.8
Melanoma of skin	5,712	31.0	25.0	3.4	2.6	5.0	2.5
Breast	7,066		65.6		7.3		20.8
Cervix	1,058		10.2		1.0		3.2
Other uterus	1,059		9.6		1.2		1.8
Ovary	984		8.9		1.0		5.8
Prostate	5,405	47.8		5.4		17.8	
Bladder	2,126	14.6	4.2	1.7	0.5	4.4	1.4
Kidney	1,456	8.6	5.0	1.0	0.6	3.8	2.0
Brain	1,066	6.2	4.7	0.6	0.5	5.0	3.6
Non-Hodgkin's lymphoma	2,227	12.2	8.2	1.4	2.4	6.0	3.8
Leukaemia	1,629	9.9	6.1	1.0	0.6	6.0	3.5
All (except nonmelanocytic skin cancers)	59,512	308.0	238.0	35.5	26.6	160.2	100.8

[a] Rates are per 100,000 person years and are standardised to the world population[4].
[b] Cumulative rates are from 0 to 74 years of age and assume survival to 75 years of age.

Table 1.3 Estimated or projected cancer incidence trends: a comparison of Australia, England and Scotland, and the white population of the USA[8,13].

Cancer site or type	Australia (change per year projected from 1982–1990 trend)		England and Scotland (trend 1973 to 1987)		USA (white) (trend 1973–1987)	
	Males	Females	Males	Females	Males	Females
Lip	+0.8%	+7.4%	Down	–	Down	–
Head and neck	+0.8%	+2.0%	Up	Variable	Up	Variable
Oesophagus	+1.5%	+3.0%	Up	Up	Up	Down
Stomach	-4.2%	-5.6%	Down	Down	Down	Down
Colon and rectum	+0.4%	-0.6%	Up	Down	Up	Variable
Pancreas	-2.4%	-1.3%	Down	Up	Down	Variable
Lung	-3.1%	+1.5%	Down	Up	Up	Up
Melanoma of skin	-0.5%	0.0%	Up	Up	Up	Up
Breast		+1.8%		Up		Up
Cervix		-1.2%		Up		Down
Other uterus		+0.1%		Up		Down
Ovary		-1.4%		Up		Down
Prostate	+17.5%		Up		Up	
Bladder	-4.0%	-1.6%	Up	Up	Up	Up
Kidney	+0.8%	+2.0%	Up	Up	Up	Up
Brain	+0.1%	+0.4%				
Non-Hodgkin's lymphoma	+2.6%	+0.6%	Up	Up	Up	Up
Leukaemia	+0.4%	+0.3%	Up	Up	Variable	Variable
All (except nonmelanocytic skin cancer)	+1.0%	+0.8%				

all cancers diagnosed in South Australia (excluding non-melanocytic skin cancers) in 1977 to 1994 were 46% in men and 57% in women. Generalising these figures, it can be said that about 52% of Australians diagnosed with an internal cancer, cancer of the lip or melanoma of the skin will not die from cancer over the following 5 years. Ninety percent of those who survive five years will avoid death from cancer altogether; at both 10 and 15 years after diagnosis, the relative survival proportions were 47%[10]. The most notable exception to this generality is breast cancer in which more than 20% of those who survive to five years will die from breast cancer over the next 10 years[10].

For all types of cancer for which comparisons could be made, 5-year relative survival in South Australia from cancers diagnosed in 1977–94 exceeded that in England from cancers diagnosed in 1983–85[11] (Table 1.4). However, the South Australian data related to people of all ages while the English data related only to people 15 years of age and over. As a result, comparisons of brain cancer and leukaemia at least will be biased in favour of South Australia (because of appreciable numbers of these cancers in children in whom survival is better). Inclusion of childhood cancers in the English figures increased the estimated 5-year relative survival to 17% for brain cancers and 25% for leukaemias; thus the English figures are still lower.

Table 1.4 Comparisons of estimated 5-year relative survival proportions after diagnosis of cancer in South Australia, England (people 15+ years of age), and the population covered by the SEER cancer registries in the USA[10–12]

Cancer site or type	South Australia 1977–94		England (age 15+) 1983–85		USA (SEER) 1986–92	
	Males	Females	Males	Females	Males	Females
Lip	96%	97%			95%	100%
Head and neck	43%[a]	54%[a]	40%	42%	49%	61%
Oesophagus	10%	18%	6%	8%	11%	10%
Stomach	22%	21%	10%	12%	18%	24%
Colon	52%	54%	39%	38%	63%	61%
Rectum	52%	56%	39%	40%	60%	60%
Pancreas	4%	3%	3%	3%	3%	4%
Lung	10%	13%	6%	6%	12%	16%
Melanoma of skin	86%	92%			84%	91%
Breast		76%		64%		84%
Cervix		72%		60%		69%
Corpus uteri		90%		72%		84%
Ovary		35%		29%		46%
Prostate	67%					87%
Bladder	64%	56%			84%	74%
Kidney	50%	46%	37%	36%	59%	58%
Brain	22%	24%	14%	13%	26%	28%
Non-Hodgkin's lymphoma	54%[a]	50%[a]			48%	56%
Leukaemia	46%	47%	22%	22%	43%	40%
All (except nonmelanocytic skin cancer)	46%	57%			54%	61%

[a] Estimated from site- or type-specific results reported by the South Australian Cancer Registry[10].

Comparisons with the SEER population in the United States, on the other hand, suggest generally higher relative survival rates in the USA than in South Australia[12] (Table 1.4). The SEER (Staging, Epidemiology and End Results) cancer registries cover about 10% of the total population of the USA. The population covered is fairly representative of the US except that blacks and rural residents are under-represented. The US survival rates were appreciably higher than the South Australian rates for cancers of the head and neck, colon and rectum, breast, ovary, prostate (probably because of greater screening 'lead time'), bladder and kidney. Part of each of these differences could be due to the later average diagnosis period covered by the US data (midpoint 1989) than the South Australian data (midpoint 1985). SEER data suggest that this difference in time could add about 4 percentage points to the 5-year relative survival rates.

REFERENCES

1. Parkin, D.M., Pisani, P. and Ferlay, J. (1993) Estimates of the worldwide incidence of eighteen major cancers in 1985. *Int J Cancer,* **54**, 594–606.
2. Parkin, D.M., Pisani, P. and Ferlay, J. (1993) Estimates of the worldwide mortality from eighteen major cancers in 1985. Implications for prevention and projections of future burden. *Int J Cancer,* **55**, 891–903.
3. Armstrong, B.K. and Kricker, A. (1995) Skin cancer. *Dermatologic Clinics,* **13**, 583–94.
4. Parkin, D.M., Whelan, S.L., Ferlay, J., Raymond, L. and Young, J. (1997) *Cancer Incidence in Five Continents Volume VII.* Lyon: International Agency for Research on Cancer.
5. Coates, M. and Armstrong, B. (1997) *Cancer in New South Wales Incidence and Mortality 1994.* Sydney: NSW Cancer Council.
6. Marks, R., Staples, M. and Giles, G.G. (1993) Trends in non-melanocytic skin cancer treated in Australia: the second national survey. *Int J Cancer,* **53**, 585–90.
7. South Australian Cancer Registry (1997) *Epidemiology of Cancer in South Australia. Incidence, mortality and survival 1977 to 1996, incidence and mortality 1996 analysed by type and geographical location - Twenty years of data.* Adelaide: South Australian Health Commission.
8. Coleman, M., Esteve, J. and Damiecki, P. (eds) (1993) *Trends in Cancer Incidence and Mortality.* Lyon: International Agency for Research on Cancer.
9. Giles, G.G., Armstrong, B.K., Burton, R.C., Staples, M.P. and Thursfield, V.J. (1996) Has mortality from melanoma stopped rising in Australia? Analysis of trends between 1931 and 1994. *BMJ,* **312**, 1121–5.
10. South Australian Cancer Registry (1996) *Epidemiology of Cancer in South Australia. Incidence, mortality and survival 1977 to 1995, incidence and mortality 1995 analysed by type and geographical location - nineteen years of data.* Adelaide: South Australian Health Commission.
11. Berrino, F., Sant, A., Verdecchia, R., Capocaccia, R., Hakulinen, T. and Esteve, J. (eds) (1995) *Survival of cancer patients in Europe: the EUROCARE study.* Lyon: International Agency for Research on Cancer.
12. Ries, L.A.G., Kosary, C.L., Hankey, B.F., Harras, A., Miller, B.A. and Edwards, B.K. (eds) (1996) *SEER Cancer Statistics Review, 1973–1993: Tables and Graphs.* Bethesda: National Cancer Institute.
13. Jelfs, P., Coates, M., Giles, G., Shugg, D., Threlfall, T., Roder, D., Ring, I., Shadbolt, B. and Condon, J. (1996) *Cancer in Australia 1989–1990 (with projections to 1995).* Canberra: Australian Institute of Health and Welfare.

CHAPTER 2

TUMOUR PATHOLOGY

Jeremy R. Jass

DIAGNOSIS OF CANCER

The diagnostic histopathologist participates at two steps in the management of a patient with cancer: (1) the handling of the initial biopsy specimen to derive a tissue diagnosis, and (2) the reporting of the definitive surgical specimen.

The tissue diagnosis of cancer is achieved by relatively non-invasive techniques such as fine needle aspiration or incisional biopsy. Formal diagnosis of cancer may not be straightforward as some benign lesions may closely mimic cancer.

Overdiagnosis of cancer is a potentially serious error because it may lead to unnecessary treatment. Wise pathologists err on the side of caution, knowing that underdiagnosis will be corrected by time and further investigation.

The diagnosis of cancer is achieved through the integration of clinical history, macroscopic appearance of tumour (including X-ray appearances in the case of bone and breast tumours) and microscopic examination. The histological features of malignancy include loss of normal architecture pattern, cytological changes including nuclear enlargement and hyperchromatism and, most importantly, invasion of normal tissue by malignant cells.

The entire process of receiving a biopsy, preparing slides for histological diagnosis and reporting back to the clinician takes at least 24 hours. The exercise is facilitated by the provision of relevant clinical details.

TYPING OF CANCER

When a certain diagnosis of cancer has been achieved, the tumour is classified according to its histogenesis. This is based on the type of tissue constituting the cancer.

The most common forms of malignancy are those derived from epithelial surfaces or glandular organs. They include adenocarcinoma (gland forming), squamous cell carcinoma and transitional cell carcinoma.

The other major types of cancer are leukaemia and lymphoma, malignant tumours of connective tissues (sarcoma), and germ cell tumours.

At this point the pathologist must also determine if the tumour is primary (arising at the site of biopsy) or secondary (when the biopsy specimen represents metastatic spread to a distant organ). The distinction between primary and secondary cancers is based on a knowledge of the types of primary and secondary cancers that may present in a particular organ. This is important because it is generally inappropriate to treat secondary cancer by radical surgery.

Some cancers are difficult to type because they are poorly differentiated. Electron microscopy and immunohistochemistry are valuable special techniques for typing poorly differentiated tumours. This is of considerable clinical importance because the various types of cancer are managed by different forms of therapy and have different outcomes. Most cancers can be typed successfully using modern histological techniques.

The second step of pathological management follows the surgical excision of the tumour. Since the entire primary lesion is usually included in such a specimen, the pathologist can provide more detailed information by studying material that is fully representative. Hopefully the diagnosis and type of malignancy will be confirmed. Two additional activities remain, namely the grading and staging of cancer. We can reiterate that the three forms of classification of a primary cancer encompass:

1. typing,
2. grading, and
3. staging.

GRADING OF CANCER

Grading is a measure of the biological aggressiveness of a cancer. Grading can be attempted in an incisional biopsy sample, but this is frequently non-representative and misses more aggressive subclones in the deeper parts of the lesion. However, the diagnosis of a high grade (aggressive) cancer in an incisional biopsy sample is useful since it is the worst area that determines prognosis and this fact may influence treatment options.

There are different approaches to grading. The first and most well known relates to how well differentiated the cancer is. A well-differentiated cancer resembles the tissue of origin and behaves less aggressively than a poorly differentiated cancer that shows little resemblance to the normal tissue counterpart. Moderately differentiated cancers are an intermediate category. Secondly, grading is achieved by studying the infiltrative pattern. A well-circumscribed or pushing type of growth has a better prognosis than a diffusely infiltrative pattern. A third feature is nuclear pleomorphism or the degree to which nuclei vary in size, shape and staining pattern. A fourth feature is the mitotic count providing an indication of the rate of proliferation. The final approach is an evaluation of lymphocytic infiltration indicating an immune response by the host that helps to reduce the aggression of the tumour.

These features may be more useful in some cancers than others. They may be combined in certain cancers to give an overall prognostic index (for example, differentiation, mitotic count and nuclear pleomorphism in breast cancer). Newer techniques, including flow cytometry, immunohistology and molecular biology, have rarely been found to add important and independent prognostic information, particularly after the stage has been established.

STAGING OF CANCER

Pathological staging defines the extent of spread within the surgical specimen, whereas clinicopathological staging goes beyond this and establishes the extent of spread within the patient. Clinicopathological staging provides more prognostic information than pathological staging, but requires close liaison between surgeon and pathologist. Each form of cancer is staged by a specific system (or systems) and these are described in detail elsewhere. The elements of staging include tumour size, extent of local spread, lymph node spread and distant spread. Vascular invasion (venous or lymphatic) is noted but does not feature in staging systems.

One crucial aspect of staging is establishing whether or not there is a clear margin of normal tissue around the cancer or conversely whether the surgeon has transected cancer of one at one or more points. The demonstration of tumour transection implies incomplete cancer excision and hence the presence of residual tumour in the patient. This is recognised by the symbol R1 in modified versions of the TNM staging system. Documentation of the completeness of excision by the pathologist represents a most important form of audit that is highly relevant to clinical outcome.

CONCLUSION

The histopathologist plays a fundamental role in the management of cancer by establishing the tissue diagnosis of malignancy and classifying the tumour in terms of type, grade and stage. Such reporting should occur in a standardised manner. Cancer classification influences management directly and provides information of prognostic importance.

REFERENCES

1. Fletcher, C.D.M. (1995) *Diagnostic Histopathology of Tumours*, vols 1 and 2. Edinburgh: Churchill Livingstone.

CHAPTER 3

MOLECULAR BASIS
OF CARCINOGENESIS

Robert L. Sutherland

INTRODUCTION

The essential characteristic of a cancer cell is a change in gene expression that confers a growth advantage over its normal cellular neighbours. This acquired property of uncontrolled growth is the hallmark of the broad spectrum of diseases collectively known as cancers.

Despite major differences in biological properties, diverse tissues of origin and distinct mechanisms for subverting growth control, all cancers share this basic underlying initiating event which is followed by further genetic changes that allow the cancer cells to invade into local tissues and eventually metastasise to distant sites. It is these latter events that often result in patient death, but these properties arise as a direct consequence of the initial genetic changes.

Thus, cancer is a genetic disease where mutations in DNA lead to consequent changes in gene expression which change the properties of the cell. The central question of what initiates this often fatal process is one that has attracted the attention of cancer researchers for decades, but it is only in the relatively recent past that significant progress has been made in identifying the molecular basis for the critical events in tumourigenesis.

MOLECULAR CHANGES ASSOCIATED WITH THE EVOLUTION OF CANCER

The culmination of recent research in molecular oncology is the appreciation that normal growth control is regulated by two distinctly different types of genes: oncogenes, whose normal cellular function is to accelerate cell proliferation, and tumour suppressor genes, which function to inhibit or retard cell proliferation.

Under normal physiological conditions the relationship between these two essentially opposing processes is delicately balanced such that cells undergo highly regulated patterns of proliferation and differentiation. In cancers, gain-of-function mutations in oncogenes or loss-of-function mutations in tumour suppressor genes disturb this balance in favour of cell proliferation.

Cancer development is associated with an accumulation of mutations in a number of different oncogenes and tumour suppressor genes in a multi-step process which differs markedly for different tumour types but is becoming increasingly well defined for several different human cancers. Each mutation results in further cellular proliferation associated with increased tumour size, increased genomic disorganisation and increased malignancy. Several such mutations are required to complete the process and the number appears to vary with different tumour types.

The common molecular mechanisms that underpin these changes involve point mutations, gene amplification, chromosomal translocations and rearrangements and gene truncations and deletions, the net result of which is dysregulated expression or function of the corresponding gene product. Identifying the particular oncogenes and tumour suppressor genes involved and determining the functional consequences of their aberrant expression is a major ongoing priority in cancer research with very significant advances occurring in recent times as detailed below.

ONCOGENES

The development of oncogene research evolved from the study of the biology of tumour viruses. These studies provided the initial concept of oncogenes or 'cancer causing genes' when it was demonstrated that cultured cells infected with these viruses acquired the characteristics of cancer cells. Further studies on the viral genome led to the discovery that retroviral oncogenes were derived from normal cellular genes or proto-oncogenes, i.e. during the evolution of the viral genome, genes were captured from the cellular host that conferred an evolutionary advantage.

From these observations evolved the central concept that the genome of higher vertebrates contains a multitude of proto-oncogenes that can be converted to oncogenes by specific genetic changes which lead to the production of abnormally active gene products, or to the inappropriate expression of the normal gene product. Although this model has now been supported for dozens of genes, only a minority of normal cellular genes are proto-oncogenes and thus have the potential to be oncogenic.

Perhaps not surprisingly in retrospect, it is now clear that oncogenes and their cellular antecedent proto-oncogenes play important functions in the control of normal cell proliferation and differentiation. Thus there is compelling evidence that proto-oncogenes encode: cellular receptors and their ligands; signalling molecules that transmit growth stimulatory signals from cell surface receptors to the cell nucleus; nuclear transcription factors that control rates of gene expression; and molecules intimately involved in the molecular control of cell cycle progression, cell proliferation, cell differentiation and apoptotic cell death.

Examples of oncogenes from these various functional classes of molecules are listed below.

- Growth factors — The c-*sis* oncogene encodes the B chain of the platelet derived growth factor, while the INT-2, KS3 and HST genes encode members of the fibroblast growth factor family.
- Receptors — Several oncogenes encode receptor tyrosine kinases, the cell surface receptors for a number of common cellular growth factors, e.g. a broad spectrum of tumours overexpress members of the c-*erb*B family including the epidermal growth factor receptor (c-*erb* B1) and the HER-2/*neu* oncogene or c-*erb* B2, while others overexpress *bek* and *flg*, two fibroblast growth factor receptors, *fms*, the receptor for colony stimulating factor-1, and *trk*, a nerve growth factor receptor.
- Signalling molecules — These fall into several classes including: membrane associated protein tyrosine kinases, e.g. *src* and *lck*; cytoplasmic protein tyrosine kinases, e.g. *fes* and *abl*; membrane

associated G proteins of which the *ras* family is prototypic; cytoplasmic protein serine-threonine kinases, e.g. *raf* and *mos*; and adaptor molecules in signalling pathways, e.g. *crk*.

- Transcription factors — The most studied of these is the *myc* family which plays a major role in the control of cell proliferation and cell death and components of the AP-1 transcription complex *fos* and *jun*. Additionally some members of the steroid hormone/thyroid hormone/retinoid family of ligand-activated nuclear transcription factors are implicated in some tumours most notably retinoic acid receptor and *erb*-A, a thyroid hormone receptor.

- Cell cycle regulators — these emerging families of oncogenes include the cyclins, particularly cyclins D1, D2 and E, and the cyclin-dependent kinases that control progression through key checkpoints in the cell cycle thus determining rates of cell proliferation.

TUMOUR SUPPRESSOR GENES

The early emphasis in the field of molecular oncology was on the dominant expression and action of cellular oncogenes that act as positive regulators of cell proliferation. Data from these studies were compatible with cytogenetic studies identifying amplification of specific loci within chromosomes and well-defined chromosomal translocations segregating with particular tumour types.

Such data, however, were incompatible with cell fusion experiments which demonstrated that the normal phenotype was dominant over the cancer phenotype when the two cell types were fused. This implied that the cancer cell was deficient in factors essential for normal function and that these could be supplied by the normal cell resulting in the suppression of the cancer phenotype.

The genes responsible for these traits were termed tumour suppressor genes and illustrated that recessive genetic damage could lead to the formation of cancer. Although the experimental approach employing cell hybrids identified the existence of such genes and their assignment to specific chromosomes, their identity ultimately came from studies of inherited cancers.

The vast majority of human cancers are sporadic, i.e. there is no evidence of inherited susceptibility and they arise as a consequence of mutations in somatic cells. Mutations inherited from parents through the germ cells contribute to a minority of human cancers, but these diseases have been extremely informative in identifying potential tumour suppressor genes. Studies of familial cancers have established genetic linkage to specific chromosomal sites which subsequently allowed the identification of the gene responsible through positional cloning.

It is now recognised that many of these genes also play a major role in the development of sporadic cancers where loss-of-function mutations occur in somatic cells. However, tumour development requires disruption of both copies of a tumour suppressor gene within the normal genome. If one disrupted copy is inherited from a parent, only one further disabling mutation is required, and cancer will occur at an earlier age.

The prototypic tumour suppressor gene is the retinoblastoma gene, RB, which in its mutated form is responsible for retinoblastoma in children and osteosarcoma later in life. Similarly, the APC gene is responsible for an inherited form of colon cancer, WT1 for Wilm's tumour of the kidney and BRCA1 and BRCA2 for breast cancer. In contrast to these genes, which result in tumours that are confined to specific tissue sites, the inherited mutant versions of the p53 found in families with Li-Fraumeni syndrome, and the INK4A/CDKN2 gene encoding the p16 cell cycle inhibitor, cause tumours at multiple sites.

Like oncogenes, tumour suppressor genes demonstrate a diversity of cellular functions, some of which fit into defined families of molecules, e.g. p53, RB and INK4A are all inhibitors of cell cycle progression, p53 and WT1 are transcription factors, while NF1 regulates signalling pathways including the *ras* pathway.

Finally, a more recently defined function of some tumour suppressor genes is in the control of DNA repair. Given that mutations are continuously occurring in DNA as a result of changes in the intracellular environment and to a lesser extent exposure to environmental carcinogens including ultraviolet radiation, the cell is equipped with enzymes that are able to repair these defects such that mutations do not accumulate. However, some inherited defects result in decreased function of such genes allowing mutations to accumulate with consequent effects on cancer incidence. To date several putative tumour suppressor genes, including those of the mismatch repair genes MLH1 and MSH2, and the ATM gene, are believed to contribute to tumourigenesis in this way.

IMPLICATIONS FOR CLINICAL MEDICINE

The recent rapid developments in our understanding of the molecular basis of cancer from studies on oncogenes and tumour suppressor genes have direct application to the clinical management of human cancer. Successful management is critically dependent on an accurate diagnosis and identification of markers of prognosis which aid in identifying the likely natural progression of the disease and probable response to different therapeutic modalities.

Knowledge of the role of the specific chromosomal translocations in leukaemias and lymphomas has led to the use of molecular hybridisation techniques to more accurately diagnose the disease. Similarly, poor prognosis groups within several tumour types can now be identified by amplification and/or overexpression of several oncogenes including members of the *myc*, *erb*B and cyclin families. Identification of point mutations in specific codons of the *ras* genes and p53 also identify subgroups with poor prognosis which in turn aids in the choice of therapy.

One of the more exciting recent developments relates to the ability to identify inherited mutations in genes like BRCA1 which predispose to the development of particular tumour types. Perhaps, more importantly, defining the molecular basis of cancer causation provides new and potentially more specific targets for therapeutic development and preventative intervention.

REFERENCES

Bishop, J.M. (1995) Cancer: The rise of the genetic paradigm. *Genes and Development,* 9, 1309–1315.

Haber, D. and Harlow, E. (1997) Tumour-suppressor genes: evolving definitions in the genomic age. *Nature Genetics,* 16, 320–322.

Hunter, T. (1997) Oncoprotein networks. *Cell,* 88, 333–346.

Knudson, A.G. (1993) Antioncogenes and human cancer. *Proc. Natl. Acad. Sci. USA,* 90, 10914–10921.

Vogelstein, B. and Kingler, K.W. (1993) The multistep nature of cancer. *Trends in Genetics,* 9, 138–141.

Weinberg, R.A. (1996) How cancer arises. *Scientific American,* 275, 62–70.

CHAPTER 4

GENETIC CHANGES IN CANCER

Ronald J. Trent

GENES INVOLVED IN THE DEVELOPMENT AND TREATMENT OF CANCER

Genetic (DNA) changes in cancer are found in a number of genes which include the following.

Proto-oncogenes

Proto-oncogenes play a role in normal cellular growth and differentiation. These genes encode for proteins which work via the signal transduction pathway, eg. *RAS*, *MYC* families. Mutated proto-oncogenes are called oncogenes and they express in a dominant fashion, i.e. only 1 of the 2 proto-oncogenes needs to be mutated, to produce a gain of function in terms of the cell's growth potential. Genetic mechanisms leading to oncogene transformation include: point mutations, deletions, chromosomal translocations and duplications[1].

Tumour Suppressor Genes

Tumour suppressor genes, on the other hand, play an inhibitory role in the normal cell's growth and differentiation, e.g. retinoblastoma *RB1* and *P53* genes. Loss of both *RB1* genes is required before tumours develop. The 2 hit model proposed by Knudson in the early 1970s explains how this can occur (see below). Loss of heterozygosity is one manifestation of tumour suppressor gene inactivation[1].

Cell Cycle Regulator Genes

Cell cycle genes, such as the D-type cyclins and their associated kinases and inhibitors, are more recent arrivals into the field of cancer genetics. The cell cycle is finely tuned by a number of inhibitory and stimulatory signals, perturbation of which can lead to cell dysfunction and ultimately cancer. Genes encoding cell cycle regulators are numerous, and mutations in these genes have been implicated in a range of human tumours such as breast, head and neck, oesophageal, hepatocellular, sarcomas, gliomas and familial melanoma[2].

Housekeeping Genes

Housekeeping genes include those involved in DNA repair, e.g. the mismatch repair genes which, when mutated, produce the autosomal dominantly inherited colon cancer known as HNPCC (hereditary nonpolyposis colon cancer)[1]. Another class of genes in the housekeeping category are those involved in cellular growth through their ability to program cells for death, i.e. apoptosis. An example of this is the *BCL2* proto-oncogene which overexpresses following a chromosomal translocation. This interferes with apoptosis which results in the development of a lymphoma (entry no. 151430 in ref. 3).

Metastasis Genes

The least well-described genetic changes in cancer are those involved in metastasis. The metastatic phenotype has been associated with both metastasis-producing genes and metastasis suppressor genes. An example of the latter is *KAI*1, which belongs to a structurally distinct family of cell surface glycoproteins involved in a range of biological functions including cellular adhesion, migration and invasiveness (entry no. 600623 in ref. 3).

Drug Resistance and Susceptibility Genes

Treatment failures in cancer occur for many reasons, e.g. the development of drug resistance. *MDR1* is the best characterised of the drug resistance genes. It encodes P-glycoprotein, which is involved in the extrusion of a variety of drugs across the plasma membrane (entry no. 171050 in ref. 3). Increased activity of *MDR1* will impair a drug's effectiveness.

In contrast, reduced levels of the thiopurine S-methyltransferase (TPMT) are found in approximately 10% of individuals who carry a deficiency in the gene encoding TPMT, with 1 in 300 having no activity as both alleles are mutated (i.e. autosomal recessive transmission). Since TPMT is involved in the inactivation of cytotoxics such as azathioprine and thioguanine, a deficiency of this enzyme can produce potentially fatal treatment complications, if drug doses are not reduced in those with reduced TPMT activity (entry no. 187680 in ref. 3).

HYPOTHESES EXPLAINING CANCER AS A FORM OF GENETIC DISEASE

The genetic component of a cancer comprises a wide spectrum, from a sporadic condition to one which follows the traditional mendelian inheritance pattern within a family. In between, are cases which demonstrate familial clustering that cannot be completely explicable by chance or environmental exposure.

The genetic risk for cancer is clearly seen in a number of disorders, many of which are rare and have an onset in childhood. These exhibit classical autosomal recessive or dominant inheritance patterns. For example, the gene for Bloom syndrome (*BLM*) (entry no. 210900 in ref. 3) was isolated in 1995 and shown to have helicase activity. Like many of the defects found in tumour suppressor genes, the majority of mutations in *BLM* produce truncated proteins, thereby leading to a loss of function. Because of its autosomal recessive mode of transmission, parental consanguinity becomes a risk factor in this rare condition.

Familial retinoblastoma develops from mutations in the tumour suppressor gene *RB1* and is transmitted as an autosomal dominant condition (entry no. 180200 in ref. 3). Early-onset tumours of retinal cells, which are usually bilateral, are produced. As a consequence of improved detection and more aggressive treatment, a cohort of affected children has survived to adult life. However, the underlying genetic mutation in *RB1*, which they continue to carry, can manifest as an increased predisposition to osteosarcoma.

A unifying hypothesis which explains the typical inheritance pattern in the genetic cancers described, as well as the less obvious mendelian transmission in related but sporadic tumours, was proposed by Knudson. This followed from his observations of the familial and sporadic forms of retinoblastoma. His statistical model proposed that 2 'hits' were required to develop a tumour. In the familial form, one hit (mutation) was inherited and so it was present in all cells. Therefore, it was relatively easy to undergo a second hit in a somatic cell, and so an early-onset tumour which was frequently bilateral developed. On the other hand, sporadic retinoblastoma occurred because the 2 distinct hits had to involve the same somatic cells. Because the probability of this occurring was considerably less, a unilateral tumour, of later-onset, was found in sporadic cases (ref. 1 and entry no. 180200 in ref. 3).

More recently, the 2 hit model has been expanded to include up to 4 hits. This follows from the proposition that genes can function as *gatekeepers* or *caretakers* (entry no. 600185 in ref. 3). Gate-keepers are genes that directly regulate tumour growth through effects on growth or apoptosis, e.g. *RB1* gene. Each cell has a very limited number of gatekeepers. Inactivation of both gatekeeper alleles produces a tissue-specific tumour. Caretaker genes, on the other hand, have a more subtle and indirect effect, since mutations in them enable the development and accumulation of other defects, which might involve a range of genes including gatekeepers and those required for DNA repair. Thus, a mutation in a caretaker gene, e.g. *BRCA1*, *BRCA2* and one of the HNPCC genes described earlier, is unlikely to be found in sporadic cancers because up to 4 hits would be required, i.e. 2 caretaker and 2 gatekeeper genes. The two breast cancer genes mentioned are considered examples of caretakers because of their complex functional domains.

EPIGENETIC MECHANISMS IN CANCER

An additional complexity in the inheritance of cancer or its predisposition, arises from epigenetic modifications. These are changes which affect the phenotype but not the genotype. The changes are inherited but they do not involve an alteration in the DNA. The best studied of these is genomic imprinting and its associated DNA methylation[4].

Imprinting refers to reversible modification of DNA that leads to differential expression of maternally and paternally transmitted DNA or homologous chromosomes. Thus, in some autosomal loci the contributions from both parents is not equal since the maternal or paternal allele is silenced, i.e. imprinted.

A model for imprinting in cancer is found in the paraganglioma tumour (entry no. 168000 in ref. 3). Molecular genetics studies have identified that there is a locus for this neoplasm on chromosome 11q. However, it is only the paternally transmitted gene which is functional, and so mutations will have a differential effect depending on their parent of origin, i.e. a mutated gene coming from the mother will not lead to tumour formation, but offspring with the mutant gene will be carriers.

Development of the tumour only occurs if transmission of the mutant gene has come from the father. As well as confusing the inheritance pattern so that clinically it would be difficult to reconcile with traditional mendelian inheritance, the presence of imprinting at a specific locus (and so the silencing of a parental allele) is an epigenetic change by which 1 of the 2 hits can be present without a specific mutational event having occurred.

Epigenetic changes also highlight the importance of carefully determining family histories in the investigation of patients with cancer.

CANCER GENETIC MODELS AND RESEARCH

P53 Gene and the Li-Fraumeni Syndrome

Although rare, this dominantly inherited cancer syndrome, caused by germline mutations in the *P53* gene, has provided a model to understand further the pathogenesis of genetic cancers. Unlike the truncating mutations which characterise the tumour suppressor genes, the majority of defects in *P53* involve missense changes, and so they can work either through loss of function, e.g. failure to arrest in G_1/S or G_2, or the defects involve a gain of function or a dominant-negative effect. In the latter, a mutant *P53* gene can be shown to inhibit its wild-type allele through oligomeric complexing between mutant and normal proteins.

Another observation to emerge from the Li-Fraumeni syndrome is that carriers of *P53* mutations appear to be more sensitive to damage from X irradiation. Hence, the potential in these circumstances to cause harm through the development of second malignancies has identified the necessity to re-evaluate some screening and therapeutic strategies if there are underlying *P53* mutations[1,5].

Genes and Breast Cancer

A genetic predisposition to breast cancer has long been recognised. A positive family history of breast cancer can increase the overall relative risk by 2–3 depending on the closeness of the relationship. It remains to be determined if known risk or protective factors operate equally in those with or without a positive family history.

What has emerged from genetic studies is that there are breast cancer genes, e.g. *BRCA1* and *BRCA2*, which are highly penetrant, but are relatively rare (with some population exceptions) in terms of their frequency. On the other hand, other genes, e.g. *ATM* (ataxia telangiectasia) and a polymorphism found with the *HRAS* gene, are of low penetrance but they are relatively common in the community. Thus, the genetic basis of breast cancer remains to be fully determined, a task which is made more difficult by the multiplicity of genes and the heterogeneity of mutations present[1,6].

Predictive Testing

Predictive testing can now be sought through DNA mutation analysis and has opened up a new potential approach to prevention, particularly in at-risk families. The clinical value of predictive testing has been shown in familial adenomatous polyposis through mutation analysis of the *APC* gene. However, there is general agreement that mutation testing in breast cancer should, for the present, be undertaken as part of a research protocol, so that the full implications of this development in management can be adequately evaluated[1,6].

REFERENCES

1. Ponder, B.A.J. (ed) (1994) Genetics of malignant disease. *British Medical Bulletin*, **50**, 517–752.
2. Hall, M. and Peters, G. (1996) Genetic alterations of cyclins, cyclin-dependent kinases and cdk inhibitors in human cancer. *Advances in Cancer Research*, **68**, 67–108.

3. Online Mendelian Inheritance in Man, OMIM™. Center for Medical Genetics, Johns Hopkins University (Baltimore, MD) and National Center for Biotechnology Information, National Library of Medicine (Bethesda MD), (1997). URL: http://www.ncbi.nlm.nih.gov/Omim/

4. Laird, P.W. and Jaenisch, R. (1996) The role of DNA methylation in cancer genetics and epigenetics. *Annual Review of Genetics,* 30, 441–64.

5. Varley, J.M., Evans, D.G.R. and Birch, J.M. (1997) Li-Fraumeni syndrome: A molecular and clinical review. *British Journal of Cancer,* 76, 1–14.

6. Greene, M..H. (1997) Genetics of breast cancer. *Mayo Clinic Proceedings*, 72, 54–65.

CHAPTER 5

GENETIC COUNSELLING
FOR CANCER RISK

Kelly-Anne Phillips

INTRODUCTION

Family history has long been recognised as an important risk factor for the majority of common cancers, such as breast, colon, ovarian and prostate cancer. More recently, studies of families with many individuals affected with malignancy have resulted in the identification and cloning of numerous cancer susceptibility genes (see Table 5.1).

These advances in the understanding of the molecular basis of hereditary cancer syndromes have had, and will continue to have, a significant impact on the management of individuals with a strong family history of cancer. In addition, many cancer susceptibility genes identified in 'cancer families' have subsequently yielded important information on the molecular pathogenesis of sporadic cancers. Examples are the involvement of the APC gene in sporadic colon cancer, and the RB1 gene in sporadic retinoblastoma.

The increased focus on inherited cancer syndromes has prompted the development of multidisciplinary familial cancer risk clinics. In such clinics comprehensive genetic counselling is tailored to the needs of individual participants. Genetic and other risk factors, options for genetic testing and their limitations, lifestyle and medical management, and psycho-social issues are addressed, with an emphasis on participation in research protocols where appropriate.

IDENTIFICATION OF INDIVIDUALS AT INCREASED RISK FOR HEREDITARY CANCER

The compilation of a detailed family history is essential, and should include at least all first- and second-degree relatives of the proband. When evaluating a pedigree, the number of affected individuals is clearly important. However, there are several other cardinal features of high risk families[1]. These include:

- unusually early age of cancer onset, e.g. breast cancer before age 40;

- bilateral or multifocal cancer, e.g. bilateral breast cancer, multifocal renal carcinoma;
- multiple separate primary cancer sites in an individual;
- rare cancer types, e.g. male breast cancer, phaeochromocytoma;
- clustering of cancers within a family, consistent with a syndrome, e.g. a family with colon, ovarian and endometrial cancers, suggests HNPCC;
- associated physical stigmata, eg. café au lait spots and neurofibromas in neurofibromatosis.
- specific ethnic background known to have an increased incidence of 'cancer gene' mutations, e.g. Ashkenazi Jews (BRCA1 and BRCA2), Icelandic kindreds (BRCA2);
- Mendelian pattern of inheritance, although there can be marked variability in gene penetrance.

Family size and the age and sex distribution within the family are also of relevance when assessing genetic risk. For example, the significance of three cases of breast cancer in a small family with only a few women may be much greater than the same family history in a pedigree with many post-menopausal women.

Pathologic confirmation of the primary site of cancer cases reported in the family should be sought, if possible, as discrepancies may dramatically alter the assessment of the pedigree. For example, when a family with multiple cases of breast cancer describes an individual with 'stomach cancer', the pathology report may in fact reveal primary ovarian cancer. This increases the likelihood of hereditary breast-ovarian syndrome.

COMPREHENSIVE COUNSELLING

Accurate genetic counselling for cancer may be facilitated by genetic testing. Unlike other medical tests, genetic tests provide information not only about the individual being tested but also about that individual's parents, siblings and children. Testing is only performed after comprehensive counselling, which provides information regarding:

- the specific test being performed and its technical accuracy;
- the possibility that the test will not be informative, e.g. single base pair change of uncertain significance in the gene of interest (i.e. polymorphism versus a mutation associated with disease);
- implications of a positive and negative result;
- risks of psychological distress;
- risks of insurance or employer discrimination;
- issues of confidentiality;
- risk of passing the mutation to children;
- options and limitations of medical surveillance and interventions following testing;
- options for risk estimation without genetic testing[2].

RECOMMENDATIONS FOR GENETIC TESTING

Recommendations for genetic testing will likely change over time as more information becomes available. Currently none of the available tests for cancer susceptibility genes is appropriate for screening of asymptomatic individuals in the general population. The American Society of Clinical Oncology

Table 5.1 Selected inherited cancer predisposition syndromes

Syndrome	Characteristic tumour types[a]	Gene with germline mutation	Gene type	Mode of inheritance
Hereditary breast/ovarian cancer	Breast carcinoma Ovarian carcinoma	BRCA1/BRCA2	Tumour suppressor	Dominant
Familial adenomatous polyposis (FAP)	Colon carcinoma Upper GI carcinomas	APC	Tumour suppressor	Dominant
Turcot's syndrome	Colon carcinoma Cerebellar medulloblastoma			
Gardner syndrome	Colon carcinoma Osteoma, Desmoid tumours			
Hereditary non-polyposis colorectal carcinoma (HNPCC, Lynch Syndromes)	Colon carcinoma Endometrial carcinoma Ovarian carcinoma Gastric carcinoma Small bowel carcinomas Carcinoma of ureter or renal pelvis Pancreatic carcinoma	MSH2/MLH1 PMS1/PMS2	Mismatch repair	Dominant
Li-Fraumeni	Sarcomas, Breast carcinoma Brain tumours, Leukaemia Adrenocortical carcinoma	p53	Tumour suppressor	Dominant
Familial medullary thyroid tumour	Medullary thyroid carcinoma	RET	Protooncogene	Dominant
Multiple endocrine neoplasia type 2	Medullary thyroid carcinoma Phaeochromocytoma			
Hereditary retinoblastoma	Retinoblastoma, Osteosarcoma	RB1	Tumour suppressor	Dominant
Von Hippel-Lindau	CNS hemangioblastomas Renal cell carcinoma Phaeochromocytomas	VHL	Tumour suppressor	Dominant

Table 5.1 Continued

Syndrome	Characteristic tumour types[a]	Gene with germline mutation	Gene type	Mode of inheritance
Hereditary melanoma	Malignant melanoma	p16/CDK4	Tumour suppressor	Dominant
Gorlin syndrome	Basal Cell carcinomas Brain tumours	PTCH	Tumour suppressor	Dominant
Hereditary Wilms' tumour	Nephroblastoma, Hepatoblastoma	WT1	Tumour suppressor	Dominant
Hereditary prostate cancer	Prostate cancer	HPC1 linked to Chr 1q		
Bloom syndrome	Leukaemia Carcinoma of the tongue Esophageal carcinoma Wilms' tumour, Colon carcinoma	BLM	Putative DNA helicase	Recessive
Fanconi anaemia	Leukaemia Esophageal carcinoma Skin carcinoma, Hepatoma	FAA FAC	DNA repair	Recessive

[a] Does not include all reported associations.

Source: Mulcahy, G.M., Goggins, M., Willis, D., Decker, R.A., Luce, M.C. and Parsons, R. (1997) Pathology and genetic testing. *Cancer,* **80(3)**, 636–648.

has, however, defined two categories for which testing for germline mutations may be acceptable outside of research protocols[3]:

1. Families with well-defined hereditary cancer syndromes, for which either a positive or negative result will change medical management, and for whom genetic testing may be considered part of routine medical care. For example:

    (a) Familial adenomatous polyposis

        (i)   FAP mutation positive: consider prophylactic colectomy.

        (ii) FAP mutation negative: cease regular sigmoidoscopic surveillance for polyps.

    (b) Multiple Endocrine Neoplasia Type 2a

        (i)   RET mutation positive: consider prophylactic thyroidectomy.

2. Individuals within a hereditary cancer syndrome family, where a negative result (in the context of a known mutation within the family) may confer psychological advantage, and where there is a presumed, but not yet proven, benefit of medical intervention for gene carriers. For example:

    (a) Hereditary breast-ovarian syndrome

        (i)   BRCA1 positive: consider ovarian screening or prophylactic oophorectomy and increased mammographic screening, or mastectomy.

ASSESSMENT AND DISCLOSURE OF CANCER RISK

Assessment of cancer risk involves using available epidemiological data to quantify the statistical probability of an individual developing cancer. It may or may not include testing for cancer predisposition genes.

At the time of disclosure of the risk estimate, the information must be conveyed in a way that is sensitive to the individual's personality, cognitive level and pre-existing perceptions of risk. The information may be described in a variety of ways, to account for different preferences for information processing between individuals. For example, descriptive (high, moderate, etc.) versus percentage lifetime risk, versus relative risk when compared with the general population.

The intrinsic uncertainty of risk estimates is communicated, and individuals given low risk estimates are informed of their continued risk for sporadic cancers and the importance of continuing routine population-based cancer screening (e.g. mammography, pap smears)[3].

RISK MANAGEMENT

At the present time there are insufficient data regarding the effectiveness of most intervention strategies for individuals determined to be at higher risk of cancer because of family history, indicating the importance of including these patients in research protocols where possible. Potential options vary depending on the cancer syndrome, but in general they may include:

- lifestyle changes, e.g. dietary changes, cessation of smoking;
- chemoprevention trials, e.g. Tamoxifen, non-steroidal anti-inflammatory drugs, vitamins, retinoids;
- cancer screening, e.g. mammography, transvaginal ultrasound, CA-125, PSA; and
- prophylactic surgery.

CONCLUSION

The potential opportunity for early detection or prevention of cancer in individuals at increased risk because of genetic factors should not be neglected. Physicians should be familiar with the features of hereditary cancer syndromes, and obtaining a family history should be a routine part of the initial oncology consultation. Ideally, individuals suspected to be at increased genetic risk should be offered a referral to a familial cancer risk clinic for risk assessment, genetic counselling and risk management recommendations.

REFERENCES

1. Lynch, H.T., Fusaro, R.M., Lemon, S.J., Smyrk, T. and Lynch, J. (1997) Survey of cancer genetics. *Cancer,* **80**(3), 523–32
2. Offit, K., Biesecker, B., Burt, R.W., Clayton, E.W., Garber, J., Kahn, M.J.E., et al. (1996) Statement of the American Society of Clinical Oncology: Genetic testing for cancer susceptibility. *J Clin Oncol,* 14,1730–6
3. Bottorff, J.L., Ratner, P.A., Johnson, J.L., Lovato, C.Y. and Joab, S.A. (1996) Uncertainties and challenges: communicating risk in the context of familial cancer. A report to the National Cancer Institute of Canada. School of Nursing, University of British Columbia.

CHAPTER 6

CANCER PREVENTION, SCREENING AND EARLY DETECTION

Robert C. Burton and Graham G. Giles

CAUSES OF CANCER

Of the 9–10 million new cancers diagnosed around the globe each year, 53% could be prevented given our current knowledge.

Tobacco

For example, one-third of all fatal male cancers in most developed and many developing countries are tobacco related. The scale of the tobacco problem is enormous. The World Health Organization (WHO) estimates that there are 1.1 billion smokers in the world: 42% of men and 24% of women smoke in developed countries, and 48% of men and 7% of women in the developing countries. Tobacco is estimated to be responsible for about 2.6% of the total world burden of death and disease; this is projected to increase to 9% by the year 2020. For every 1,000 tonnes of tobacco produced, about 1,000 people will eventually die, and an estimated 250 million humans will perish in this way between 1965 and 2025.

Diet

Doll and Peto (1981) have estimated that diet is as important in cancer causation as smoking. Total dietary intake of fat is positively associated with mortality from cancers of the colon, breast, endometrium, ovary and prostate.

  Dietary intake of fruit and vegetables is found to be protective in most case control and cohort studies in cancers of the lung, larynx, oro-pharynx, oesophagus, stomach, colon and rectum, and pancreas. In respect of colorectal cancer, dietary fibre and vitamin C have consistently been shown to be protective. These findings have led to large intervention studies on diet for the prevention of colorectal cancer, which are now in progress.

Infection

It is likely that as much as 20% of the global burden of cancer is caused by infection, and is thus susceptible to prevention by vaccination. Over 700,000 cancers of the stomach and 400,000 cancers of the cervix are diagnosed annually worldwide. Most of these would vanish if infection with Helicobacter-pylori, in the case of stomach cancer, and human papilloma virus, in the case of cancer of the cervix, could be prevented. Primary liver cancer, the seventh commonest cancer in developing countries, is largely caused by the hepatitis B virus for which a vaccination program is now in progress.

Solar Radiation

Each year, more than a million new skin cancers are caused by solar radiation in white populations. Australia is notable for its high incidence of skin cancer with over 1,000 per 100,000 person years in 1995. A significant, but unknown, proportion is attributable to occupational exposure to ultraviolet radiation.

Other Causes

Whilst, tobacco, diet, viruses, and ultraviolet light are major causes of cancer, it is estimated that approximately 5% of cancers in the developed world are due to occupational exposures. Over 300 chemicals have now been confirmed as carcinogens by the International Agency for Research on Cancer. Very small percentages of cancer are attributed to ionizing radiation, iatrogenic causes and other possible risks such as environmental pollution.

CANCER PREVENTION AND EARLY DETECTION

Chemo-prevention

Chemo-prevention of cancer is a recent addition to strategies of cancer control. It has been estimated that the regular use of non-steroidal anti-inflammatory drugs (NSAIDs) has the potential to prevent 40–50% of all deaths from colorectal cancer (O'Brien, 1996). Tamoxifen, an anti-oestrogen agent, is currently under trial for the prevention of breast cancer in women at more than normal risk, and a number of vitamins have been trialled as cancer prevention agents in high risk population groups.

Behavioural Change

Most prevention strategies rely on behavioural change by individuals and populations, as do many of the strategies for screening and early diagnosis. Behaviour change has not been easy to obtain, although the reduction in male smoking rates in Australia from an estimated high of 70% at the end of 1960s to 25% in the 1990s is a notable success. The potential for prevention strategies to change the face of fatal cancer in Australia can well be appreciated when one considers cancer mortality trends since 1950, and the numbers of new cases and deaths in 1995 illustrated in Figures 6.1 and 6.2.

Cancer Screening

Screening and early detection of cancer are terms which are often confused. Early detection means detecting a cancer at a stage when it is still curable. Screening is 'the examination of asymptomatic people in order to classify them as likely, or unlikely, to have the disease that is the object of screening' (Morrison, 1992).

The aim of screening is to reduce mortality, and perhaps morbidity, from the disease. For a screening program to be effective it must adhere to the following criteria:

- The screening test must be valid and reliable.

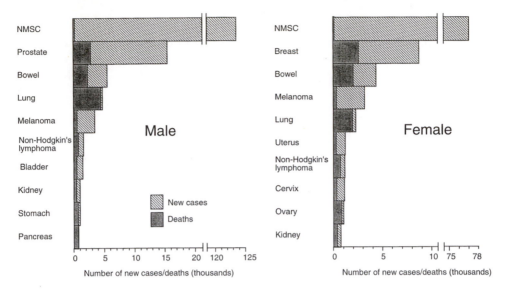

Figure 6.1 Cancer incidence and mortality in Australia 1995: Leading sites of new cancers and cancer deaths

Source: Jelfs, P., Coates, M., Giles, G. et al, (1996) *Cancer in Australia 1989–1990* (with projections to 1995). Australian Institute of Health and Welfare and the Australasian Association of Cancer Registries, Canberra; Australian Institute of Health and Welfare.

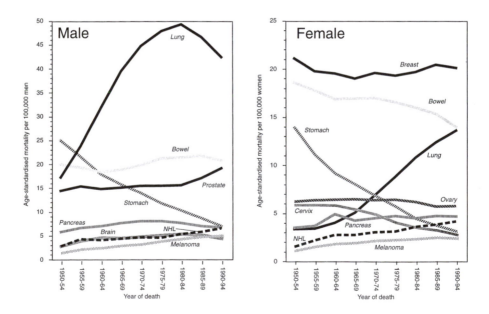

Figure 6.2 Australian cancer mortality 1950–1994: Leading causes of death for men and women

Source: Giles, G. and Thursfield, V. (1997) Trends in cancer mortality, Australian 1910–1994. Canstat No. 24. Melbourne: Anti-Cancer Council of Victoria.

- The natural history of the disease should be understood.
- The screening test must detect disease at an earlier stage than it would be detected if people presented with symptoms.
- Effective treatment should be available.
- Treatment at an earlier stage must confer advantage over treatment at a later stage.
- The program should be acceptable to the 'target' population and the program must be cost effective.

A screening program is likely to be most effective when there is an organised approach to screening. In this situation there is a uniform policy regarding:

- the target population (the mechanisms of recruitment of the target group)
- adequate facilitates
- agreed mechanisms for the interpretation of tests
- agreed follow-up of positive screening tests

Opportunistic screening is screening that occurs in an ad hoc way, such as a general practitioner recommending a PSA test; it is unlikely to produce reductions in mortality from the screened disease.

Mammographic Screening

Population-based screening is expensive and it is now expected that large randomised controlled trials (RCTs) must show that screening reduces mortality before new programs can be introduced. Thus, three RCTs of mammography in the diagnosis of asymptomatic breast cancer had been reported in the mid 1980s before the decision was taken to introduce a national screening program for Australian women aged 50 to 69. A fully functioning national program, screening 70% of all eligible 50–69 year old women should be in place before the year 2000. However, we do not expect mammographic screening to reduce breast cancer mortality in Australia until the end of the century.

Bowel Cancer Screening

There is a long lead time for introducing evidence-based screening. Three RCTs of faecal occult blood screening for bowel cancer were begun in the mid 1970s to early 1980s and the results are only just to hand, each revealing a reduction in cause-specific mortality. A bowel cancer screening program for all Australians aged over 50 is likely to be introduced in the near future. It will take some years to fully implement, and mortality reductions will take at least a decade to appear.

Cervical Cancer Screening

The current Pap screen program was not based on RCTs. However, case-control studies show that two to three yearly Pap smears can reduce mortality from cervical cancer by over 90%. In the near future, we should have a HPV vaccine to prevent carcinoma of the cervix, and so by the end of the next century it should have disappeared in the same way that polio, measles and other infectious diseases have been controlled. There are, however, generations of women infected with HPV and, therefore, at risk of cervix cancer, so the national Pap screen program will be needed for at least another 50 years.

Early Detection

Population publicity campaigns to detect cancer early, such as the seven early warning signs of cancer, have been undertaken in Australia since the 1960s. Biologically, cancers produce symptoms in the last quarter of their life span, so early clinical diagnosis can rarely be an early biological diagnosis. Nonetheless, reporting any change in a mole, one of the seven signs, can lead to an earlier diagnosis of melanoma. The prognosis of melanoma is related to its thickness and those less than 0.76 mm virtually never kill. The proportion of melanomas less than 0.76 mm has increased to over 50% in Australia in recent decades, leading to a fall in melanoma mortality in women and a plateauing of melanoma mortality in men.

In the UK and the USA breast cancer mortality is now falling. Over the last two decades the median diameter of breast cancers diagnosed in symptomatic women has more than halved. The most likely explanation for the current downturn in mortality is that women themselves have detected their breast cancers significantly earlier. Therefore, earlier symptomatic diagnosis of melanoma and breast cancer has been shown to effect mortality, and one would predict that organised screening for these cancers would build on that success.

CONCLUSION

When we know the cause of a cancer, then prevention should be our primary strategy. When we do not know the cause of a cancer, or have not identified significant avoidable risk factors, then early detection and screening are our fall-back positions. Prostate cancer stands out in this regard, since we simply do not know its cause(s), and we do not have a screening test which has been shown to reduce mortality. In this situation, screening for prostate cancer using the PSA test, combined with the high morbidity associated with available treatments, might do more harm than good.

The current genetic and molecular biology revolution holds great promise for improved early detection and treatment strategies for cancer, together with much more accurate prediction of prognosis at the time of diagnosis. Today, the emphasis for some cancers must be on fundamental biomedical research, for others on RCTs of early detection and treatment. However, all aspects of the prevention, screening and early detection of cancer require increased commitment to biological, epidemiological, behavioural and educational research.

REFERENCES

Coldritz, G., DeJong, W., Hunter, D., Trichopoulos, D. and Willett, W. (eds) (1996) Harvard Report on Cancer Prevention. *Cancer Causes and Control,* 7 (suppl. 1), 1–59.

Doll, R. and Peto, R. (1981) The causes of cancer: quantitative estimates of avoidable risks of cancer in the United States today. *JNCI,* **66**,1191–308.

Morrison, A.S. (1992) *Screening in Chronic Disease.* New York: Oxford University Press.

O'Brien, P. (1996) The use of NSAIDs in chemoprevention of colorectal cancer. *Cancer Forum,* **20**, 281–4.

Trichopoulos, D. and Willett, W. (eds) (1996) Nutrition and Cancer. *Cancer Causes and Control,* **7(1)**, 3–180.

World Health Organisation (1996) Tobacco Alert, Internet edition, No. 4. URL: http://www.who.org/psa/toh/Alert/4–96/E/index.htm

PART II

THE PRINCIPLES OF
CANCER TREATMENT

CHAPTER 7

RADIOBIOLOGY: ITS RELEVANCE TO TREATMENT

Andrew A. Miller and John H. Kearsley

INTRODUCTION

The understanding of the biological effects of radiation on molecules, cells, tissues, organisms and populations is based on laboratory investigation and clinical observation. The science is not exact because the molecular ionisation events from radiation and the various expressions of damage may be separated by years.

The aim of radiation treatment is to deliver a precisely measured dose of ionizing radiation to a defined tumour volume with as little damage as possible to surrounding healthy tissues, resulting in eradication of the tumour, a high quality of life and prolongation of survival at reasonable cost.

RADIOBIOLOGY OF RADIATION DAMAGE

Ionizing radiation (photons or X-rays, electrons, protons, neutrons) causes the formation of free radicals within the cell. Free radical damage to renewable molecules (RNA, membranes, proteins, single-strand DNA breaks) is rarely significant, while damage to non-renewable molecules (double-strand DNA breaks) is significant.

The DNA damage caused by a single radiation dose depends on the size of the dose (measured in centiGray (cGy) which is equivalent to the old unit, the 'rad'), the dose rate and the radiation's LET (linear energy transfer; a measure of ionization density). The outcome of this ionization event includes accurate repair, immediate cell death by apoptosis, or inaccurate repair. Inaccurate DNA repair may be inconsequential in an inactive part of the genome, or produce cell death in mitosis because of chromosome cross-linking, or produce a non-fatal genetic mutation that may predispose to carcinogenesis.

Currently, radiobiologists model radiation damage using the linear-quadratic formalism which is based on cell survival curves and current molecular biological theories of DNA damage and repair mechanisms. From the LQ formalism derives an equation for comparing early and late side effects from differing radiation therapy regimens (Figure 7.1).

$$\textbf{BED} = \textbf{n.d.} \left(1 + \frac{\textbf{d}}{\alpha/\beta} \right)$$

BED = Biological Effective Dose
n = number of fractions
d = dose per fraction (in gray)
α/β = a ratio derived from cell survival curves
α/β = 10 for early responding tissues
α/β = 2 for late responding tissues in late effects

Figure 7.1 The linear-quadratic equation

Source: Modified from Barton, M. (1995) Tables of equivalent dose in 2 Gy fractions: a simple application of the linear quadratic formula. *Int J Radiat Oncol Biol Phys*, **31(2)**, 371–378.

In radiobiological terms, the aim of curative treatment is the eradication of tumour clonogens with subclinical or tolerable damage to surrounding normal structures.

RADIOBIOLOGY OF THE THERAPEUTIC RATIO

Modern curative radiation therapy uses fractionated treatments, with the total dose is split into smaller fractions (usually 180–200 cGy/day, i.e. 1.8–2.0 Gy/day) and repeated every day for several weeks. As a reasonable estimate, one fraction will reduce tumour cell survival by 50%. A similar dose the next day will further reduce survival by 50%, that is to 25% of the original population. Repeated doses result in a logarithmic decline in total surviving tumour cell numbers. The majority of radiation side effects occur within the area of irradiation.

Radiosensitivity

Different tumours are affected by radiation differently. One fraction of radiation may reduce tumour cell survival by 10% in one cell type such as some melanomas, and by 90% in another cell line, such as some lymphomas. More total radiation is needed to remove the first tumour than the second. Therefore, the second tumour has a greater radiosensitivity.

Repair

In the time between radiation doses, DNA damage is repaired. The extent of repair is not equal in all tissues. Late responding normal tissues have greater repair capacity than malignant or early responding normal tissues. The logarithmic cell killing effect means that the differences of a single day are exponentially magnified: if the cell survival in a tumour is 50%, and in a late responding normal tissue is 60% because of a greater repair capacity, then after 30 dose fractions the relative survival ratio will be $(60/50)^{30}$ which equals 237! (see Figure 7.2). Thus, fractionation exploits a difference in repair.

Repopulation

Although the repair capacity of malignant and early responding normal tissues is similar, the response of these tissues to cell loss is different. Early responding normal tissues, such as epithelial tissues and

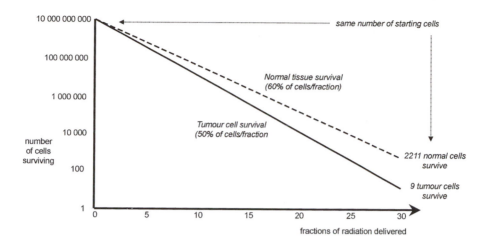

Figure 7.2 Repair differences are exploited by fractionation appliction of the linear quadratic formula

Source: Adapted from Peters, L.J. et al. (1990) Radiation biology at clinically relevant fractions. *Important Adv Oncol*, 65–83.

bone marrow, have a homeostatic response to cell depletion, responding with accelerated repopulation after 10 daily dose fractions. When established, normal tissue repopulation can repair the daily dose fraction damage, that is, replacement of the 50% of cells killed. Tumours also undergo a similar response but are slower, taking 4 weeks to occur, and are less exuberant since they can soak up 60 cGy of radiation damage each day. To exploit this difference, treatments need to be completed promptly before tumour repopulation 'wastes' radiation damage.

Oxygenation

Tumour radiosensitivity is affected by the tissue oxygenation levels. Oxygen is very important to the radiochemical process of free radical generation by ionizing radiation and tissue hypoxia can increase cell survival. Some experiments suggest a two to three times increase in radioresistance in hypoxic tumour cells. Hypoxia results when cells reach the diffusion limit of oxygen from capillaries at about 150 mm. Killing oxygenated cells near capillaries will permit some hypoxic cells undergo re-oxygenation. These cells can become more radiosensitive.

Cell Cycle

Tumour radiosensitivity is also affected by the large changes in cellular radiosensitivity that occur at different phases in the cell cycle. The most radiosensitive phases are M and G_2, and the most radioresistant is the S phase. A daily dose will selectively kill sensitive cells leaving a partly synchronized cell population. The next day, some of the cells that survived in the radioresistant phases will have progressed to radiosensitive phases. This self-sensitizing effect of cell cycle redistribution occurs in both tumours and early responding normal tissues.

Geographical Miss

Achieving the aim of clonal eradication by radiation also depends on physical factors. If a radiation field does not include all the locoregional tumour, a failure is guaranteed by a geographical miss. To prevent this happening the radiation oncologist draws on anatomical knowledge to predict lymphatic drainage patterns, clinical ability in radiological interpretation and physical examination to define the full extent of the tumour and understanding of the technical limitations of beam definition, patient positioning and immobilization. Since a treatment course may consist of 30 dose fractions, reproducibility and quality assurance are essential.

Radiation Heterogeneity

When the radiation dose to a defined tumour volume is uneven or heterogeneous, the therapeutic ratio is reduced. The highest dose in the volume determines the early and late side effect rates, while the lowest dose determines the likelihood of cure. For this reason, radiation oncologists are obsessive about quantifying and minimizing heterogeneity so that the delivered treatment reflects the planned treatment.

The clinical reality is that the probability of both late side effects and cure are similar. There is a threshold dose below which no tumour is cured. As the dose increases, control improves rapidly. A similar curve applies to late effects which, through the factors mentioned above, is displaced to a lower dose. The greater the difference, the greater the therapeutic ratio (Figure 7.3).

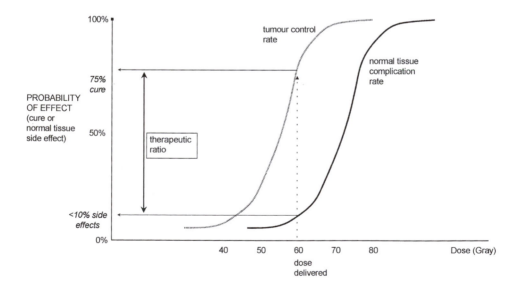

Figure 7.3 The therapeutic window between tumour control and tissue complications

Source: Modified from Peters, L.J. et al. (1990) Radiation biology at clinically relevant fractions. *Important Adv Oncol* 65–83.

RADIOBIOLOGY OF ACUTE EFFECTS

Deterministic Effects

Acute radiation responses are inflammatory in type and vary with tissue type. They may occur early in treatment or near the end of treatment. These responses are called 'deterministic' effects because their incidence and severity are directly proportional to the radiation dose.

Early Responding Tissues

Epithelial surfaces, skin, mucosa and bone marrow are the early responding tissues that react within days of receiving radiation. These 'hierarchical' tissues have a fast turnover time. The transition time from stem cell to functional cell produces a fixed latent period for onset of side effects. The turnover rate of functional cells fixes the rapidity of onset of side effects. However, the severity and duration of side effects are related to dose. The recovery time is also rapid for the same reasons (Figure 7.4).

Late Responding Tissues

Mesenchymal tissues, liver, muscle, heart and lung are late responding tissues. These 'flexible' cells turn over more slowly. It is unusual to see these cells react during a 6 week radiation course, but reactions typically last weeks to months. The latent period, rapidity of onset, severity and prevalence of the side effect are all dose related (Figure 7.5).

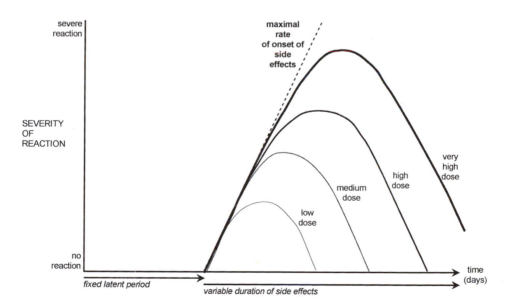

Figure 7.4 The time course of acute reactions in early responding tissues

Source: Modified from Awwad, H.K. (1990) *Radiation Oncology: Radiobiological and Physiological Perspectives: The Boundary-Zone Between Clinical Radiotherapy and Fundamental Radiobiology*, pp.109–127. Dordrecht: Kluwer Academic.

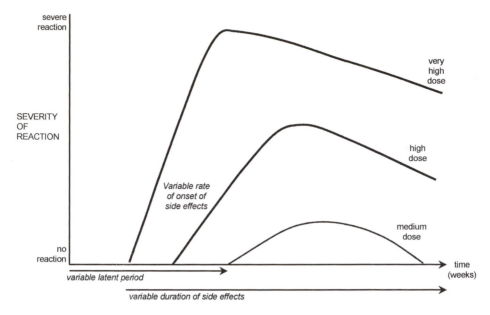

Figure 7.5 The time course of acute reactions in late responding tissues

Source: Modified from Awwad, H.K. (1990) *Radiation Oncology: Radiobiological and Physiological Perspectives: The Boundary-Zone Between Clinical Radiotherapy and Fundamental Radiobiology*, pp.109–127. Dordrecht: Kluwer Academic.

RADIOBIOLOGY OF LATE EFFECTS

Late radiation effects are generally of the atrophic or insufficiency variety. They usually take months to develop and represent the loss of parenchymal cell and vascular supply to the irradiated area. Once they have developed they are permanent. As a matter of convention, radiation oncologists regard a 5% late effect as acceptable when treating malignant disease.

RADIATION PROTECTION

The experience of early radiation workers, radium dial painters and two atomic bomb explosions has taught us that large acute doses of radiation kill quickly, and small slow doses can induce cancers.

Radiation carcinogenesis is a 'stochastic' effect of radiation as only the incidence is linked to dose. Even if it only happens to one person in a million, that person gets a 100% cancer!

For this reason radiation protection is paramount and governed by the ALARA principle — As Low As Reasonably Achievable — given social, economic and clinical practice. This recognizes the usefulness of radiation as well as its detriment.

When dealing with radiation, four factors which reduce exposure are lessening the time exposed, increasing distances to the radiation source, interposing shielding and limiting exposure through measurement.

REFERENCES

Awwad, H.K. (1990) *Radiation Oncology: Radiobiological and Physiological Perspectives: The Boundary-Zone Between Clinical Radiotherapy and Fundamental Radiobiology*, pp.109–127. Dordrecht: Kluwer Academic.

Barton, M. (1995) Tables of equivalent dose in 2 Gy fractions: a simple application of the linear quadratic formula. *Int J Radiat Oncol Biol Phys,* **31**(2), 371–378 .

Peters, L.J., Brock, W.A. and Travis, E.L. (1990) Radiation biology at clinically relevant fractions. In *Important Advances in Oncology,* edited by V. Devita, S. Hellman, S.A. Rosenberg, pp. 65–83. · Philadelphia: JB Lippincott.

CHAPTER 8

PRINCIPLES OF RADIOTHERAPY

Michael Barton

THE PHYSICAL BASIS OF RADIOTHERAPY

The biological basis of radiotherapy has been discussed in a preceding chapter. It is not possible to understand the action and effects of radiotherapy, however, without a knowledge of the physical properties of radiotherapy and how these are use to improve the therapeutic ratio.

Planning

Radiation beams are aligned from many different directions using a simulator and aligned so that they overlap on the cancer. This gives a high dose to the cancer with relative sparing of surrounding normal tissues. The choice of radiation type and quality is also critical.

X-rays

External Beam or Teletherapy

Tele (distant) therapy uses sources of radiation such as X-ray tubes or radioisotopes to produce X-rays for radiotherapy. About 95% of radiotherapy is given this way.

Orthovoltage Therapy

This is the deep X-ray therapy (DXRT) of the pre-modern era. These X-rays are made by high voltage vacuum tubes similar to diagnostic X-rays. They only penetrate short distances and are not used commonly because most tumours are too deep-seated.

Megavoltage (MV) Therapy

Linear accelerators (LinAcs) make X-rays with energies of several million volts. These X-rays are highly penetrating and at the same time spare the skin from high doses. Megavoltage radiation is the workhorse of modern radiotherapy.

Brachytherapy

Before MV, the best way to treat to a high dose was by putting radioactive sources directly into cancers. As the dose is determined by the inverse square law (dose = $1/$distance^2), the cancer gets a high dose but the normal tissues get much less. In cervix cancer this gives an advantage over teletherapy.

Electrons and Other Particles

Electrons penetrate only a short distance depending upon their energy. This property is useful for treating superficial regions of the body that overlie critical and sensitive normal tissues, e.g. spinal cord. Other particles such as neutrons, protons and heavy charged particles are used in research facilities. Routine use has been hampered by high cost and limited clinical applications.

CLINICAL APPLICATIONS OF RADIOTHERAPY

Curative Intent

About half of all cancers are cured. Radiotherapy and surgery are the major curative modalities of cancer treatment. Over 80% of cures are by local therapy alone. The choice between radiotherapy and surgery is often made on the basis of organ preservation and patient preference. All therapeutic decisions are a balance between anti-tumour effect and complications.

Radiotherapy Alone

Modality of Choice

Radiotherapy is the modality of choice where it offers the highest chance of cure for a minimum of side effects. For nasopharyngeal cancers and low-grade non-Hodgkin's lymphomas, radiotherapy is the only curative modality available. Early Hodgkin's disease can be cured by radiotherapy or chemotherapy but radiotherapy has a lower rate of complications.

Organ Preservation

Where radiotherapy and surgery give similar cure rates, radiotherapy may be preferred if surgery is ablative such as with mastectomy for breast cancer. Lumpectomy and radiotherapy produce equivalent survival rates to mastectomy and are often chosen because the breast is not removed. Similar results are achieved in sarcomas, anal cancers and head and neck cancers.

Even when control is not as good as surgery radiotherapy may be preferred if salvage treatment is available. Radiotherapy for larynx cancer preserves the voice in 60–80% with laryngectomy reserved for salvage. Overall the survival rates of radiotherapy and surgical salvage are identical to laryngectomy alone but the majority of patients keep their voice box intact.

Combined Modality Therapy

Radiotherapy is frequently used in combination with other cancer treatments because the different modalities have different strengths and side effects.

Radiotherapy and Surgery

Surgery is excellent at removing large tumour masses. Radiotherapy can treat larger areas where microscopic cancer cells may remain after surgery. Combined surgery and radiotherapy allows more limited surgery and higher cure rates may be achieved.

- Preoperative radiotherapy. Pre-operative radiotherapy reduces tumour bulk, reduces the risk of implantation at the time of operation and treats tumours that are not subject to postoperative hypoxia or accelerated repopulation. Lower doses can frequently be used. Randomised studies have shown an advantage in rectal cancer. Radiotherapy may delay wound healing though the evidence of any significant effect is sparse.
- Intra-operative radiotherapy. Intra-operative radiotherapy is rarely given because of logistic problems with linear accelerators and operating theatres. The intra-operative placement of brachytherapy applicators has increased local control of limb sarcomas and improved limb preservation rates.
- Postoperative radiotherapy. Radiotherapy is frequently given postoperatively to treat residual microscopic cancer. It has the advantages of better definition of disease extent and better selection of patients who may benefit. Disadvantages are the larger treatment field required to encompass the operative site and the potential for increased tumour resistance due to hypoxia or repopulation.

Radiotherapy and Chemotherapy

There are several potential advantages to using radiotherapy and chemotherapy together. These include the following.

- Spatial co-operation. Radiotherapy works locally while chemotherapy affects the entire body but usually only achieves modest cytoreduction. Radiotherapy and chemotherapy combined are successful when there is a moderately chemosensitive cancer with a high risk of spread. Examples include bulky Hodgkin's disease, childhood cancers and adjuvant rectal cancer.
- Independent toxicities. When chemotherapy and radiotherapy have different side effects, their use in combination may allow effective dose intensification, with improved cancer cure. Examples where this applies include anal cancer and oesophagus.
- Enhanced tumour response. Chemotherapy may enhance radiation response. Specific hypoxic cell sensitisers increase radiosensitivity and have improved tumour control in head and neck cancers.
- Radioprotection. Theoretically, it may also be possible to improve the therapeutic ratio by selectively reducing normal tissue radiosensitivity. Sulfhydryl compounds such as WR 2721 that scavenge free radicals may increase normal tissue tolerance. They may also reduce chemotherapy toxicity.

Palliative Intent

Its selective effect and high tumour kill rate are characteristics which makes radiotherapy a major modality for the palliation of incurable cancer. Radiotherapy is the most effective treatment for bone metastases with response rates of 70–80% following short courses of treatment. Radiotherapy is the treatment of choice for spinal cord compression unless the diagnosis is not certain, there is progression during radiotherapy or the spine has been previously treated to tolerance. Radiotherapy is also highly effective in palliating brain metastases.

COMPLICATIONS

'Every therapeutic rose has its thorns' — Sir William Osler

Radiotherapy complications are dose related with high doses, and larger volumes, giving higher risks of complications.

Acute Side Effects

Acute side effects occur during or shortly after a course of radiotherapy. Their nature depends on the body site being treated. For instance, alopecia occurs with brain radiotherapy but not with lung. Nearly all acute side effects are reversible, though that may take anything from weeks to months to resolve. Acute side effects may be permanent only when the organ is especially sensitive (e.g. parotid) or when the dose is high (e.g. accelerated hyperfractionation of head and neck cancers).

Late Side Effects

Complications from radiotherapy may occur months to years after treatment. These complications are usually irreversible, and therefore the art of clinical radiotherapy is to minimise their incidence while aiming for the maximum cure rate (Figure 8.1). Larger doses per fraction of radiotherapy cause more late side effects. Hence radiotherapy is usually given in multiple small doses.

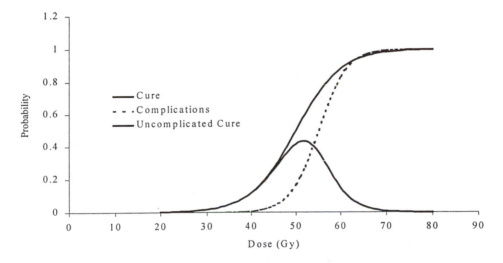

Figure 8.1 Theoretical dose response for tumour cure and normal tissue compliations illustrating the concept of therapeutic ratio. The aim of optimum treatment is to define the level of the maximum rate of uncomplicated care.

REFERENCES

1. Perez, C.A. and Brady, L.W. (1987) *Principles and Practice of Radiotherapy*. Philadelphia: JB Lippencott.

CHAPTER 9

PRINCIPLES OF CHEMOTHERAPY

James F. Bishop

INTRODUCTION

The theoretical advantage of a systemic treatment for cancer is that it will be delivered throughout the body to attack cancer at all metastatic sites simultaneously. Thus, patients with widely disseminated chemo-sensitive metastatic cancer, or those with early stage cancer at risk from undetectable micrometastasis, could be treated by this method. In the latter case, we know that a proportion of early stage breast cancer patients, and limited stage small cell lung cancer patients, have cancer cells in bone marrow detectable by sophisticated methods.

However, it is surprising that chemotherapy is successful as it is, given some obvious obstacles that arise with this concept. Such obstacles include intrinsic or acquired tumour drug resistance, lack of complete knowledge on optimal doses, schedules and routes of administration, and significant dose-limiting toxicity in normal tissues with these drugs.

The modern era of chemotherapy was ushered in during the Second World War with an accidental explosion in Bari Harbour and exposure of US seaman to nitrogen mustard gas. The alkylating agent caused marrow and lymphoid hypoplasia and was quickly adapted for clinical trials in advanced lymphomas at Yale University in 1943.

Early excitement with dramatic results in haematological and lymphoid tumours was followed by initial disappointment with the return of tumours and lack of activity in epithelial cancers. Over the last 50 years, we have seen the value of new chemotherapy agents demonstrated in childhood malignancies, germ cell cancers, palliation of epithelial cancers and their use in the adjuvant therapy of breast and colon cancers. Chemotherapy has developed a special place in cancer management in marrow transplantation conditioning, concurrently with radiation and in an optimal sequence in combined modality treatment. A number of new agents have recently shown surprising activity in lung, breast and colon cancers.

WHEN TO CONSIDER CHEMOTHERAPY

- Surgery, radiotherapy and chemotherapy represent the major, successful modalities currently available for cancer treatment. In all cancer patients, each modality and their sequence must be at least considered at each decision point for optimal cancer management.
- The decision to use chemotherapy should be following a histologically proven cancer diagnosis and a complete, appropriate staging work-up.
- The use of chemotherapy can then be placed in the framework of worldwide evidence available for its likely benefits and risks for that type of cancer, at the stage established in the patient. The oncologist's experience, and knowledge of the evidence, then allows a recommendation to be made.
- Patients must be physically well enough to undergo chemotherapy. Oncologists frequently use a performance status score to determine general fitness (see appendix I) before recommending chemotherapy. Age appears less important than performance status. Concurrent serious non-malignant medical conditions such as heart, renal, CNS or lung disease should be considered.
- The patient's phase of the disease must be taken into account. Such obvious phases include first presentation, localised or locally advanced, metastatic to particular organs and within weeks of death from cancer.
- The likely benefits or goals of treatment and the duration of therapy must be quite clear and understood by the medical advisers, the patient, house staff and relatives before embarking on treatment.
- Chemotherapy can only be considered when an informed patient, fully conversant with the likely benefits and risks, gives consent to have chemotherapy. If the patient is unwilling to undergo chemotherapy it cannot and should not be given. If such chemotherapy could be curative, the medical obligation is that the patient and relatives or friends should be fully aware of the consequences of their decisions. Following the patient's decision they should be medically supported in the treatment path they have chosen.

WHICH CHEMOTHERAPY TO USE

Which Specific Chemotherapy

The exact type of standard chemotherapy for each condition is well established in the literature, based on evidence from clinical trials. The specifics for each cancer are covered elsewhere in this text. For example, the standard drugs for diffuse intermediate large cell non-Hodgkin's lymphoma is cyclophosamide, doxorubicin, vincristine, prednisone (CHOP).

Combination Chemotherapy versus Single Agent Therapy

- The rationale for combination chemotherapy is that several anti-cancer drugs have different mechanisms of cytotoxic action on cancer cells. Therefore, different classes of drugs may be more effective at killing cancer cells which could have acquired some drug resistance (see Chapters 10 and 13). In addition, drugs are frequently combined that have different toxicities and thus can be given close to full dose in the combination.

- This principle of combination chemotherapy is most frequently applied to cancers potentially curable with chemotherapy such as lymphoma, leukaemia, germ cell tumours and childhood malignancies.
- In reality, the use of combinations or a single agent must be based on clinical trial evidence of benefit on a case by case basis.
- The doses of cytotoxic drugs in combination may be substantially less than as single agents. This can compromise efficacy especially if some of the drugs in the combination are ineffective.
- In general, combinations may produce a higher response rate and sometimes a longer duration of response but with less proven impact on survival when used in palliative setting.
- Recently, there has been new evidence of benefit of blocks of 3 or 4 courses of single agents or combinations then switching to other single agents or combinations in a pre-planned sequence.

When There is No Proven Standard Therapy

The use of chemotherapy in this setting is a matter of judgement and a joint decision between the patient and their medical adviser following a frank discussion of the risks and benefits. The options are often for new anti-cancer drugs or a standard approach valuable in a similar clinical situation.

It is the role of the oncologist to honestly attempt to weight the likely benefits compared to side effects, listening to the goals of the patient, before making any recommendations.

HOW TO USE CHEMOTHERAPY

Chemotherapy is best delivered in a chemotherapy suite with appropriately designed pharmacy facilities for cytotoxic containment, with nursing expertise in patient education, drug extravasation, drug side effects and cytotoxic handling, spills and waste disposal.
In general, chemotherapy should be:

- given at the maximum tolerated dose for optimal cancer control;
- given by the optimal schedule and route of administration based on pharmacokinetic studies and clinical evidence of efficiency;
- given on time, especially if the intent is cure or long term cancer control;
- assessed for toxicity at each visit by:
  — a full discussion of toxicity;
  — a full blood examination, urea and electrolytes and liver function tests before each repeat dose of chemotherapy; and
  — a full blood examination at the likely nadir, at least with the first cycle of chemotherapy;
- dose reduced by about 25% for:
  — nadir neutrophil counts $< 0.5 \times 10^6/L$;
  — nadir platelet counts $50 \times 10^6/L$;
  — World Health Organisation (WHO) Grade 3 or 4 non-haematological toxicity (see references); and
  — mucositis on standard dose therapy;
- delayed until neutrophil counts are $> 1.5 \times 10^6/L$ and platelets $> 100 \times 10^6/L$ and WHO Grade 3 non-haematological toxicity has cleared;

- re-assessed for efficiency clinically at each visit or by imaging at every 2 or 3 visits;
- stopped in the presence of clearly progressive disease based on WHO criteria or unacceptable toxicity following dose reduction;
- stopped at any time on the patient's request;
- stopped, or considered for stopping, two or three courses after the maximum response has been achieved based on evidence in each specific clinical setting.

SIDE EFFECTS OF CHEMOTHERAPY

The patient will often contemplate chemotherapy with the question: 'Is the treatment worse than the disease?' Discussion of the risks, side effects and benefits of chemotherapy is best approached with a sympathetic understanding of this underlying anxiety.

There is good evidence that uncontrolled metastatic cancer is associated with more symptoms and poorer quality of life than disease well controlled with chemotherapy. However, if unsuccessful, the patient may experience both uncontrolled disease and the side effects of chemotherapy. Several studies have compared best supportive care and chemotherapy in palliative settings such as metastatic lung or breast cancer. Surprisingly, almost all of these studies have shown better quality of life and symptom control overall with chemotherapy.

If there is a realistic hope of tumour control, even in the palliative setting, many patients will choose chemotherapy, at least as a short-term trial of therapy.

When chemotherapy is given with curative intent or for long-term cancer control, most patients and their oncologists will readily accept the usual chemotherapy side effects for a longer term benefit.

The side effects of specific chemotherapy drugs are covered elsewhere (see Chapters 10 and 16). Most side effects are dose dependent. Most patients tolerate side effects surprisingly well with sensitive dose adjustment and patient education. Major side effects include the following:

- Nausea and vomiting: In general, both are now well controlled in over 90% of patients.
- Alopecia: Dependent on the drug(s) used, is temporary, begins at 4–6 weeks after initiation of therapy and returns in 6–9 weeks of cessation.
- Mucositis: Mucositis on standard outpatient chemotherapy usually means the dose given is too high and requires a minimal dose reduction. It is a potent portal for systemic infection, causes severe pain and should be avoided.
- Myelosuppression: Is a side effect (WHO Grade 2 or 3, neutrophils $> 0.5 \times 10^6$/L) monitored to ensure adequate doses are delivered. More severe myelosuppression (WHO Grade 4, neutrophils $< 0.5 \times 10^6$/L) is more common than appreciated in most standard regimens. It will inevitably result in episodes of febrile neutropenia unless nadir counts are monitored on the first course. All patients should be fully conversant with how they should seek medical help if they develop fevers while on chemotherapy.
- Neurotoxicity: Common with vinca alkaloids, platins and taxanes. The general principle is that chemotherapy should be modified or stopped if motor function is affected by peripheral neuropathy. Predisposing risk factors for neurological toxicity includes pre-existing neurological deficits, such as motor neurone disease or diabetic peripheral neuropathy, and concomitant or prior use of other neurotoxins.

- Cardiac toxicity: Uncommonly seen with anthracyclines, left sided chest irradiation, concomitant cardiac disease or fluid overload such as intravenous cisplatin hydration.
- General lethargy: Is more common than generally appreciated with many drugs and should be asked for specifically.

The side effects of all anti-cancer drugs have been documented, and are well known by treating oncologists. Thus, patient education is important to provide detail on the possible side effects of each cytotoxic drug to be given. Such individualised information is an important requirement for safe, tolerable and efficient delivery of chemotherapy.

HIGH-DOSE CHEMOTHERAPY AND DOSE INTENSITY

High-dose chemotherapy and bone marrow or peripheral stem cell transplantation have established roles in haematological and relapsed germ cell malignancies. The place of this technique in adult solid tumours needs further evidence from randomised clinical trials (see chapters by Alan Coates and Ken Bradstock).

The intensity of treatment may have some impact on treatment outcome. It seems clear, in a number of cancers, that inadequate or sub-optimal doses are inferior. Hence the recommendation that treatment should be delivered close to the maximum tolerated dose. However, the case for a very high dose or a more intense dose of chemotherapy is not well established and is based on retrospective data largely showing the inadequacy of low-dose therapy. Transplants with high-dose treatment have been successful in leukaemia and lymphoma and high-dose cytarabine in acute myeloid leukaemia. However, more intense therapy schedules have not yet proven to improve outcomes in small cell lung cancer, breast cancer or lymphomas and this concept requires more clinical trial evidence.

CHEMOTHERAPY USE AND SECOND CANCERS

Some chemotherapy drugs can induce second cancers. Such second malignancies are seen in long-term survivors of curable cancers such as Hodgkin's disease. Hopefully, in the future, we will be more successful in producing long-term cancer survivors. Thus, this may become an increasingly important issue.

Chemotherapy-induced second cancers are predominantly acute myeloid leukaemias. Some factors which predispose to second cancers after chemotherapy include:

- The use of drugs acting on DNA rather than anti-metabolites.
- The long-term use of alkylating agents.
- Some alkylating agents, such as melphalan, chlorambucil or CCNU, are more likely to induce malignancy than others, such as cyclophosphamide. Cumulative doses of cyclophosphamide greater than 20 g do not appear to confer an appreciable leukaemia risk. Controversy exists with other drugs such as procarbazine.
- The use of topoisomerase II inhibitors.
- Concomitant or sequential use of radiation and chemotherapy may increase risk but this remains controversial.
- Certain chemotherapy associated with chromosomal abnormalities, such as abnormalities of chromosome 5 or 7 by alkylating agents or the translocation t(11q23) by epipodophyllotoxins.

REFERENCES

De Vita, V.T. (1997) Principles of cancer management: Chemotherapy. *In Cancer: Principles and Practice of Oncology* (5th edn), edited by V. DeVita, S. Hellman and S.A. Rosenberg, pp. 333–346. Philadelphia: Lippincott-Raven Pulo.

Miller, A.B., Hoogstraten, B., Staquet, M. and Winkler, A. (1981) Reporting results of cancer treatment. *Cancer*, 47, 207–214.

Perry, M.C. (ed.) (1997) *The Chemotherapy Source Book* (2nd edn). Baltimore: Williams and Wilkins.

Smith, G.A. and Henderson, I.C. (1995) High dose chemotherapy with autologous bone marrow transplantation (ABMT) for the treatment of breast cancer: The jury is still out. In *Important Advances in Oncology 1995*, edited by V. Devita, S. Hellman and S.A. Rosenberg, pp. 201–214. Philadelphia: JB Lippincolt.

Levine EG, Bloomfield CD. (1992) Leukaemias and myelodysplastic disorders secondary to drug, radiation and environmental exposure. *Semin Oncol,* 19, 47–55.

Van Leeuwen, F.E., Chorus, A.M.J., VanderBelt-Dusebout, A.W., Hagenbeek, A., Noyon, R. van Kerkhoff, E.H.M., Pinedo, H.M. and Somers, R. (1994) Leukemia risk following Hodgkin's Disease: Relation to cummulative dose of alkylatory agents, treatment with teniposide combinations, number of episodes of chemotherapy and bone marrow damage. *J Clin Oncol,* 12, 1063.

CHAPTER 10

ACTIONS OF ANTI-CANCER DRUGS

Stephen J. Clarke and Laurent P. Rivory

INTRODUCTION

Chemotherapy plays an integral part in the treatment of cancer. In the setting of paediatric malignancy, it is frequently given with curative intent. This is also the case with some solid tumours such as germ cell tumours and some types of lymphoma.

Chemotherapy may be administered prior to surgery (i.e. neoadjuvant) to facilitate resection and prevent metastasis or after surgical debulking (adjuvant) to reduce the risk of distant relapse. It improves the rates of survival from advanced disease in a number of situations where radiotherapy and/or surgery are no longer appropriate. The value of chemotherapy in improving the quality of life of patients, by palliating symptoms and pain, even in the absence of a survival advantage, is increasingly recognised.

Drugs used in cancer chemotherapy represent an enormous range of structural diversity. The spectrum of processes which they target, is just as impressive (see Table 10.1). For some drugs, their exact mechanism(s) of action are still being elucidated.

In most cases, these drugs:

- cause DNA damage, e.g. anthracyclines, bleomycin, alkylating agents;
- directly inhibit enzymes;
- deplete vital cofactors, e.g. antifolates and precursors, e.g. asparaginase;
- produce a combination of any of the above, e.g. 5-FU, gemcitabine.

Cells which are actively growing and dividing are, in general, more sensitive to these interferences and this gives chemotherapy some selectivity for cancer cells. Compromised cells will either stop growing as seen with cytostatic agents, or initiate the cascade of programmed cell death known as apoptosis as with cytotoxics.

Table 10.1 Mechanism of action and principal toxicities of commonly used cytotoxic agents

Agent	Cytotoxic mechanism	Principal toxicity
Antimetabolites		
Methotrexate	Inhibition of DHFR and effects of polyglutamates on *de novo* purine biosynthesis	Schedule dependent Mucositis and myelosuppression Nephrotoxic in high dose
Tomudex	TS inhibition	Myelosuppression, malaise, GI toxicity
5-FU	TS inhibition Incorporation into RNA/DNA	GI toxicity and myelosuppression (bolus) Plantar/palmar syndrome (infusion)
Ara-C	Inhibition of DNA polymerase α Ara-CTP incorporation into DNA	Myelosuppression, GI toxicity
Gemcitabine	Inhibits ribonucleotide reductase	Myelosuppression
6-MP/6-TG	DNA incorporation Inhibition of *de novo* purine biosynthesis	Myelosuppression, GI toxicity
Hydroxyurea	Inhibition of ribonucleotide reductase	Myelosuppression
Edatrexate (10-EDAM)	as per methotrexate	Mucositis and myelosuppression
Pentostatin (deoxycoformycin)	Inhibition of adenosine deaminase	Immunosuppression
Fludarabine monophosphate	Incorporation of F-ara-ATP into DNA	Myelosuppression
2'-chlorodeoxyadenosine	DNA strand breaks (++ causes)	Myelosuppression
Alkylating agents		
Mustard derivatives: Mechlorethamine, chlorambucil, busulfan, cyclophosphamide, ifosfamide	DNA alkylation	Cumulative myelosuppression Nausea and vomiting Haemorrhagic cystitis with cyclophosphamide and ifosfamide
Nitrosoureas: BCNU, CCNU and methyl CCNU	DNA alkylation	Delayed myelosuppression
Mitomycin C	DNA alkylation	Myelosuppression

Table 10.1 *Continued*

Agent	Cytotoxic mechanism	Principal toxicity
Procarbazine	DNA alkylation	Nausea and vomiting
		Myelosuppression, Neurotoxicity
Dacarbazine (DTIC)	DNA alkylation. Inhibition of purine nucleoside incorporation into DNA	Delayed myelosuppression
Platinum derivatives		
Cisplatin	DNA-Pt adduct formation	Emesis, nephropathy, neuropathy
Carboplatin	DNA-Pt adduct formation	Myelosuppression
Anthracyclines and like		
Doxorubicin, epirubicin, daunorubicin, idarubicin	Topoisomerase II inhibition or free radical induced DNA strand breaks	Nausea and vomiting
		Myelosuppression and alopecia
		Cardiac toxicity
Mitoxantrone, amsacrine	Topoisomerase II inhibition	Myelosuppression
Plant alkaloids		
Vincristine	Tubulin binding	Neuropathy
Vinblastine	Tubulin binding	Myelosuppression
Vinorelbine	Tubulin binding/ DNA strand breaks	Myelosuppression, Neuopathy, Phlebitis
Etoposide/Teniposide	Topo II strand breaks	Myelosuppression
Paclifaxel/Docetaxel	Stabilization of tubulin	Myelosuppression
Others		
Actinomycin D	Inhibition of RNA and protein synthesis via DNA binding	Myelosuppression and GI toxicity
L-asparaginase	Depletes circulating L-asparagine inhibiting protein synthesis	Decreased protein synthesis
		Hypersensitivity
CPT-II (Irinotecan)	Topoisomerase I inhibition	Diarrhoea, Myelosuppression, Alopecia
	Single strand breaks in DNA	
Topotecan	Topo I inhibition	Myelosuppression

CLASSES OF CYTOTOXIC AGENTS

Antimetabolites: Inhibitors of Ribonucleic Acid (RNA, DNA) Synthesis

Antimetabolites are structurally similar to some of the necessary cofactors and building blocks required for cell growth and division. This similarity leads to competition with the natural substrates resulting in a variety of effects such as inhibition of vital enzymes and the incorporation of fraudulent bases into RNA and DNA.

Methotrexate

Methotrexate is a folate-based inhibitor of the enzyme dihydrofolate reductase (DHFR) which is essential for the production of reduced folate cofactors. Reduced folates are required in enzymatic reactions in the *de novo* synthesis of purines and the conversion of dUMP to dTMP by thymidylate synthase (TS). Methotrexate thus impairs the production of (d)ATP, (d)GTP and TTP which impacts on RNA and DNA synthesis.

Tomudex

Tomudex is a new folate-based anticancer drug designed to inhibit TS and have effects solely on TTP production, thereby specifically impairing DNA synthesis.

5-Fluorouracil

5-Fluorouracil (5-FU) is a uracil analogue with multiple putative sites of action. It is activated by conversion to FdUMP which, in turn, forms a ternary complex with TS and 5,10-methylene tetrahydrofolate, resulting in inhibition of *de novo* synthesis of dTMP. The stability of the ternary complex is enhanced by increased concentrations of reduced folates, such as folinic acid. In addition, FUTP and FdUTP are incorporated into DNA and RNA, respectively, in place of their non-fluorinated analogues with consequent effects on cellular metabolism.

Cytarabine

Cytarabine (Ara-C) is a deoxycytidine analogue which when phosphorylated to ara-CTP is a potent inhibitor of the enzyme DNA polymerase α. This enzyme plays a critical role in DNA replication and repair. Other possible mechanisms of cytotoxicity associated with the use of ara-C are the incorporation of ara-CTP into DNA, inhibition of the enzyme ribonucleotide reductase and inhibition of the synthesis of some components of cell membranes. Ara-C also has the capacity to down-regulate the expression of the c-myc oncogene.

Gemcitabine

Gemcitabine (2′,2′-difluorodeoxycytidine) is another deoxycytidine analogue with multiple modes of action. As with ara-C, the activated diphosphate form is an inhibitor of ribonucleotide reductase which leads to a depletion of intracellular pools of dCTP and dATP. The triphosphate may be incorporated into DNA by the enzyme DNA polymerase followed by a futher deoxynucleotide. Gemcitabine, in this penultimate position, is resilient to exonucleases and this leads to 'masked' DNA chain elongation termination. Gemcitabine has other self-potentiating effects such as inhibiting CTP synthetase. Also, dCTP is a required cofactor for dCMP deaminase, which converts gemcitabine to the essentially inactive 2′,2′-difluorodeoxyuridine. The depletion of the dCTP pools should reduce the inactivation of the drug.

6-Mercaptopurine (6-MP) and 6-Thioguanine (6-TG)

6-MP and 6-TG are both antipurine agents which bear structural similarity to guanine. Both compounds are metabolised to triphosphated nucleotides which are incorporated into DNA as fraudulent bases, leading to DNA strand breaks. In addition, the monophosphated nucleotides inhibit *de novo* purine biosynthesis.

Alkylating Agents

The alkylating agents, as their name suggests, alkylate a variety of macromolecules, including proteins and DNA. The N-7 nitrogen of deoxyguanylic acid in DNA is particularly prone to this reaction and bifunctional alkylating agents, those having two reactive groups, can cause the cross-linking of adjacent strands in G-X-C sequences. The extent of this effect correlates well with the cytotoxicity of the individual agent and bifunctional alkylators are, in general, much more active than monofunctional ones. Nevertheless, some monofunctional agents (e.g. dacarbazine, procarbazine) have interesting activities which are probably mediated through the depurination of alkylated deoxyguanylic acid residues, leading to the formation of DNA single-strand breaks.

Cyclophosphamide and Ifosfamide

Cyclophosphamide and ifosfamide are pro-drugs which require activation by hepatic microsomal enzymes to aldo- and hydroxy-phosphamide. The latter exist in equilibrium. The aldophosphamides degrade spontaneously to cytotoxic phosphoramide mustards. These alkylating agents are relatively well tolerated because many of the traditional organs of toxicity of alkylating agents, primitive hematopoietic cells, gastrointestinal mucosa cells, contain high activities of aldehyde dehydrogenase. This enzyme converts the reactive aldophosphamide to inactive carboxy forms.

Platinum Derivatives

The platinum complexes, cisplatin and carboplatin, both exert cytotoxicity by the formation of platinum-DNA adducts which may be formed within or between DNA strands. The exact contribution of each type of platinum-DNA adduct toward cytotoxicity is uncertain. There is some evidence to suggest that as little as two platinum adducts per genome is sufficient to inhibit replication. Much like the alkylating agents, the platinum compounds are more reactive towards the N-7 nitrogen of deoxyguanylic acid.

Topoisomerase Inhibitors

Topoisomerases are involved in resolving the complex DNA topological problems which arise during DNA processing, such as transcription, replication and daughter strand separation. This is done by both unknotting, as with topoisomerase II, and unwinding, as with topoisomerases I and II, manoeuvres. Some of the more established anticancer drugs are now recognised as being topoisomerase II inhibitors. These include anthracyclines and epipodophyllotoxins. On the other hand, the camptothecins are newly developed topoisomerase I inhibitors.

It should be pointed out that although the term 'inhibitor' is used for these compounds, they do not act by inhibiting the catalytic activity of these enzymes but rather by stabilizing nicked DNA enzyme complexes. These normally transient complexes interfere with DNA processing and eventually lead to double-stranded DNA breaks. Therefore, in general, cancer cells containing higher concentrations of active topoisomerase are *more* prone to cytotoxicity.

Anthracyclines

The anthracyclines doxorubicin, idarubicin, daunorubicin and epirubicin are potent topoisomerase II inhibitors. Although they are strong intercalating agents, the anti-topoisomerase II activity of these and other anthracyclines does not appear to be correlated with the degree of intercalation. Additionally, anthracyclines undergo redox cycling leading to the production of free radicals and subsequent damage to cell membranes. This latter mechanism has been proposed as being the causative factor in anthracycline-related cardiotoxicity. Other important intercalating topoisomerase II inhibitors are amsacrine and mitoxantrone.

Epipodophyllotoxins

The epipodophyllotoxins VP-16 (etoposide) and VM-26 (teniposide) are semi-synthetic derivatives of podophyllotoxin which is a tubulin binder. However, these compounds are principally non-intercalating topoisomerase II inhibitors.

Bleomycin: A Class of its Own

Bleomycin is in fact a mixture of related glycopeptides initially isolated as a fermentation product of the yeast *Streptomyces verticillus*. Bleomycin forms a complex with oxygen and Fe(II) which then binds with high affinity to DNA. Local production of radicals from the redox cycling of this complex leads to the production of single- and double-stranded DNA breaks.

Tubulin Binders

Vinca Alkaloids

The *Vinca* alkaloids and their derivatives (vincristine, vinblastine, vinorelbine and vindesine) are avid binders of tubulin and prevent microtubule assembly. It is generally assumed, therefore, that the principal mechanism of cytotoxicity of these agents is the disruption of the formation of the mitotic spindle. However, microtubules are implicated in a wide variety of other activities including the transport of vesicles. Since microtubules are very dynamic structures in a constant flux of assembly and disassembly, it is likely that the *Vinca* alkaloids, and indeed, other tubulin binding agents, will have a range of other effects on cells.

Taxanes

The taxanes, paclitaxel (Taxol) and docetaxel (Taxotere), are plant alkaloids derived from the Yew tree species. Unlike the *Vinca* alkaloids, these compounds enhance microtubule assembly when they bind to tubulin. This results in the formation of abnormal spindle asters and cell cycle arrest in mitosis. The tubulin binding site of the taxanes is distinct from those of colchicine, *Vinca* alkaloids and podophyllotoxin.

REFERENCES

Chabner, B.A. and Collins, J.M. (1990) *Cancer Chemotherapy: Principles and Practice*. Philadelphia: JB Lippincott.

De Vita, V., Hellman, S. Rosenberg, S. (1997) *Cancer: Principles and Practice of Oncology*. Philadelphia: JB Lippincott-Raven Publishers.

Dorr, R.T. and van Hoff, D.D. (1994) *Cancer Chemotherapy Handbook*. Connecticut: Appleton & Lange.

Perry, M.C. (ed.) (1997) *The Chemotherapy Source Book*. Philadelphia: JB Lippincott.

Tannock, I.F. and Hill, R.P. (1992) *The Basic Science of Oncology*. USA: McGraw-Hill.

CHAPTER 11

NEW ANTI-CANCER DRUGS

Michael J. Millward

INTRODUCTION

Advances in chemotherapy have resulted in the ability to cure certain cancers, particularly germ cell tumours, leukaemias and paediatric malignancies, that were otherwise fatal. However, the outlook for many patients with the common adult cancers has not changed significantly in recent years.

Adjuvant chemotherapy after initial surgical resection has led to better survival for patients with breast and colorectal cancer. However, these and other common cancers, such as non-small cell lung cancer, prostate cancer, melanoma and upper gastrointestinal and pancreatic adenocarcinomas, are incurable with existing chemotherapy when recurrence or metastases occur.

Thus, there is an urgent need to find better anti-cancer drugs. This chapter will outline the steps in this process.

STEP 1: ACQUISITION AND SCREENING

The identification of potentially active drugs has largely depended on the 'screening' of large numbers of compounds either obtained from nature or made synthetically. The ability of a potential drug to kill one or more of a panel of tumour cell lines is investigated and the availability of automated assays for cell kill allows rapid screening of literally tens of thousands of compounds per year.

Murine Tumour Screens

This approach led to the identification of several drugs now in routine use such as mitoxantrone, deoxycoformycin and some nitrosureas. However, many potential drugs ound in the older screening systems did not ultimately prove to be effective in humans. This failure partly reflects the use of murine leukaemia cell lines as the main cell type in this screening. This approach had limitations in assessing the activity of drugs against human solid tumours. This was particularly noted with paclitaxel, which showed only limited activity in initial screenings. However, once its unique mechanism of action was elucidated, it proceeded to further pre-clinical evaluation and subsequently has entered clinical practice.

Human Tumour Cell Lines

In recent years, screening systems have changed to emphasise panels of human tumour cells lines with clearly defined molecular abnormalities, such as the presence or absence of mutated p53. Sophisticated computer programs allow the comparison of differential cytotoxicity against various cell lines in the screen to be performed between candidate new drugs and existing agents. This gives clues to the mechanism of action of new agents that show profiles different to existing agents can be identified and become important lead compounds for clinical development.

Rational Drug Design

The greatly increased knowledge about the biochemical and molecular differences between malignant and normal cells have also led to more rational drug design. Specific inhibitors of metabolic enzymes can be designed using computer modelling of protein structure derived from knowledge of the amino acid sequence. Antisense oligonucleotides can be designed to block expression of genes of known sequences involved in the malignant process. Drugs can be messengers that link growth factor activation to other intracellular pathways. These approaches hold great promise for providing novel drugs for clinical trials.

Analogue Development

New drugs can also be designed by modifying the structure of known cytotoxics. Such modifications were first performed to reduce toxicity, such as renal impairment, rather than to improve the activity of the drug. Current knowledge about the mechanisms of resistance to chemotherapy has meant that it is possible to design analogues of existing drugs that may be able to circumvent such resistance mechanisms.

STEP 2: PRE-CLINICAL PHARMACOLOGY AND TOXICOLOGY

A new drug is administered to animals to determine a safe starting dose for clinical trials in humans and the toxicities likely to occur. LD_{10}, the dose that is lethal to 10% of animals treated, is determined in mice and toxicity determined by observation, biochemical testing, and autopsy.

Toxicity testing in higher animals has now largely been abandoned. Toxicity testing in dogs is sometimes assessed where it is thought that a particular action or metabolism of the drug is more analogous to man in the dog than in rodents. Determination of the drug's pharmacology in animals is important as a guide to future trials in humans.

STEP 3: PHASE I TRIALS

A Phase I trial is the initial administration of the drug to humans. The aims are to determine the optimal dose for therapeutic studies and investigate the drug's pharmacology and toxicity. To be considered for Phase I trials, patients:

- must give informed consent;
- must have cancers that have not responded to established cytotoxics;
- have cancer where existing drugs are ineffective;
- should be in good general medial condition; and
- have normal or near normal hepatic and renal function, since these are the major pathways of drug metabolism and elimination.

Potential toxicity is determined by frequent clinical examination, haematological and biochemical testing and assessment of cardiac, neurological and other organ system function as appropriate. Frequent blood sampling is performed to establish the new drug's pharmacology in humans.

Traditionally the starting dose of the drug in Phase I trials has been $^1/_{10}$ the LD_{10} in rodents. Cohorts of 3–6 patients are entered at doses that are progressively increased by successively smaller percentages above the previous dose until significant toxicity is seen. Toxicity is graded by established international criteria, usually that of the WHO. For each organ system or haematological/biochemical parameter, toxicity is graded from 0 (no toxicity) to 4 (life threatening or irreversible toxicity). The maximum tolerated dose (MTD) is defined as that which causes WHO Grade III (severe but reversible) or Grade IV toxicity in ≈2/3 or ≈4/6 patients. The dose level below that is generally chosen for further Phase II trials.

This method of performing Phase I trials is now recognised to have several drawbacks. Typically 6–12 dose escalations are required to reach the MTD, which means most patients receive doses that are well below that ultimately determined to be potentially therapeutic. A way around the problem is to escalate the dose based on the pharmacokinetic results at the previous dose level, using the known pharmacokinetics of the drug at the LD_{10} in animals as a guide to those drug levels that are likely to produce toxicity in humans. This approach, termed 'pharmacokinetically guided dose escalation' has been successful in some Phase I trials in reducing the number of dose escalations.

A second problem is that the MTD is dependent not only on drug dose but on the ability to prevent toxicity. Thus, the use of recombinant colony-stimulating factors (CSFs) to prevent neutropenia has meant that for many cytotoxics, where neutropenia is the dose limiting toxicity, a substantially higher MTD can be reached using CSFs. Other agents being developed are able to reduce thrombocytopenia and non-haematological toxicity such as peripheral neuropathy and cardiotoxicity.

STEP 4: PHASE II TRIALS

Phase II trials are therapeutic trials using the optimal dose found from Phase I trials. Patients with a specific tumour type at the same stage are entered, for example, metastatic bowel cancer. A new drug therefore undergoes many different Phase II studies in different types of cancer. As in Phase I trials, patients must give informed consent, be reasonably medically fit and not have major abnormalities of organ function. Additionally, they must have lesions that can be assessed to determine if a response (see Chapter 13) to the new drug occurs.

A minimum of 14 patients are treated in a Phase II trial. If no responses occur then there is a > 90% chance that the true response rate to the new drug is < 20%. A drug with a response rate of < 20% is generally considered inactive and not worth further testing. In addition to anti-tumour activity, Phase II trials generate considerable additional data on toxicity. Pharmacokinetics of the new drug are usually now measured in Phase II trials to explore possible relationships between drug levels and toxicity and, if appropriate, response.

STEP 5: PHASE III TRIALS

Occasionally a new drug is so effective in Phase II studies that these studies alone are sufficient to establish its role in that cancer. Paclitaxel for ovarian cancer that has relapsed after other chemotherapy is one recent example.

Although Phase II studies provide information on the drug's anti-tumour activity, they generally do not determine whether it has clinical usefulness as a treatment. This is done by a larger randomised Phase III trials where patients are allocated to either the new drug or standard chemotherapy.

The endpoints are response rate, survival, toxicity and patient quality of life which can be measured using standardised questionnaires. Such trials require many cooperating institutions and are frequently national or multinational in scope to provide the statistical power needed.

STEP 6: FURTHER TRIALS

Results of Phase III trials generally determine whether a drug will be granted a licence to be marketed as an anti-cancer treatment by the responsible government regulatory agencies. However, finding the optimal way to use the new drug requires further trials. Its potential to be combined with other drugs or radiation therapy is explored through the same type of early clinical trials as discussed above for the drug alone. The use of the new drug as an adjuvant therapy may be explored. Finally post-marketing surveillance may reveal rare side effects not detected in Phase III trials or unexpected long-term problems in cancer survivors.

ETHICAL ISSUES IN CLINICAL TRIALS OF NEW ANTI-CANCER DRUGS

Patients participating in trials of new anti-cancer drugs have incurable diseases for which no satisfactory treatment exists. Media publicity about 'wonder drugs' creates unrealistic expectations and pressure to participate in such trials. It is essential that patients are fully informed about the nature of the trials and that they give written informed consent. All clinical trial protocols and consent forms must be approved by an appropriate ethics committee.

Developing a new anti-cancer drug may take 10 years and cost $100 million. Such investment is generally undertaken by the private sector pharmaceutical industry. Therefore, nearly all new drug trials are done in cooperation with industry. Doctors involved in trials must ensure their primary responsibility is the welfare of patients in the trial. Anything that gives a perception of a conflict of interest, particularly holding shares or other financial interests in sponsoring companies, should be avoided.

REFERENCES

Newell, D. (1990) Phase I clinical studies with cytotoxic drugs: Pharmacokinetic and pharmacodynamic considerations. *Br J Cancer*, **61**, 189–191.

Schwartsmann, G. and Workman, P. (1993) Anticancer Drug Screening and Discovery in the 1990's: A European Perspective. *Eur J Cancer*, **29A(1)**, 3–14.

Williams, C.J. (ed) (1992) *Introducing New Treatments for Cancer: Practical, Ethical and Legal Problems.* Chichester: Wiley.

CHAPTER 12

HORMONAL THERAPY OF CANCER

Robin Murray

BREAST CANCER

Since George Beatson demonstrated in 1896 that some breast cancers respond to oophorectomy, hormonal therapy of breast cancer has become one of the two major methods of treating early and late disease, in both pre- and post-menopausal women.

The majority of hormonal therapies act mainly by either blocking the binding of oestradiol to its specific intracellular receptor, or by decreasing plasma and intracellular oestrogen. If cell growth is oestrogen dependent, the cell will be unable to divide and eventually die. If resistance to one hormonal manoeuvre develops, the cell may still be sensitive to a different hormonal manoeuvre. Thus, a series of different hormonal manoeuvrers can be used sequentially.

When used in an adjuvant setting, hormonal therapy has been shown to delay recurrence, reduce the incidence of contralateral breast cancer and to prolong survival. When used therapeutically in advanced disease approximately 30% of unselected women will experience a remission which has a median duration of around 18 months. If only women whose tumours are ER-positive are treated the remission rate increases to around 60%.

Likelihood of response to a hormonal therapy is increased in the following circumstances:

1. The tumour is oestrogen or progesterone receptor positive (ER+/PR+).

2. The tumour is slow growing (free interval > 3 years).

3. The tumour is well differentiated.

4. A response has occurred with a prior hormonal therapy.

Commonly Used Hormone Treatments

Pre-menopausal Women

Oophorectomy

Oophorectomy may be induced surgically by radiation or medically using an LHRH analogue (such as Zoladex 3.6 mg s/c 4 weekly) which cause depletion of pituitary LH and FSH leading to shut down of gonadal sex steroid synthesis. Oophorectomy produces a premature menopause and its side effects are those of the menopause and include hot flushes, decreased libido, vaginal dryness, irritability.

Anti-oestrogens

Substances such as tamofifen compete with oestradiol for the oestrogen receptor and thus block oestrogenic activity. Tamoxifen has a number of other actions including increasing TGF-B levels. While it is an anti-oestrogen in breast tissue tamoxifen has oestrogenic activity in some tissues. Thus, bone mass is preserved and tamoxifen has beneficial cardiovascular effects in post-menopausal women. Tamoxifen is well tolerated, although it may produce menopausal symptoms in pre-menopausal women. Nausea occurs in < 5% of cases.

Post-menopausal Women

Tamoxifen

Tamoxifen is the hormonal drug of first choice for both early (Stage I & II) and advanced (Stage III & IV) disease in post-menopausal women. The standard dose is 20 mg per day.

Aromatase Inhibitors

These drugs act by inhibiting the enzyme aromatase which is responsible for converting adrenal androgens into oestrogen. They are ineffective in pre-menopausal women.

Aminoglutethimide has been the standard aromatase inhibitor used after tamoxifen in patients with advanced disease. In high doses, it also inhibits the adrenal enzyme desmolase and therefore inhibits adrenal synthesis of cortisone and aldosterone. It should not be given in a dose greater than 250 mg twice daily and at that dose physiological steroid replacement should also be given (cortisone acetate 25 mg twice daily). Treatment should start with 125 mg twice daily and the dose should be increased to 250 mg twice a day (bd) after 2 weeks. Aminoglutethimide causes a temporary, generalised erythematous rash which may be associated with systemic symptoms of fever and malaise in approximately 15% of patients. This usually occurs within 14 days of starting treatment and lasts for about 1 week. The drug should not be stopped but the patient should be reassured that the rash will disappear completely. Other side effects such as dizziness and drowsiness are rare if the dose used is 500 mg/day or less. Very rarely exfoliative dermatitis or thrombocytopenia may occur — in these circumstances the drug must be stopped.

A new group of specific aromatase inhibitors (triazoles) are becoming available, including anastrozole (Arimidex®), letrozole (Femara®), vorozole (Rivizor®). These are potent, pure aromatase inhibitors that are given as a single daily dose and have very few side effects. Early studies suggest they are better tolerated than aminoglutethimide and that they may induce a longer progression-free survival time than progestogens.

Progestogens

These drugs have a complex method of action which includes down regulation of oestrogen receptors, glucocorticoid effects and possibly an effect through the progesterone receptor. Their side effects tend to be dose related and include nausea, fluid retention, significant weight gain (up to ten kilos), and thrombosis.

The evidence that 'more is better' is unconvincing. The dose of medroxy-progesterone (Provera, Farlutal®) should not exceed 500 mg per day while that of megestrol (Megace®) should not exceed 160 mg/day. If the patient experiences excessive weight gain or has glucocorticoid side effects, the dose should be reduced.

Oestrogen

It is paradoxical that while oestrogen is clearly a growth factor in some cases of breast cancer, pharmacological doses of it can induce a remission in some instances in post-menopausal women. There is uncertainty about the minimum effective dose and little information about bioequivalence between different oestrogens. Conjugated equine oestrogen (Premarin) 1.25 mg/day is usually reasonably well tolerated. Side effects include nausea, PV bleeding and thrombosis.

Recommended Therapeutic Regimens

1. Adjuvant therapy for Stage I or II disease
    (a) Pre-menopausal patients: ER+ only
        (i)   Oophorectomy—surgical, radiation or medical (treat for at least 5 years), or
        (ii) Tamoxifen 20 mg/day for 5 years. (See Chapter 24 for recommendations on chemo-therapy.)
    (b) Post-menopausal patients
        (i)   Tamoxifen 20 mg/day for 5 years with or without chemotherapy depending on clinical circumstances.
2. Advanced disease: Stage III or IV
    (a) Pre-menopausal patients: ER+ only
        (i)   Oophorectomy — surgical, radiation or medical, or
        (ii) Tamoxifen 20mg/day
    (b) Post-menopausal patients
        (i)   Tamoxifen 20 mg/day, followed by on relapse
        (ii) An aromatase inhibitor, triazole if available, otherwise
        (iii) Aminoglutethimide, followed by on relapse
        (iv) Progestogen (Megace® 40 mg qid), followed by on relapse
        (v)   Oestrogen (Premarin 1.3 mg/day).

PROSTATE CANCER

Huggins demonstrated that prostate cancer was androgen dependent in 1941, when he showed that bilateral orchidectomy caused tumour shrinkage. Since that time orchidectomy has become the 'gold standard' in the hormone treatment of advanced prostate cancer (Stage C or D). Sixty to eighty percent of patients with advanced disease will achieve a remission following orchidectomy with a median duration of 18 months.

Hormonal Agents in Prostate Cancer

In recent years a number of new drugs have been developed that either inhibit the production of testosterone or its metabolites, or block its action by competing for the intra-cellular androgen receptor.

1. LHRH analogues: Zoladex®, Lucrin®. These are administered subcutaneiously or intramuscularly 4 weekly and lead to depletion of pituitary LH and FSH and secondarily to shutdown of synthesis of testosterone by the testes thus producing a 'medical orchidectomy'. LHRH analogues produce identical results to surgical orchidectomy and have the same side effects including hot flushes, loss of libido and impotence.

2. Antiandrogens: Cyproterone acetate (Androcur®), Flutamide (Eulixon®) and Casodex. These all compete with testosterone for the intra-cellular androgen receptor. It's claimed that libido and potency are retained in approximately 50% of patients if they are used as single agents. Cyproterone will inhibit hot flushes in orchidectomised patients. Up to 20% of patients will have gastric intolerance with flutamide. Casodex is a derivative of flutamide and has less toxicity.

3. 5 alpha reductase inhibitors: Finesteride. These drugs inhibit the enzyme responsible for converting testosterone to its more active metabolite dihydrotestosterone. Potency and libido are preserved and they have few side effects. However, early studies suggest that finesteride alone is not as effective as orchidectomy.

Conflicting results have been obtained in studies comparing medical or surgical orchidectomy with an additional antiandrogen. This approach is known as maximum androgen blockade. A recent meta-analysis showed that if there was any benefit for the combined treatment, it was small.

Until recently, early disease (Stage A or B) has not been treated hormonally. However, with availability of new medical agents, trials are underway to assess the effects of adjuvant and neo-adjuvant therapy, using 5 alpha reductase inhibitors and anti-androgens or LHRH analogues respectively. At this stage neo-adjuvant therapy has shown a reduction in the percentage of tumours that have positive margins on resection but this has not translated into prolongation of disease-free survival.

In advanced disease, there are few effective options when relapse occurs. If the patient has been taking an anti-androgen this should be stopped as a withdrawal response is sometimes seen. It is essential to continue with an LHRH analogue if the patient has been receiving this, in order to maintain testicular suppression.

Treatment with aminoglutethimide, 250 mg twice daily, and cortisone acetate, 25 mg bd, to cause suppression of adrenal androgens will induce a further remission in approximately 30% of patients for a median duration 12–18 months.

Second line treatment with anti-androgens is useful in < 10% of cases.

REFERENCES

Motta, M. and Serio, M. (1994) *Sex Hormones and Antihormones in Endocrine Dependent Pathology*. Amsterdam: Elsevier.

Prostate Cancer Trialists Collaborative Group (1995) *Lancet*, **346(8970)**, 265–269.

CHAPTER 13

DRUG RESISTANCE

Stephen J. Clarke

INTRODUCTION

Tumour resistance to the action of currently available cytotoxic agents is the principal reason for the failure of chemotherapy to cure cancer. The resistance mechanisms may be present *ab initio* as a feature of a particular tumour type or develop after exposure to chemotherapy. The former situation is exemplified by lack of tumour response to initial therapy whilst the latter is usually demonstrated by a failure of tumour response to further chemotherapy on relapse, in spite of having shown initial chemosensitivity.

The study of cytotoxic drug resistance has attracted much research attention because of a relative dearth of new agents with enhanced activity which might override mechanisms of drug resistance. By characterising the mechanisms of drug resistance it is envisaged that new agents may be developed which are either not subject to drug resistance or able to impair the resistance mechanisms, and thereby re-establish sensitivity to existing agents.

The majority of mechanistic studies of drug resistance are performed in *in vitro* models using tumour cell lines derived from human or animal malignancies. These models enable the biochemical and molecular characterisation of drug resistance and the identification of markers which may then be used to assess the prevalence of similar mechanisms in tumour samples from patients in the clinic. Resistance is induced in tumour cell lines by repeated or continuous exposure to low doses of drug, usually commencing at half the dose which results in a 50% cell kill (IC_{50}). This dose is gradually escalated and the degree of resistance induced is compared to the parent line in multiples of the IC_{50}. Aliquots of cells are taken for freezing at each stage of this process to ensure the perpetuation of the model. Once resistance has been achieved, screening of other compounds with known mechanisms of action can be performed to characterise the resistance. Biochemical and genetic parameters which might accompany the resistance can also then be assessed.

The known mechanisms of resistance for most currently available cytotoxic agents are summarised in Table 13.1. It is evident from this list that resistance can occur at multiple sites for an individual agent and relates to the metabolism and mechanism of action of the agent.

Table 13.1 Causes of cytotoxic drug resistance per class of compound

Class of Compound	Resistance Mechanism(s)
Antimetabolites	
1. Methotrexate	Defect in active transportation
	Polyglutamation defect
	Increased DHFR
2. 5-FU	Alterations in activating enzymes
	Increased TS
	Increased dUMP
3. Ara-C	Impaired cellular uptake
	Decreased activation (deoxycytidine kinase)
	Increased catabolism (deoxycytidine deaminase)
	Increased dCTP
4. 6-MP/6-TG	Decrease in activating enzyme activity (HGPRT)
	Increased catabolism (alkaline phosphatase)
Alkylating agents	
1. Mustard derivatives	
(a) General	Decreased cellular uptake
	Increased cellular glutathione
	Enhanced DNA repair
(b) Specific cyclophosphamide	
	Increased catabolism (aldehyde dehydrogenase)
2. Nitrosoureas	Enhanced DNA repair via guanine-O^6-alkyl transferase
	Decreased cellular uptake
Platinum derivatives	Increased cellular glutathione
	Enhanced DNA repair
Anthracyclines and like agents	P-glycoprotein
	Altered topoisomerase-II activity
	Increased cellular glutathione
Bleomycin	Enhanced DNA repair
Natural alkaloids:	Decreased binding to tubulin
Vinca alkaloids	P-glycoprotein
	Alternations in tubulin
Epipodophyllotoxins	Altered topoisomerase-II activity
	Enhanced DNA repair
	P-glycoprotein
Taxanes	Alterations in tubulin
	P-glycoprotein

Many agents require intracellular transportation to reach their target and thus cellular mutations which result in impairments of these transport mechanisms can lead to drug resistance. Drugs such as cyclophosphamide and 5-FU also require metabolic activation to cytotoxic forms to exert their activity. Cells which have decreased levels of the activating enzymes may not be sensitive to these compounds. For agents such as methotrexate and 5-FU which inhibit specific enzymes to exert their cytotoxic action, tumour cells which over express the target enzyme will be less sensitive to these compounds than those with lower levels of the same enzyme.

A variety of compounds such as the alkylating agents, anthracyclines, epipodophyllotoxins and platinum derivatives exert at least part of their cytotoxicity through damage to DNA. Naturally occurring mechanisms exist for the repair of DNA damage, and tumour cells with enhanced levels of DNA repair capacity would be unlikely to show sensitivity to these classes of compound. Tumour cells demonstrating enhanced ability to detoxify and catabolise cytotoxic agents could also be drug resistant.

Thus, it is obvious that there is not a single cause of cytotoxic drug resistance. However, some mechanisms of resistance affect multiple drugs of differing structures and class, including drugs to which the cell lines have not been previously exposed. These patterns of cross-resistance, of which several have been delineated, are termed multidrug resistance or MDR.

CLASSIC MULTI-DRUG RESISTANCE (P-GLYCOPROTEIN MEDIATED RESISTANCE)

Classic multi-drug resistance is principally associated with the use of anti-cancer agents obtained from natural sources which include the anthracyclines, vinca alkaloids, dactinomycin, mitomycin C, epipodophyllotoxins, taxol and colchicine. Cross-resistance is usually not seen to anti-metabolites, alkylating agents or platinum derivatives. One of the major features associated with this form of resistance is reduced intracellular drug accumulation due to the action of a membrane bound, energy dependent, unidirectional efflux pump which is composed of 170 kD glycoprotein known as P-glycoprotein (P-gp).

Although discovered through analysis of resistant tumour cell lines, the establishment of monoclonal antibodies to this protein and the identification of the mRNA encoding it, with use of the polymerase chain reaction (PCR), have permitted the analysis of clinical tumour and normal tissue specimens to determine the breadth of expression of P-gp. P-gp is normally expressed on cells on the gastrointestinal epithelium in the colon and jejunum, in the lining of the biliary tree, the proximal tubule in the kidney, in small ductules of the pancreas, and capillary endothelial cells in the brain and testis. A variety of other organs also have some structural expression of P-gp. The action of the pump, its specificity for natural products and its locations, which include the major organs associated with absorption and excretion, suggest P-gp has a normal role in the detoxification of foreign substances.

The gene encoding P-gp, the MDR 1 gene, is located on chromosome 7 and transfection of this gene into previously drug sensitive cell lines induces drug resistance. In some *in vitro* models there is a linear correlation between the degree of drug resistance and the expression of MDR 1. Recent evidence suggests that P-gp may be responsible for other malignant cell functions apart from drug efflux. The presence of increased levels of P-gp expressing cells at the edges of tumours with a high metastatic potential suggests a possible role for P-gp in invasion and metastasis.

In clinical samples, P-gp has been demonstrated in a range of tumours including ovarian, breast, cervical and renal cell cancers, acute and chronic leukaemias, multiple myeloma, soft tissue sarcoma and neuroblastoma. Correlations with outcome suggest that patients with tumours positive for P-gp are chemotherapy resistant and have a worse survival rate than those whose tumours are negative.

In *in vitro* models a number of non-cytotoxic agents can reverse the expression of P-gp and reverse cytotoxic drug resistance. These agents include verapamil and diltiazem and related calcium antagonists, the phenothiazines, reserpine and related indole alkaloids, tamoxifen and like compounds, dipyridamole, dihydropyridine and cyclosporine A. The proposed mechanism of action is through binding to P-gp. These findings have led to clinical trials of these agents used in combination with cytotoxic compounds aimed at modulating drug resistance.

MULTI-DRUG RESISTANCE ASSOCIATED WITH ALTERED TOPOISOMERASE II

Multi-drug resistance (MDR) associated with altered topoisomerase II occurs across a range of compounds with different structures which all have Topoisomerase II as their locus of action. There is no associated expression of P-gp and no cross-resistance to agents such as the vinca alkaloids which would normally occur if MDR 1 was the causative genetic alteration. Drug classes affected by this form of MDR include the anthracyclines and the closely related anthracenediones (e.g. mitozantrone), the epipodophyllotoxins and actinomycin-D. The resistance is thought to be due to alteration in the activity of topoisomerase II which principally results in fewer drug induced DNA strand breaks.

OTHER POSSIBLE FORMS OF MULTI-DRUG RESISTANCE

The distinctions between the above forms of multi-drug resistance are not always clear cut, for instance, resistant cell lines have been characterised which display a mixture of the features of classic MDR and altered topoisomerase II. In addition, other resistant cell lines have been developed which show all the features of classical multi-drug resistance, but without the expression of either P-gp or MDR-1.

There is also some preliminary evidence to suggest that increased levels of enzymes responsible for detoxification of certain classes of cytotoxic compounds may also contribute to multi-drug resistance. The thiol containing glutathione S-transferases (GSTs) are important in the detoxification of a variety of cytotoxic agents including the alkylating agents, cisplatin and doxorubicin. Thus, it is possible that an over-expression of the genes responsible for the production of these enzymes could cause cross-resistance to these various classes of cytotoxic agents.

MOLECULAR MECHANISMS OF DRUG RESISTANCE

Programmed cell death or apoptosis appears to be a frequent cytotoxic endpoint of anti-cancer drugs. This is a complex process affecting the cell cycle involving interactions between a number of genes, especially p53, but also including p21, p27, GADD 45, BAX and BCL-2. It is increasingly apparent that genetic abnormalities in these pathways may impair programmed cell death and result in drug resistance. One example of this occurs with lymphomas where tumours overexpressing BCL-2 are resistant to chemotherapy.

REFERENCES

Beck, W.T., Dalton, W.S. (1997) Mechanisms of drug resistance. In *Cancer: Principles and Practice of Oncology* (5th edn), edited by V. Devita, S. Hellman and S.Rosenberg. Philadelphia: Lippincott-Raven Publishers.

Filipits, M., Suchomel, R.W., Zochbauer, S. Malayeris, R. and Pirker, R. (1996) Clinical relevance of drug resistance genes in malignant disease. *Leukemia*, **10**(Suppl. 3), 510–517.

Kaye, S.B. (1995) Clinical drug resistance: The role of factors other than P-glycoprotein. *Am J Med*, **99**(64), 40–44.

Kaye, S.B. (1993) P-glycoprotein and drug resistance: Time for reappraisal. *Cancer*, **67**(4), 641–643.

Patel, N.K. and Rothenberg, M.L. (1994) Multidrug resistance in cancer chemotherapy. *Invest New Drugs*, **12**(1), 1–13.

CHAPTER 14

PRINCIPLES OF SURGICAL ONCOLOGY

John F. Thompson

INTRODUCTION

Surgical procedures are performed in cancer patients for a variety of reasons. The objective may be to achieve a permanent cure, but it may instead be only for staging purposes, or to obtain local disease control and thus prevent the pain or inconvenience associated with local recurrence. Often the appropriate surgery will be major and radical, involving en bloc resection of the primary tumour and any regional disease. Sometimes, however, a more conservative surgical operation which preserves function and reduces disfigurement may be the preferable option, if its effectiveness as a cancer operation has been established. Alternatively, a purely palliative procedure may be all that can reasonably be undertaken, to relieve symptoms or prevent interference with important bodily functions. In some circumstances surgery may be undertaken simply to enhance the likelihood of other treatment modalities being successful, by reducing tumour bulk. The surgical oncologist must not only have the training and experience to be able to undertake these cancer operations, but must also have the judgement and oncological knowledge to determine which treatment option is likely to achieve the most satisfactory outcome in a given clinical situation.

DISTINCTIONS BETWEEN SURGICAL ONCOLOGY AND ONCOLOGICAL SURGERY

Fifty years ago surgery offered the only possibility of cure for most patients with malignant disease. The disciplines of medical oncology and radiation oncology were still in their infancy, and the value of chemotherapy and radiotherapy as supplementary or alternative treatments for patients with cancer had not been established. Even today, many malignancies, such as early stage gastric or colorectal cancers, are able to be treated effectively by surgery alone. Such conditions are likely to be well managed by surgeons who may have received no formal training in surgical oncology, but who have specialised operative experience in treating that particular form of cancer, and are competent and effective oncological surgeons[1].

There are, however, many malignancies which are best treated in an integrated, multidisciplinary fashion, and the oncologist with surgical expertise is an important member of the partnership of clinicians from different specialities who form the effective multidisciplinary team. In such a team, the distinctions between surgical oncologist, gynaecological oncologist, medical oncologist and radiation oncologist may be blurred. Every oncologist, from any background, must have a sound knowledge of the biology of malignant diseases, must be aware of the range of therapies available for particular tumour types, and must be capable of formulating an appropriate combination and sequence of cancer treatments for the individual patient.

Every oncologist also has responsibilities in the fields of basic and clinical research, and in the education of medical undergraduates and postgraduates about the principles and practice of oncological treatment. Yet, the surgical oncologist must have the skills, knowledge and judgement to recommend and safely apply appropriate surgical treatment options ranging from conservative to radical. At the same time the surgical oncologist must fully understand the indications, risks and benefits of adjuvant chemotherapy, hormonal therapy, immunotherapy and radiotherapy, and be aware of the evidence for such benefits as demonstrated by properly conducted clinical trials.

LOCOREGIONAL CONTROL OF MALIGNANT DISEASE

There is a group of malignant diseases for which radical operative surgery, radiotherapy or systemic chemotherapy all give poor results, and in which the pattern of failure is usually locoregional. Such diseases include advanced cancer of the head and neck and some tumours of the gastrointestinal tract. There are other malignant diseases which have a propensity for widespread dissemination but which in some patients show a tendency to locoregional patterns of recurrence, such as soft-tissue and bone sarcomas, locally advanced breast cancers, and melanomas in a limb. Still other malignancies have characteristic patterns of spread, such as to the liver or peritoneal cavity, which tend to be associated with terminal illness yet are frequently seen without more widespread dissemination, such as colorectal, gastric, pancreatico-biliary and ovarian cancers.

All the diseases cited above are usually only partially sensitive to radiotherapy or chemotherapy. They present some of the most difficult problems in oncology. It is the regional nature of these diseases which makes it desirable for their management to be carried out by practitioners who can plan and initiate appropriate multi-modal regional therapy, part of which is surgical. This is the particular role of surgical oncologists who can provide integrated regional cancer management.

Operative surgery thus represents only one facet of surgical oncology. The American Board of Surgery recognised this when it defined surgical oncology as 'coordinated multidisciplinary care of the cancer patient, including screening, diagnosis, surgical treatment, adjunctive therapy, rehabilitation and follow up'[2]. It must be emphasised that surgical oncology is not a discipline in competition with medical oncology or radiation oncology, rather its role is to complement them. The specific expertise of the surgical oncologist may be required for successful treatment of other locoregionally advanced or recurrent tumours, and of solid tumours which have complex or unusual features.

REGIONAL CHEMOTHERAPY BY INTRA-ARTERIAL INFUSION AND VASCULAR ISOLATION TECHNIQUES

Regional cancer treatment has been largely the province of surgical oncologists, because they are particularly concerned with the management of locoregional disease by surgery alone or in combination with regional chemotherapy and/or radiotherapy and the development and implementation of new techniques. Following the observation, by Klop in 1950, that accidental injection of nitrogen mustard into an artery rather than a vein resulted in a greatly increased tissue reaction in the distribution of the artery, it was postulated that intra-arterial delivery of an effective anticancer agent had the potential to achieve a greater local effect than its systemic administration.

Subsequent clinical experience has confirmed this hypothesis in many clinical situations. Examples of important advances in cancer treatment using regional chemotherapy include isolated limb perfusion for melanoma, the management of locally advanced breast cancer, the management of limb sarcoma, hyperthermic cytotoxic perfusion of the isolated pelvis for recurrent pelvic malignancy, and the management of liver metastases by hepatic artery drug infusion, chemoembolisation or isolated liver perfusion.

The surgical oncologist must draw on his or her skills as a surgeon in implementing all these techniques. For example, intra-vascular drug delivery systems often require very precise operative placement of catheters, and isolated regional perfusion techniques for limbs or organs such as the liver require considerable skill and experience in vascular surgery.

INDUCTION (NEO-ADJUVANT) CHEMOTHERAPY

In many regional cancer treatment techniques, the regional therapy is not the definitive treatment but is given with the aim of reducing tumour bulk and destroying as many malignant cells as possible, prior to radical surgery or radiotherapy, and possibly systemic chemotherapy. A most important principle of induction chemotherapy is that the treatment should be given before a tumour and its blood supply have been disturbed by operative surgery or radiotherapy. For some tumour types, preoperative induction with systemic chemotherapy can be effective, but in many situations the much higher local drug concentrations which can be achieved using regional chemotherapy techniques result in considerably higher rates of tumour cell kill.

APPLYING THE PRINCIPLES OF SURGICAL ONCOLOGY

Ways in which the principles of surgical oncology are applicable to the management of specific tumours in the various surgical subspecialities are well documented in other chapters of this book and elsewhere in the medical literature[3]. Over the past decade the discipline of surgical oncology has become a more clearly defined entity, with basic tumour biology and fundamental surgical principles as its foundation stones, and the various components of multidisciplinary clinical cancer management as complementary, interlocking building blocks.

Surgical procedures, sometimes complex, sometimes simple, are coordinated with regional and systemic chemotherapy, external beam and stereotactic radiotherapy, brachytherapy, immunotherapy and a range of other forms of treatment with the goal of maximising benefits for cancer patients whilst minimising morbidity and side effects. Meanwhile, new techniques for achieving locoregional control of malignant disease are being explored, and important unanswered questions in surgical oncology are being addressed through appropriately designed clinical trials.

REFERENCES

1. Stephens, F.O., Storey, D.W., Thompson, J.F. and Marsden, F.W. (1992) Surgical oncology and the role of regional chemotherapy. *Aust NZ J Surg,* **62**, 691–696.

2. Editorial (1994) What is a surgical oncologist? *Ann Surg Oncol,* **1,** 2–4.
3. Allen-Mersh, T.G. (ed.) (1996) *Surgical Oncology.* London: Chapman & Hall Medical.

CHAPTER 15

PRINCIPLES OF PALLIATIVE CARE

J. Norelle Lickiss

DEFINITION OF PALLIATIVE CARE

Palliative care focuses on those last years or months of life when death is foreseeable rather than merely a possibility. There is emphasis on the pattern of physical, emotional, social and spiritual distress which may be present, and which should and can be relieved.[1] Palliative care should be available for every patient with incurable cancer, whether or not specific anti-cancer treatment is available or appropriate, or is being currently used.

WHO (National Cancer Control Programmes, 1995) notes that relief from suffering and improvements in the quality of life, both for cancer patients themselves and their families, can be achieved more immediately through palliative care than through any other approach for cancer control.

The principles of palliative care should be pervasive in all situations including the hospital, nursing home or home. For some patients specialist palliative care services may be necessary. WHO recommends that resources for palliative care should equal resources available for all anti-cancer measures such as surgery, radiotherapy and chemotherapy in developed countries. Further, that the vast majority of all cancer related resources in the developing world should be focussed on palliative care.

Palliative care is concerned with the facilitating of the central human task of fashioning and achieving a human life in accord with one's personal, unique potential, priorities, hopes and existential situation. This task must continue to be central, even if cancer is obviously incurable.

THE PATIENT AS THE SUBJECT

Palliative care is directed towards changing the patient's experience for the better, no matter what the context, with restoration of comfort, dignity and appropriate hope, especially when actually dying. This concept is explicitly noted in the International Association for the Study of Pain's definition of pain, 'an unpleasant sensory and emotional experience associated with the actual or potential tissue damage or described in the terms of such damage'[2].

The fact that palliative care is concerned with changing experience indicates immediately that this branch of clinical science and activity is specified by the focus on the patient as subject. This is the major philosophical and psychological theme, but in practice the concept has several practical dimensions.

The Patient's Capacities

The patient as the subject has capacities for perception, for knowledge, for formulating intentions, for setting priorities, for decision making (alone or by participation with others), and for accepting decisions made by others, such as the family in some cultures.

The Patient's Context

The patient as the subject is situated in a particular context, with a present environment including significant persons, personal bonds, resources, geographic or political features, cultural dimensions with past experience influencing the present. This past experience includes a personal history, such as the circumstances of birth, childhood, family life and occupation, experience, good or bad, of disease, authority figures and health facilities.

The Patient's Suffering

- Suffering has been defined by Cassell as a sense of impending personal disintegration.[3] Major causes of triggers of such a sensation of nearly 'going to pieces' are not predictable by clinical staff on the basis of objective medical information.

- Only the patient knows the shape of his or her suffering and what has triggered or aggravated it. The factors may be in any one of several fields of human experience, such as the loss of a supporting person, objects, or roles, bad news badly broken, unrelieved pain, the results of an investigation, the experience of chemotherapy, a self-perception as a 'treatment failure', a change in personal or clinical circumstances, or profound spiritual matters causing extreme distress.

- Some patients perceive themselves as battered by the health system or by life, and appear to revert to a state of withdrawal and apathy with an inability to respond to the staff and even to the family. Many recover if given space, time and peace, and even a brief removal from the anti-cancer treatment scene. The patient may prefer not to speak or reveal any of this, especially to a treating doctor, in case harm may result.

- One of the goals of medicine is the relief of suffering and a deeper understanding of suffering. Thus, cancer must be appropriately managed to reduce, not increase, the distress of patients and their carers and families in this precious closing phase of life.

- Current evidence indicates that decision making and care are seriously deficient in patients with a perceived poor prognosis.

- Daniel Callahan has suggested certain points at which the customary presumption to treat should be changed.[4]

  1. When there is a likely, not necessarily certain, downward course of an illness, making death a strong probability, for example, the failure of more than one organ.

  2. When the available treatments for a potentially fatal condition entail a significant likelihood of extended suffering rather than the relief of suffering.

3. When successful treatment is more likely to bring extended unconsciousness or advanced dementia than cure or significant amelioration.

4. When, whatever the medical condition, the available treatments significantly increase the probability of a bad death, even if they also promise to extend life.

APPLICATION OF PALLIATIVE CARE

Processes involved in palliative care involve a continuous cycle of assessment, clarification of the patients priorities with desirable targets for achievement, formulation of a management plan, and evaluation of the outcome desired by the patient.

Assessment

Assessment is usually the most difficult task, especially in a cross-cultural situation. It can usefully include attentive listening to the patient's narrative. It involves listening to the history of:

(a) the tumour, including the symptoms and events leading to the diagnosis;

(b) the response to the treatment undertaken;

(c) the evaluation of the patient's current high priority problems from the patient's perspective; and

(d) the pattern of response of the family or carers to the whole saga.

The use of the narrative approach for assessment, when skillfully undertaken, facilitates a process of healing for a distressed patient. It also provides crucial information leading to a comprehensive diagnosis of the current problems, including clinical, psychological, social and spiritual aspects.

Formulation of a Management Plan

Formulation of a management plan requires clear goals and objectives for the patient. The patient's priorities should be reflected in this plan.

Symptom Relief

Symptom relief is commonly an objective. There are several excellent textbooks which give detailed information concerning symptom relief within the context of comprehensive palliative care, with due regard for cultural factors (see references and Chapters 16 and 17).

COMMON PROBLEMS IN PALLIATIVE CARE

Faecal Impaction

Faecal impaction is common and very distressing. Faecal impaction can mimic tumour-related gastrointestinal obstruction with low obstruction causing constipation, noted by the patient, or high obstruction causing nausea and vomiting especially if faecal impaction is prolonged. Faecal impaction may impede effectiveness of oral medication by interference with absorption. The resulting situation may be a patient suffering preventable pain, nausea, vomiting, abdominal distension and even a confusional state.

The remedy for established faecal impaction with a loaded rectum, requires local rectal measures may have to be commenced in addition to oral laxatives. If the patient has hard faeces in the rectum, an oil retention enema overnight may be an advantage and a further retention enema of a softening agent such as docusate in the morning to assist evacuation.

Manual removal of the faecal mass should be rarely necessary but should be accompanied by sedation and/or analgesia. Faecal impaction can take two or three days to improve. Every effort should be made to prevent recurrence of this distressing symptom. Opioid drugs should not be given without oral laxatives. Dehydration of sick patients should be avoided in hot climates.

Spinal Cord or Nerve Root Compression

Moderate to severe back pain in a cancer patient should raise the suspicion of epidural tumour. This is especially true of pain in the thoracic region. Spinal cord compression as a cause should be considered and excluded. Subjective awareness of vague changes in the lower limbs may be the only symptom of spinal cord compression. Minimal neurological signs such as hesitant plantar reflexes should raise the clinical suspicion of impending compression.

Gastrointestinal Obstruction

- Gastrointestinal obstruction is a frequent complication of some forms of advanced cancer, most notably gynaecological tumours and tumours involving the retroperitoneal tissues. Precise management according to contemporary principles can yield a comfortable and peaceful final phase of life, provided that the goals of therapy are unambiguous.
- Obstruction may be due to mechanical factors associated with the tumour or a dramatic disturbance in gastrointestinal motility associated with autonomic dysfunction.
- The diagnosis of the level of obstruction will be apparent on clinical criteria.

High Bowel Obstruction

- In high bowel obstruction the surgical option should be considered. Whilst the decision is being made to consider a surgical approach, the condition of the patient should be maintained optimally and a nasogastric suction will normally be necessary, together with intravenous fluids.
- Anti-nauseant drugs may have little to offer in high obstructions but a central anti-nauseant such as haloperidol may be indicated. Metoclopramide or other gastrokinetic anti-nauseants should not be used in a high obstruction in view of the probability of worsening the situation. Corticosteroids should not be introduced during the decision making phase, while surgery is being considered.
- If a surgical approach for high bowel obstruction is not appropriate, a trial of corticosteroids can be used. Dexamethasone, 4–8 mgs, subcutaneously or IV daily for two or three days can be used. If the improvement occurs then the drug can be withdrawn and re-introduced in a pulsed fashion. If no improvement is achieved the drug should be withdrawn. Corticosteroids should be used cautiously because of potential side effects, including diabetes, infection or peptic ulcer disease, and emotional shifts which may be very distressing the patient and family.
- If corticosteroid therapy fails then the goal is comfort and quality not obstruction relief.
- Management should be changed to hyoscine hydrobromide 50–120 mgs subcutaneously per day as pulse doses or preferably by syringe driver. This reduces gut contractibility, abolishes colic and reduces the amount of fluid produced by the gut. Octreotide 100–200 micrograms three times a day (tds) or by subcutaneous infusion may be added. Once the situation has stabilised the patient may well be able to enjoy small amounts of beverages. Very high bowel obstruction may

be treated with percutaneous venting gastrostomy. It should be considered early in the course of management of end stage high bowel obstruction in some patients.

Low Bowel Obstruction

- In patients with low bowel obstruction, below the mid-small bowel, colostomy may be indicated as a terminal procedure. This may assist in the comfort and dignity of the patient.
- Abdominal distension is a major cause of discomfort in large bowel obstruction. Pain therapy with paracetamol and morphine is usually required. Oral morphine may be occasionally adequate. A trial of metoclopramide or other gastrokinetic anti-nauseant may be appropriate where the obstruction is very low to clear the stomach and upper small bowel and to improve the patients capacity to eat and drink a little.
- Intermittent or colic type discomfort is usually readily controlled by hyoscine hydrobromide subcutaneously.
- Throughout the management of end stage GIT obstruction it is inappropriate to seek to keep electrolytes in balance, and blood tests should not be undertaken.
- Emotional support is essential. The patient, with carers at home, can usually be kept at home during such management, and thus appreciate family life and home circumstances.

CARE OF THE PATIENT CLOSE TO DEATH

The proximity of death is recognised by convergence of failure of organ systems, irreversible medical changes, withdrawal of patients into the inner self, sometimes the withdrawal from close family members and a conviction on the part of the patient that death is near. Experienced nursing staff and clinicians, with special experience with care of dying patients, can recognise this stage. Once proximity of death in the next week or days is obvious, a change in treatment approach is necessary, with meticulous attention to detail.

Philippe Aries in his account of dying and death throughout the ages drew the picture of the 'tame death' as the norm in the middle ages, when death occurred fairly quickly in presence of all, with due spiritual solace. The 'wild death' can occur if therapeutic endeavours are inappropriate. In the most advanced centres in the Western world, a dignified and peaceful closure of life should be possible, with the patient not having IV infusions or drainage tubes, or the paraphernalia of intensive care units intruding between the patient and his or her loved ones.

In order to achieve dignified, peaceful and gentle dying, it is essential that the goal be clear.

- Where it is the custom, 'do not resuscitate' orders need to be clearly in place, normally discussed and understood with family and patient.
- Intrusive investigation should not be undertaken.
- Therapy given should be directed towards symptom improvement. Such therapy will include continuation of drugs already demonstrated to be essential for the control of this patient's pain and other symptoms.
- There may need to be changes in the route of administration, if the patient ceases to be able to have therapy orally. The oral route should be maintained wherever possible. The rectal route is a very useful alternative if carefully explained. The parenteral route is normally by subcutaneous

injections through an indwelling butterfly needle. IV infusion is rarely indicated.

- Antibiotics may have a place during the closing days of life but only as part of symptomatic management.

- Drugs being used for other causes of symptoms such as diabetes, heart disease or arthritis, should be continued, if the goal of comfort is clear.

- If sedation is desired to permit patients to die peacefully in their sleep, a direct sedative or hypnotic should be used rather than morphine.[5] Morphine sedates through toxic side effects and the indignity associated with myoclonus or agitation can be avoided. Midazolam 2.5–10 mg by subcutaneous injection will induce sedation, but the drug will need to be repeated every few hours or given via syringe driver because half-life is brief. Clonazepam 1–2 mg 12 hourly, is a useful alternative. Rectal chlorpromazine 50–100 mgs 2 or 3 times per day has a place for some dying patients. Similarly sublingual lorazepam 0.5–1 mg may be useful.

- As death becomes imminent bronchial secretions may accumulate. At this stage the patient may be unaware, but the family may be distressed. Hyoseine 0.4 mg 4–6 hourly may be very useful. Atropine is an alternative, but lacks the sedating effect of hyoscine which is valuable at this stage.

- Terminal crises such as massive haematemesis, haemoptysis and respiratory obstruction may occur. It is essential to relieve patients' anxiety rapidly with either midazolam 2.5–15 mg IV or IM, rectal diazepam 10–20 PR via a female catheter, or sodium phenobarbitone 200 mg SCI or IMI. Occasionally higher doses will be needed.

In the current climate created by the euthanasia controversy, it is important that patients, relatives, doctors and nurses understand that carefully used sedation is not euthanasia. To help patients to die during sleep induced by sedative drugs at normal doses is not causing death, but permitting peaceful death from other causes. Patients should have confidence that their doctors can safeguard their last hours in such a manner.

SUMMARY

Palliative care incorporates the key ideas and clinical research of the hospice movement, which originated in the UK in the middle of the twentieth century. It articulates a long tradition of care of the most vulnerable.

A hospice in the middle ages was a place of safety for travellers on a difficult journey to a sacred place. Hospice as a place, gave way in the 1970s to hospice programs and hospice philosophy. Today, it is fitting to again perceive the patient as guest in the office consultation, in the clinic, or in the hospital bed. A doctor or nurse should personally create a place where a vulnerable person, on a difficult journey, finds safety in a combination of professional competence and compassion. Palliative care offers the opportunity for correctly structured hope that life will not be disfigured, nor death deformed, by the experience of living and dying with cancer. The last phase of life, even for the most weak, may then be a time not of treatment failure but of positive achievement. It has been said by Kingsley Mortimer that 'the task of medicine is the emancipation of man's interior splendour', nothing less.

REFERENCES

1. Doyle, D., Hanks, G.W.C. and MacDonald, N. (eds) (1997) *Oxford Textbook of Palliative Medicine* (2nd edn). Oxford: Oxford University Press.
2. IASP Sub-committee on Taxonomy (1980) Pain terms: A list with definitions and notes on usage. *Pain*, **8**, 249–252.
3. Cassell, E.J. (1982) The nature of suffering and the goals of medicine. *New Eng Jour Med*, **306(11)**, 639–45.
4. Callahan, D. (1995) *The Troubled Dream of Life*. New York: Simon & Schuster.
5. Portenoy, R.K. and Cherny, N.I. (1994) Sedation in the management of refractory symptoms: guidelines for evaluation and treatment. *J Palliat Care*, **10(2)**, 31–8.

ADDITIONAL REFERENCES

Aries, P. (1981) *The Hour of our Death*. Oxford: Oxford University Press.

Chapman, C.R. and Gavrin, J. (1993) Suffering and its relationship to pain. *J Palliat Care*, **9(2)**, 5–13.

The SUPPORT Principal Investigators (1995) A controlled trial to improve care for seriously ill hospitalized patients; the study to understand prognoses and preferences for outcomes and risks of treatments (SUPPORT). *JAMA*, **274(20)**, 1591–1958.

Woodruff, R. (1996) *Palliative Medicine* (2nd edn). Melbourne: Asperula.

PART III

SYMPTOM CONTROL
AND QUALITY OF LIFE

CHAPTER 16

ANTI-EMETICS AND SYMPTOM CONTROL

Ian N. Olver

INTRODUCTION

In controlling the symptoms in patients with cancer, it is helpful to distinguish those that are directly due to the cancer, or its paraneoplastic syndromes, from those that are due to its treatment or caused by unrelated drugs or medical conditions.

Nausea and Vomiting

The use of anti-emetics is mainly associated with controlling the emesis associated with cytotoxic chemotherapy[1]. Three phases of chemotherapy-induced emesis are recognised: acute post-chemotherapy, delayed and anticipatory.

Acute Post-chemotherapy Emesis

- Acute post-chemotherapy emesis commences within six hours of administration of the cytotoxic drug and is confined to the first twenty-four hours, although it can be prolonged after cyclophosphamide and carboplatin.
- Severe emesis is associated with bolus doses of the drugs cisplatin, dacarbazine, nitrogen mustard, streptozocin and dactinomycin.
- Moderate emesis occurs with the anthracyclines, cyclophosphamide, ifosfamide, the taxanes, and cytosine arabinoside.
- Bleomycin, the vinca alkaloids, chlorambucil, 5-fluorouracil, methotrexate and mitomycin C have a low probability of causing emesis.
- Emesis is related to the dose of chemotherapy.
- Patients are more likely to vomit if they have had prior exposure to cytotoxics and a prior history of motion sickness.

- Emesis is more difficult to control in females receiving cisplatin and in younger patients.
- Patients with a long history of heavy alcohol intake experience less cytotoxic-induced emesis.

The 5 Hydroxtryptamine$_3$ Receptor (5-HT$_3$) Antagonists

The introduction of the 5 hydroxtryptamine$_3$ receptor (5-HT$_3$) antagonists, such as ondansetron, tropisetron and granisetron, have revolutionised the management of acute post-chemotherapy emesis. In combination with corticosteroids, particularly dexamethasone, control rates of up to ninety percent have been reported for cisplatin-induced nausea and vomiting. Emesis from radiation also responds well to 5-HT$_3$ antagonists. The side effects recognised include headache, constipation and mild increases in transaminases and are usually well tolerated.

The 5-HT$_3$ antagonists have largely replaced anti-emetic combinations including dopamine antagonists, the substituted benzamide, metoclopramide, and the phenothiazines such as prochlorperazine. These agents have greater side effects, particularly dystonic reactions and restlessness. For mild and moderate emesis these agents are still effective. The cannabinoids can be effective but are inferior to the 5HT$_3$ receptor antagonists. The benzodiazepine lorazepam is useful as an adjuvant to anti-emetic treatment because of its anxiolytic, sedative and amnesic properties.

Delayed Emesis

Delayed emesis is seen most often with high doses of cisplatin, commences towards the end of the first twenty-four hours and can last for several days. Delayed emesis is more likely to occur when acute emesis has not been well controlled. It is more common in women.

The mechanism of delayed emesis is not known. The 5-HT$_3$ receptor antagonists are no more effective than other classes of drugs. Corticosteroids combined with other anti-emetics are the treatment of choice, but the response rates are usually only about fifty percent.

Anticipatory Emesis

Anticipatory emesis occurs prior to a second or subsequent course of chemotherapy. It appears to be a conditioned response because it only occurs if there has been post-treatment emesis. It occurs in:

- younger patients
- patients with more severe acute emesis
- anxious patients
- patients with feelings of warmth, sweating or weakness after treatment
- patients who are prone to motion sickness

It can be difficult to treat, as desensitisation and behavioural therapy is required. It is far better to prevent anticipatory emesis from developing by preventing acute emesis using the best available anti-emetic regimen prior to the initial course of chemotherapy.

Other Causes of Vomiting in Cancer Patients

Emesis related to cancer could be the result of a bowel obstruction, secondaries or a metabolic disturbance.

- A bowel obstruction from a tumour may be relieved surgically or may settle with conservative treatment using anti-emetics, resting the bowel, allowing nothing by mouth and intravenously hydrating. Patients with inoperable obstructions may obtain some relief from a venting gastrostomy which them allows them oral intake.
- Vomiting from cerebral or liver secondaries may be alleviated by the use of corticosteroids or specific treatment of the underlying cause.
- Histamine$_2$ receptor antagonists or proton pump inhibitors can be used to reduce gastric acidity if that is exacerbating emesis.
- Metabolic abnormalities such as hypercalcaemia, either due to bone secondaries or a paraneoplastic syndrome, should always be considered as a cause for emesis.
- The opiates frequently result in emesis and anti-emetics need to be given concomitantly. Anti-emetics can be mixed with opiates in subcutaneous infusions if required.

PAIN

The symptomatic treatment of cancer-related pain will depend upon its origin. Its management is discussed elsewhere. The general principle of treating chronic pain is that dosing must occur regularly to achieve freedom from pain over twenty-four hours. The dose of opiates is titrated against the pain. Multiple approaches may be necessary to control the different types of pain[2].

Cancer-related bone pain responds very well to radiation therapy, and also to non-steroidal anti-inflammatory drugs. It can be avoided and partly controlled with bisphosphonates. Other drugs can be added to analgesics. Anti-emetics can be given concomitantly and it may also be useful to add a sedative, such as midazolam, to control associated restlessness.

Somatic Pain

- Somatic pain is in skin or deeper tissues and is well localised, and often described as dull or aching.
- The initial treatment is frequently simple analgesics such as paracetamol. For more severe pain, long acting morphine is used with short acting morphine for breakthrough pain to achieve continual pain control.
- If patients are unable to swallow tablets, morphine can be given continuously subcutaneously using an infusion pump to achieve constant analgesic cover.
- Epidural or intrathecal catheters allow very low doses of opiates in order to relieve pain without as many side effects.

Visceral Pain

Visceral pain is due to the stretching of pain fibres in organs in the abdomen, such as the liver capsule or the chest. It is often poorly localised and associated with sweating or nausea. In addition to the above analgesics, corticosteroids and non-steroidal anti-inflammatory drugs are useful for alleviating this type of pain.

Neuropathic Pain

Neuropathic pain can be due to cancer involving the nerves or the spinal cord. It is often described as a burning pain with sudden shock-like sensations. Neuralgic pain can respond to corticosteroids, systemic oral local anaesthetics such as mexiletine, anticonvulsants such as carbamazepine and tricyclic antidepressants.

MUCOSITIS

Stomatitis is often a direct toxic effect of radiation and chemotherapy drugs, particularly methotrexate, 5-fluorouracil and doxorubicin. It is difficult to prevent, although prophylactic dental care is helpful. Cooling the mucosa with ice chips during chemotherapy has been advocated and the role of growth factors is being investigated. Mucositis often presents as a burning sensation within one week of therapy and lasts for ten to fourteen days.

The treatment of mucositis is supportive, using antimicrobial mouthwashes and local anaesthetic preparations. Secondary infections are often caused by candida and treated with nystatin and amphotericin lozenges. For severe mucositis, soft or liquid diets may be needed, or if prolonged, enteral nutrition is required.

CANCER CACHEXIA

Anorexia is a common presenting symptom of cancer and over half of the patients with cancer have a history of weight loss. Cancer cachexia is also characterised by weakness and wasting which does not necessarily correlate with the tumour bulk.

The symptoms of cancer cachexia are thought to be caused by cytokines such as tumour necrosis factor, interleukin 1, interleukin 6 and gamma interferon. The body does not adapt to the malnutrition and there is equal use of fat and muscle protein for energy, leading to wasting. The use of glucose can increase and resistance to insulin has been described.

The problem can be exacerbated if the tumour causes a bowel obstruction, dysphagia or malabsorption, or if surgery requires prolonged resting of the bowel. Chemotherapy is associated with emesis, anorexia, constipation, mucositis and altered taste. Radiotherapy can cause stomatitis or enteritis depending on the site of the field. Xerostomia can also cause problems with eating and necessitates good dental hygiene. An artificial saliva or frequent sips of water may help with the symptom and some patients find pilocarpine useful.

Corticosteroids can stimulate the appetite and increase the general sense of wellbeing, alleviating some of the extreme lethargy experienced with cancer cachexia, but long-term use can be detrimental due to side effects such as proximal myopathy. Megesterol acetate has been shown to improve appetite and oral intake[3]. This is considered a side effect when it is used in endocrine sensitive cancers, but is beneficial in tumours which are not sensitive to hormones when they present with anorexia.

Patients may require counselling about oral dietary supplements. If the digestive tract is functioning enteral feeding may be helpful either via a nasogastric tube in the short term or for longer use procedures like a percutaneous endoscopic gastrostomy are required. Parenteral nutrition is only considered for those patients who cannot eat and require aggressive nutritional support during intensive anti-cancer treatment.

DYSPNOEA

Dyspnoea may be caused by a cancer obstructing an airway, lymphangitic lung infiltration, or a pleural or pericardial effusion. It may also be related to infection or pulmonary emboli.

Airways obstructions can be palliated by external beam radiotherapy or brachytherapy, bronchoscopic laser techniques or stenting. Pleural effusions can be drained using a chest tube or at thoracoscopy, then pleuradhesis with talc, tetracycline or bleomycin. Lymphangitis may symptomatically respond to corticosteroids. Specific anti-cancer chemotherapy, if appropriate, may relieve these complications.

Laboured breathing in the terminal phase of the illness may be alleviated by morphine and chlorpromazine.

PRURITUS

- Pruritus can be multifactorial with causes including cancer infiltration of the skin, paraneoplastic skin changes, cancer causing cholestatic jaundice, drug eruptions or chemotherapy causing skin dryness[4].
- Symptomatic treatment can include bathing in lanolin oils for dryness or local steroid creams.
- Premedication with antihistamines and corticosteroids may prevent hypersensitivity reactions to chemotherapy.
- Treatment of itch can involve the use of histamine$_1$ and histamine$_2$ antagonists and more recently HT$_3$ receptor antagonists, since itch can be mediated by multiple receptors.
- In cholestatic jaundice, cholestyramine and rifampicin can provide symptomatic relief.

EXTRAVASATION

Extravasation of cytotoxic agents into the tissues may cause symptoms due to increasing tissue damage over many weeks post-treatment. The most problematic drugs are the anthracyclines.

Many of the antidotes suggested are based on empirical observations. The most generally applicable recommendation for treatment is the immediate application of ice. Vincristine is the only drug where this is in doubt and hyaluronidase is suggested.

Dimethyl sulphoxide (DMSO) is a treatment for anthracycline extravasation which has been prospectively shown to decrease the tissue damage[5]. It has also been reported as useful in treating extravasations of mitomycin C.

The only other specific treatment recommended is sodium thiosulphate for nitrogen mustard extravasations. If an extravasation is neglected, or the conservative treatments fail, then surgical debridement is required.

PSYCHOLOGICAL SYMPTOMS

It is important to consider the symptoms caused by the psychological response to cancer and its treatment[6] Symptoms of anxiety and depression are common and will require intervention if they persist. Frequent problems relate to changes in body image and sexual function.

Treatment may include counselling, such as anxiety management techniques or pharmacological intervention. Simply providing information can help alleviate anxiety and return to the patients some control of their situation. It is important to allow patients to raise psycho-social issues as part of the cancer treatment consultation.

REFERENCES

1. Olver, I.N. (1996) Anti-emetic study methodology: recommendations for future studies. *Oncology*, **53**(suppl 1), 96–101.
2. Cherny, N.I. and Portenoy, R.K. (1993) Cancer pain management: current strategy. *Cancer*, (suppl)**72**, 3393–3415.
3. Beller, E., Tattersall, M., Lumley, T., Levi, J., Dalley, D., Olver, I., Page, J., Abdi, E., Wynne, E., Friedlander, M., Boadle, D., Wheeler, H., Margie, S. and Simes, R.J. (1997) Improved quality of life with megesterol acetate in patients with endocrine-insensitive advanced cancer: A randomised placebo-controlled trial. Australian Megesterol acetate Cooperative Study Group. *Ann Oncol*, **8**, 277–283.
4. Lober, C.W. (1993) Pruritus and malignancy. *Clinical Dermatology*, **11**, 125–128.
5. Olver, I.N., Aisner, J., Hament, A., Buchanan, L., Bishop, J.F. and Kaplan, R.S. (1988) A prospective study of topical dimethyl sulphoxide (DMSO) for treating anthracycline extravasations. *J Clin Oncol*, **6**, 1732–1735.
6. Harrison, J. and Maguire, P. (1994) Predictors of psychiatric morbidity in cancer patients. *Br J Psychiatry*, **165**, 593–598.

CHAPTER 17

PAIN MANAGEMENT

Paul Glare

INTRODUCTION

Pain is a common problem in cancer patients, affecting one-third of individuals at the time of diagnosis and more than two-thirds of those with advanced disease. Pain management is an important part of comprehensive cancer care, not only because of the discomfort caused but because pain interferes with function and quality of life.

Since the 1970s the mainstay of cancer pain management has been the administration of oral analgesics, as recommended by the World Health Organisation (WHO) in its 3-step 'analgesic ladder':

1. use non-opioids for mild pain
2. weak opioids for moderate pain
3. strong opioids for severe pain.

This simple approach has been shown to be effective in > 80% of cases in short-term trials. In the 1990s, oral analgesics still have a central role in cancer pain relief, but a much more sophisticated approach to pain assessment and management is now advocated.

The cornerstone of contemporary cancer pain management is comprehensive assessment of the patient's pain. Based on the outcome of the assessment, an integrated program of systemic analgesics, anti-cancer treatment and other therapies can then be offered to provide optimal pain control. Up to 95% of patients can have their pain relieved in this way. Ongoing reassessment and adjustment of treatment is then needed to maintain pain control at this level.

ASSESSMENT OF PAIN IN THE PATIENT WITH CANCER

The assessment aims to determine the likely mechanism of the pain, in the context of the natural history and prognosis of the malignancy, and the anti-tumour treatment options available to the patient. The impact of other physical symptoms and the patient's mood and pain beliefs are also considered.

An understanding of the clinical characteristics of cancer pain is essential for correct assessment to occur. Cancer pain is not a homogeneous entity. It may be due to the disease directly, a side effect of treatment, or unrelated. Many cancers present with pain, but pain at the time of diagnosis is often acute and procedure-related. Chronic cancer pain is rarely constant, but rather is characterised by day-to-day fluctuations and frequent acute exacerbations. Increasing pain does not necessarily mean that the disease is progressing.

Pain relief methods that are extremely effective initially may become less so over time and need to be supplemented or replaced by other forms of treatment. Most cancer pain responds readily to systemic analgesics. Other cancer pain may best be managed by non-pharmacological modalities from the outset, such as coeliac block for pancreas cancer pain.

There are three phases of the assessment:

1. Initial assessment aims to identify the pain mechanism and develop a management plan. Classifying cancer pain into its common syndromes hastens appropriate therapy and minimises distress.
2. Follow-up assessments form a continuing process evaluating the durability of pain relief.
3. Re-assessment with changes in pain patterns or new pain requires a new diagnostic work-up. For example, onset of radicular pain in a patient with chronic back pain from known vertebral secondaries requires consideration and exclusion of epidural disease.

Initial pain assessment, and re-assessment, consists of taking a thorough pain history of the site, intensity and other characteristics of each pain and treatment history. A focused physical examination is required, followed by appropriate investigations. A psycho-social evaluation of the patient and carer is also needed. Use of a tool such as a rating scale or brief pain questionnaire aids follow-up pain assessment and treatment, but may not be possible to use with very sick, distressed or elderly patients. It is essential that analgesic therapy be offered during pain assessment, although some adjustment of treatment may be needed once the assessment is completed.

SPECIFIC MANAGEMENT OF PAIN

Anti-tumour Therapy

Primary therapy such as surgery, radiation therapy or chemotherapy frequently produces pain relief, especially if the disease is localised. The role of anti-cancer therapy will be much more limited in advanced, incurable disease, when pain is more common, but there are notable exceptions. One third of radiation oncology practice is palliative, and radiotherapy is very effective for pain from bone metastases.

In one study, 75% of patients with advanced cancer derived partial or complete pain relief from palliative chemotherapy. Examples include painful chest wall infiltration from breast cancer, liver capsule pain due to hepatic metastases from small cell lung cancer, and back pain due to retroperitoeneal lymphadenopathy from lymphoma.

Pharmacological Therapy

Modern systemic analgesic therapy utilises the principles set out in the WHO's 'analgesic ladder'.

- Step 1. Mild pain. Non-opioids such as paracetamol or aspirin and other non-steroidal anti-inflammatory drugs (NSAIDs) are used. The usual dose of paracetamol is 1 g four hourly, although doses > 4 g/day may not be safe long term.
- Step 2. Moderate pain. Weak opioids are used. These include codeine and dextropropoxyphene, which are often combined with a non-opioid. Codeine 60 mg by mouth is approximately equivalent to 10 mg oral morphine, the preferred strong opioid for step 3.
- Step 3. Severe pain. Morphine is used. Morphine is now commercially available in several forms, including immediate release solutions and tablets, sustained release tablets and capsules, and ampoules for injection. Familiarity with the specific use of each formulation is needed. A full account is beyond the scope of this book, but guidelines for the use of morphine are shown in Table 17.1. There is no limit to the dose of morphine to be used, but most patients need < 200 mg/day for the duration of their illness. Substitution of another strong opioid (such as fentanyl or methadone) may be tried if morphine is ineffective or poorly tolerated, but pethidine should not be used for chronic cancer pain.

Adjuvant Analgesics

Adjuvant analgesics are drugs which are not normally analgesic but can provide additional analgesia independent of opioids in specific pain types, such as:

- corticosteroids and NSAIDs for inflammatory pain
- anti-depressants, anti-convulsants, anti-arrhythmics and NMDA receptor antagonists for neuropathic pain
- bisphosphonates for painful bone metastases
- benzodiazepines for skeletal muscle spasm
- hyoscine for smooth msuscle spasm
- antibiotics for pain from infections
- octreotide for bowel obstruction pain

Table 17.1 Guidelines for the correct use of morphine in chronic cancer pain

- Give by mouth, if possible.
- Give on a time-contingent, regularly-scheduled basis, not 'PRN' or as required.
- Start with immediate-release solution at a dose of 5–10 mg four-hourly; titrate dose up every 24 hours in a stepwise fashion until pain relieved or intolerable side effects occur.
- When effective dose is reached, convert to a sustained-release preparation at same total daily dose.
- Use rescue doses (100% of four-hourly dose) for 'breakthrough pain'.
- Dose may need to be adjusted up or down subsequently; dose reduction usually required if source of pain is removed or renal impairment leads to accumulation of active metabolites.
- Provide prophylaxis of side effects: laxatives usually needed; antiemetics needed infrequently.
- If parenteral administration is necessary, use the subcutaneous route. Subcutaneous morphine is twice as potent as oral morphine.
- If changing to a different opioid, the relative-potency ratio of each needs to be considered.
- Patient and carer fears about morphine addiction need to be discussed and allayed.

Issues of polypharmacy, side effects and drug interactions need to be considered when using any of these agents alone or in combination with conventional analgesics.

Invasive Techniques and Other Modalities

Chronic pain is a multidimensional phenomenon, therefore other treatment modalities can complement pharmacotherapy. For the somatic component, options include physical therapies such as TENS, hot packs, and massage. Invasive techniques such as spinal opioids, nerve blocks and neuro-ablative surgery have a role in up to 10% of cases, when systemic analgesics fail. For the other dimensions of pain, psychotherapy, relaxation techniques, support groups and pastoral care may be very effective.

PAIN IN SPECIAL POPULATIONS

Unfortunately, pain management in cancer patients remains suboptimal in many cases. Some of the reasons are listed in Table 17.2. Certain patients are at particular risk for under-treatment. These include children, the elderly, and patients with a history of substance abuse. Another group is patients in whom the spiritual/existential domain of pain predominates for them or the so-called 'total pain' patient.

Children

Attitudes to paediatric pain have changed dramatically in the last 20 years. Children do experience pain and are able to rate it, although children under 8 years can not use the rating methods used by adults. Procedure and therapy- related pain is just as common as disease-related pain in children with cancer.

Potent, rapid-acting analgesics and sedatives which can be given via novel, non-invasive routes are now available. Anaesthetic techniques are also widely used in this group.

Elderly

Many patients with cancer are over 75 years of age. This is problematic for both assessment and treatment of pain. Assessment is extremely difficult in patients with visual, hearing or cognitive impairment.

Table 17.2 Common errors in cancer pain management

- Deficits in professional knowledge and attitudes: under-estimate importance of pain relief; opiophobia.
- Errors of assessment: fail to distinguish cancer pain from pain due to other causes; fail to assess patient individually; fail to consider further disease-specific therapy; fail to address psycho-social issues.
- Errors in understanding the drugs used: fail to use morphine correctly (e.g. prescribe on wrong regimen; miscalculate dose when changing formulations or routes); fail to use co-analgesics for morphine-unresponsive pain; fail to prevent avoidable side effects.
- Errors of non-drug treatments: fail to use appropriate invasive techniques (e.g. coeliac block for pancreatic cancer pain); fail to use other modalities (e.g. massage for muscle spasm pain).
- Errors in patient carer-education: fail to allay fear of opioids; fail to ensure compliance with instructions.

Medical co-morbidities are common and frequently produce pain unrelated to the malignancy. Anti-tumour therapies are less well tolerated, so may not be a viable option for pain control in this age group.

Analgesic pharamacotherapy is complicated in the elderly by pharmacokinetic and pharmacodynamic differences. Opioids have greater peak effect and duration of effect. NSAIDs cause more gastric and renal toxicity. Anti-depressants and other adjuvants are less well tolerated. Medical co-morbidities also make drug interactions more common.

Chemical Dependence

Fear of addiction to opioids is common in health care professionals, as well as patients and carers. Although tolerance and physical dependence occur, addiction or psychological dependence is very rare and almost never occurs in patients who do not have a history of drug abuse prior to being prescribed opioids for cancer pain.

Occasionally, cancer pain needs to be managed in patients who are actively using illicit drugs. This raises difficult issues including:

- reliability of the pain report
- compliance with instructions
- tolerance
- limitation of on-going drug-seeking behaviour

Advice from a drug and alcohol service or psychiatrist can be very helpful when managing such patients. Experts in the area recommend erring on the side of believing the patient, corroborating the pain complaint with knowledge of the cancer pain syndromes. Limit-setting is often helpful in controlling drug-seeking behaviour.

Refractory Pain

In 5% patients, cancer pain becomes refractory to standard treatment. Even neuro-ablation is ineffective. Many of these patients are individuals who are truly suffering and conceptualise their existential distress as physical pain. Such individuals have been described as suffering from 'total pain'.

Ultimately, medicine can not have the answer to all the suffering of life and death. Our challenge is to understand the nature of such suffering and be empathetic to it. Suffering has been described as 'an awareness of the disintegration of self'. Our goal is to relieve the medical aspects of that sense of loss of personhood and not to contribute further to it.

CONCLUSION

The vast majority of cancer patients can have their pain adequately controlled from the time of diagnosis until cure or death. A variety of expertise may be needed to achieve this, and no one discipline can deal with all such cases alone. Oncologists, the pain clinic, palliative care, the general practitioner and the community nurse must work together to achieve this end. Only then will patients and their carers no longer fear intractable pain as the inevitable consequence of cancer.

REFERENCES

Collins, J.J. (1996) Intractable pain in children with terminal cancer. *J. Palliat. Care*, **12**(3), 29–34.

Hanks, G.W., Justins, D.M. (1992) Cancer pain:management. *Lancet*, **339**, 1031–6.

Hoffman, M., Provata, A.., Lyver, A., Kanner, R.. (1991) Pain managment in the opioid-addicted patient with cancer. *Cancer,* **68**, 1121–2.

Levy, M. (1996) Pharmacological management of cancer pain. *N Engl J Med*, **335**, 1124–32

Lipton, S. (1989) Pain relief in active patients with cancer: early use of nerve blocks. *Brit Med J*, **298**, 37–8.

Portenoy, R.K. (1992) Cancer pain: pathophysiology and syndromes. *Lancet*, **339**, 1026–31.

CHAPTER 18

MEASUREMENT OF QUALITY OF LIFE IN CANCER

Martin Stockler

INTRODUCTION

Cancer and its treatment have profound effects on the lives of those affected. The goals of anti-cancer treatment are to improve both length and quality of life. Measures of tumour shrinkage are useful to help identify treatments worthy of further evaluation, but they are at best only imperfect surrogates of patient benefit. Survival duration and health-related quality of life are the critical outcomes in the evaluation of anti-cancer treatments. The last twenty years has seen major advances in the assessment of health-related quality of life as an outcome measure for cancer clinical trials.

DEFINITION OF HEALTH-RELATED QUALITY OF LIFE

Quality-of-life (QL) is an abstract, multi-dimensional concept reflecting physical, psychological and social aspects, which includes, but is not limited to, the concept of health. It reflects an individuals perception of, and response to, their unique cirumstances[1]. The narrower concept of health-related quality of life (HRQL) reflects the more specific concerns of those interested primarily in the effects of disease and treatment on quality of life[2].

Health-related quality of life includes physical functioning but is much broader than the concept of physical performance status. An assessment of HRQL should include consideration of at least the following five domains: physical function, psychological function, social function, symptoms and global perceptions[3,4]. Table 18.1 gives examples of questions that might be used to assess these key domains. Depending on the circumstances a variety of other domains may also be of interest, including role function, financial concerns, existential concerns and satisfaction with medical care.

Table 18. 1   Examples of questions used for different domains

Domain	Questions about...
Physical Function	Walking, lifting, vitality, self-care
Psychological Function	Depression, anxiety, concentration
Social Function	Family life, social life
Symptoms	Pain, fatigue, nausea, constipation, dyspnoea,
Global Perceptions	Overall quality of life, overall wellbeing

MEASUREMENT OF HEALTH-RELATED QUALITY OF LIFE

Assessment of HRQL[5] is particularly important for clinical trials of:

- Adjuvant therapy where patients without symptoms of disease suffer the side effects of treatment to prevent or delay the recurrence of disease. For example, adjuvant radiotherapy for early breast and colo-rectal cancer.

- Treatments for diseases in which the goals of treatment are purely palliative. For example. chemotherapy for advanced lung, prostate and breast cancer.

- Treatment modalities with very different toxicity profiles. For example, chemotherapy versus radiotherapy.

- Differing durations or intensities of the same treatment modality. For example, high dose versus standard dose chemotherapy, or more radical versus less radical surgery.

- Treatments in which the expected differences will be in quality rather than duration of survival. For example. chemotherapy for advanced prostate or pancreatic cancer.

Health-related quality of life is assessed by asking the subject to answer a series of questions presented in a standardised format referred to as a quality of life instrument. The questions are usually presented as a written questionnaire to be answered on paper, but a variety of computer-based systems are under development. Quality of life is assessed best by the person in question; studies have demonstrated systematic differences between subjects' self-ratings and those of external observers such as spouses, nurses or doctors[6].

INSTRUMENTS TO MEASURE HEALTH-RELATED QUALITY OF LIFE

Many quality of life instruments or questionnaires have been developed by and for cancer researchers. These instruments have many elements in common but each was developed with a particular population and purpose in mind. Table 18.2 lists examples of HRQL instruments with a brief summary of their stated purpose and population of interest.

The instruments in Table 18.2 are ordered from most generic to most specific. Generic instruments should be applicable in a wide range of applications and therefore provide the opportunity for comparisons between groups with quite different characteristics, for example different types of cancer or even different diseases. Specific instruments should be focussed on the

Table 18.2 Examples of validated quality of life instruments

Instrument	Population	Special Features
Medical Outcomes Study Short Form 36 (MOS SF-36)[6]	People in general	Wide generalisability across diseases and populations
Cancer Rehabillitation and Evaluation Systems Inventory (CARES)[7]	People with cancer and following its treatment	Uniquely suited to cancer survivors
Functional Living Index – Cancer (FLIC)[8]	People with cancer	Generic cancer instrument focusing on functional consequences
EORTC Core Quality of Life Questionnaire (EORTC QLQ-C30)[9]	People with cancer participating in international clinical trials	Generic cancer instrument available in many languages
Functional Assesssment of Cancer Therapy – General (FACT-G)[10]	People receiving anti-cancer treatment	Generic cancer instrument available in many languages; assesses satisfaction with care
General Life Quality (GLQ-8)[11]	People receiving chemotherapy	Focus on side effects
Prostate Cancer Specific Quality of Life Instrument (PROSQOLI)[12]	Men receiving systemic therapy for advanced prostate cancer	Focus on symptoms of cancer

problems of the population for which they were developed and therefore should provide a more pertinent description than generic instruments.

KEY RESULTS FROM TRIALS ASSESSING QUALITY OF LIFE

The few studies which have assessed quality of life in cancer clinical trials have produced important counter intuitive results. Two randomised trials of chemotherapy for advanced breast cancer which assessed HRQL were based on the idea that less intense treatment might be equally effective but better tolerated than standard treatment[13,14]. These trials demonstrated that quality of life and survival duration where inferior in the women given less intense treatment.

A randomised trial assessing the addition of chemotherapy to oral prednisone in men with advanced prostate cancer demonstrated superior quality of life in the men given chemotherapy[12]. Measures of health-related quality of life have also proved to be powerful predictors of survival duration, providing prognostic information independent of conventional biological indices and physical performance status[4,12,13].

SUMMARY

These studies demonstrate that it is both feasible and worthwhile to measure health-related quality of life in cancer clinical trials. Most HRQL research to date has focused on the development and application of instruments for clinical trials. Many ongoing clinical trials include HRQL instruments as outcome measures. Simple guidelines are available for the critical appraisal of studies incorporating measures of HRQL[2].

Most anti-cancer treatment is given outside of clinical trials and much of it is given with palliative intent, aimed to improve length and/or quality of life without realistic hope of cure. It is under these circumstances that accurate assessment of HRQL is critical. The next hurdle is to translate into clinical practice the lessons learnt from clinical trials about measuring HRQL.

REFERENCES

1. Gill, T.M., Feinstein, A.R.. (1994) A critical appraisal of quality-of-life measurements. *JAMA*, **272**, 619–26.
2. Guyatt, G.H., Naylor, C.D., Juniper, E., Heyland, D.K., Jaeschke, R., Cook, D.J. for the Evidence-Based Medicine Working Group. Users' guides to the medical literature X11: how to use articles about health-related quality of life.
3. Calman, K.C. (1987) Definitions and dimensions of quality of life. In *The Quality of Life of Cancer Patients*, edited by N.K. Aaronson and J. Beckmann, pp. 1–9. New York: Raven Press.
4. Osoba, D. (1994) Lessons learned from measuring health-related quality of life in oncology. *J Clin Oncol*, 608–16.
5. Moinpour, C.M., Feigl, P., Metch, B. et al. (1989) Quality of life endpoints in cancer clinical trials: review and recommendations. *J Natl Cancer Inst*, **81**, 485–95.
6. Ware, J.E. and Sherbourne, C.D. (1992) The MOS 36-item short-form health status survey (SF-36): I conceptual framework and item selection. *Med Care*, **30**, 473–83.
7. Ganz, P.A., Schag, C.C., Lee, J.J.et al. (1992) The CARES: a measure of heath-related quality of life for patients with cancer. *Qual Lif Res*, **1**, 19–29.
8. Schipper, H., Clinch, J., McMurray, A., Levitt, M. (1984) Measuring the quality of life of cancer patients: the functional living index - cancer. *J Clin Oncol*, **2**, 472–83.
9. Aaronson, N.K., Ahmedzai, S., Bergman, B. et al. (1993) The European Organisation for Research and Treatment of Cancer QLQ-C30; A quality of life instrument for use in international clinical trials in oncology. *J Natl Cancer Inst*, **85**, 365–76.
10. Cella, D.F., Tulsky, D.S., Gray, G. et al. (1993) The Assessment of Cancer Therapy Scale: development and validation of the general measure. *J Clin Oncol*, **11**, 570–9.
11. Butow, P., Coates, A., Dunn, S., Bernhard, J., Hurny, C. (1991) On the receiving end IV: Validation of quality of life indicators. *Ann Oncol*, **2**, 597–603.
12. Tannock, I.F., Osoba, D., Stockler, M.R. et al. (1996) Chemotherapy with mitoxantrone plus prednisone or prednisone alone for symptomatic hormone-resistant prostate cancer: a Canadian randomized trial with palliative end points. *J Clin Oncol*, **14**, 1756–64.
13. Coates, A., Gebski, V., Bishop, J.F. et al. (1987) Improving the quality of life during chemotherapy for advanced breast cancer: a comparison of intermittent and continuous treatment strategies. *N Engl J Med*, **317**, 1490–5.
14. Tannock, I.F., Boyd, N.F., DeBoer, G. et al. (1988) A randomized trial of two dose levels of cyclophosphamide, methotrexate, and fluorouracil chemotherapy for patients with metastatic breast cancer. *J Clin Oncol*, **6**, 1377–87.

PART IV

LUNG CANCER

FAST FACT SHEET 1

LUNG CANCER

R. Supramaniam and Bruce K. Armstrong

WORLD IMPACT

In 1985, some 896,000 new cases of lung cancer were diagnosed worldwide[1]. In the same year, an estimated 785,000 cancer deaths were due to lung cancer[2].

Incidence rates of lung cancer vary about 10-fold worldwide in both sexes [3]. In 1988–92, the highest male rates were in US blacks, New Zealand Maoris and Canadians and the highest female rates were in New Zealand Maoris, US blacks and US whites. The lowest incidence rates were in males and females in West and East Africa.

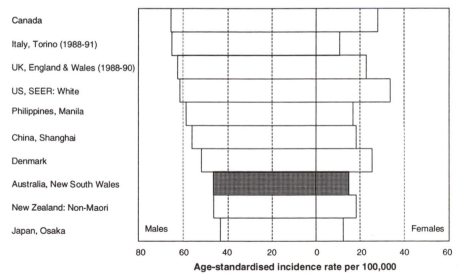

Figure FFS 1.1 Age-standarised incidence rates of lung cancer in selected countries, 1988–1992[3]

103

IMPACT IN AUSTRALIA

In 1990, 6,772 new cases of lung cancer were recorded in Australia accounting for 11.2% of all new cancers[4]. In 1994, lung cancer was the fifth most common cancer in all people in New South Wales, after nonmelanocytic skin cancer and cancers of the prostate, colon and rectum and breast. It was fourth in men and fifth in women.

In 1995, 6,689 people died from lung cancer in Australia. It was the most common cause of death from cancer. Lung cancer was the leading cause of cancer death in males and the third most frequent in females after cancers of the breast and colon and rectum[5]. See Table FFS 1.1.

INCIDENCE BY AGE AND SEX

In New South Wales in 1990–94, lung cancer was rare in people aged less than 40 years. Rates rose steeply in males over 50 years of age and steadily but much less steeply in females of the same ages. The peak incidence rates were in males 80–84 years of age and females 75–79 years of age[6].

INEQUALITIES IN INCIDENCE AND MORTALITY

In 1987–91, incidence of lung cancer in urban NSW increased steeply with decreasing socioeconomic status. This pattern was evident in both sexes and for both incidence and mortality. Rates in males in the lowest quintile of socioeconomic status exceeded those in the highest by 74%. For females in the lowest socioeconomic status quintile, the excess was 24% for incidence and 32% for mortality[7].

Compared to Australian-born people, migrants from the United Kingdom and Ireland had higher mortality rates from lung cancer in 1979–1988. Males born in Northern Europe and Malta and females born in New Zealand also had higher mortality rates. Lower mortality rates were experienced in males born in New Zealand, Hungary and Asia and females from the Netherlands, the former Yugoslavia, Southern Europe and Vietnam[8].

Table FFS 1.1 Australian lung cancer statistics

Statistics	Males	Females
Crude incidence 1990	57.4 per 100,000	21.3 per 100,000
Age adjusted incidence 1990	45.8 per 100,000	15.2 per 100,000
Cumulative incidence to 75 years of age 1990	5.8%	2.0%
Crude mortality 1995	52.3 per 100,000	22.0 per 100,000
Age adjusted mortality 1995	38.0 per 100,000	13.8 per 100,000
Person years of life lost to 75 years of age 1990	29,228 years	11,847 years
Trend in age adjusted incidence 1972–94 in New South Wales	−0.7% p.a.	+2.8% p.a.
Trend in age adjusted mortality 1972–94 in New South Wales	−0.8% p.a.	+2.9% p.a.
Five-year relative survival 1977–94 in South Australia	10.1%	12.6%

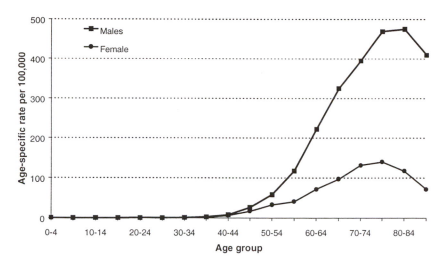

Figure FFS 1.2 Age-specific incidence rates of lung cancer in New South Wales, 1972 to 1994[6]

INCIDENCE AND MORTALITY TRENDS

Incidence and mortality of lung cancer in New South Wales showed parallel trends between 1972 and 1994. In males, the incidence and mortality rates have fallen about 18% since their peak in the early to mid 1980s. In females incidence rates have increased 82% and mortality rates 89% since 1972[6].

SURVIVAL RATES

The 5-year relative survival rates from lung cancer in South Australia improved from 9.1% in people diagnosed in 1977–85 to 11.2% in those diagnosed in 1986–94. The five-year relative survival rate was 10.1% in males and 12.6% in females in 1977–94. Those diagnosed before the 55 years of age had a five-year survival rate of 16.7% compared with only 5.1% in those aged 75 years or older[9].

RISK FACTORS

Cigarette smoking is the strongest risk factor for lung cancer and has been estimated to cause 84% of lung cancers in males and 77% in females in Australia[10]. Lifelong non-smokers passively exposed to cigarette smoke at home have been estimated to have a 20–30% increase in the risk of lung cancer compared with those not so exposed[11].

Occupational exposures associated with an increased risk of lung cancer include exposure to arsenic, asbestos, chloromethyl ethers, hexavalent chromium compounds, nickel compounds, polycyclic aromatic hydrocarbons, radon and silica. These exposures may account for as much as 15% of lung cancers in men. Other significant risk factors include ionising radiation from sources other than radon (e.g. medical irradiation and atomic explosions) and air pollution. There is substantial evidence that a diet high in fruit and vegetables reduces the risk of lung cancer.

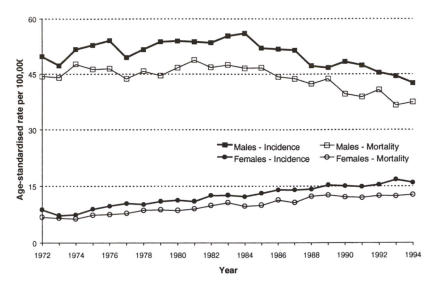

FFS 1.3 Trends in annual age-standardised incidence and mortality rates of lung cancer in New South Wales, 1972 to 1994[6]

There is familial aggregation of lung cancer that may be due to inherited factors. A number of studies suggest that risk of lung cancer varies with polymorphism in different cytochrome p450 genes, possibly as a result of variation in ability to metabolise particular carcinogens or pro-carcinogens. Deletion of the CDKN2 gene is common in non-small cell lung cancer and an increased risk of non-small cell lung cancer has been found in families with a high incidence of melanoma associated with mutation of the CDKN2 gene[12].

REFERENCES

1. Parkin, D.M., Pisani, P. and Ferlay, J. (1993) Estimates of the worldwide incidence of eighteen major cancers in 1985. *Int J Cancer,* 54, 594–606.
2. Pisani, P., Parkin, D.M. and Ferlay, J. (1993) Estimates of the worldwide mortality from eighteen major cancers in 1985. Implications for prevention and projections of future burden. *Int J Cancer,* 55, 891–903.
3. Parkin, D.M., Whelan, S.L., Ferlay, J., Raymond L. and Young, J. (1997) *Cancer Incidence in Five Continents Volume VII.* Lyon: International Agency for Research on Cancer.
4. Jelfs, P., Coates, M., Giles, G., Shugg, D., Threlfall, T., Roder, D., Ring, I., Shadbolt, B. and Condon, J. (1996) *Cancer in Australia 1989–1990 (with projections to 1995).* Canberra: Australian Institute of Health and Welfare.
5. Australian Bureau of Statistics (1996) *Causes of Death Australia 1995.* Canberra: Australian Government Publishing Service.
6. Coates, M. and Armstrong, B.(1997) *Cancer in New South Wales Incidence and Mortality 1994.* Sydney: NSW Cancer Council;

7. Smith D, Taylor R, Coates M. (1996) Socioeconomic differentials in cancer incidence and mortality in urban New South Wales, 1987–1991. *Australian & New Zealand Journal of Public Health,* **20**, 129–37.

8. Giles, G., Jelfs, P. and Kliewer, E. (1995) *Cancer mortality in migrants to Australia 1979–1988.* Canberra: Australian Institute of Health and Welfare.

9. South Australian Cancer Registry (1996) *Epidemiology of Cancer in South Australia. Incidence, mortality and survival 1977 to 1995, incidence and mortality 1995 analysed by type and geographical location – nineteen years of data.* Adelaide: South Australian Health Commission.

10. English, D.R., Holman, C.D.J., Milne, E., Winter, M.G., Hulse, G.K., Codde, J.P., Bower, C.I., Corte, B., de Klerk, N., Knuiman, M.W., Kurinczuk, J.J., Lewin, G.F. and Ryan, G.A. (1995) *The quantification of drug caused morbidity and mortality in Australia 1995 edition.* Canberra: Australian Government Publishing Service.

11. Blot, W.J. and Fraumeni, J.F. (1996) Cancers of the lung and pleura. *Cancer Epidemiology and Prevention,* edited by D. Schottenfeld and J.F. Fraumeni, pp. 637–65. New York: Oxford University Press.

12. Yarbrough, W.G., Aprelikova, O., Pei, H., Olshan, A.F. and Liu, E.T. (1996) Familial tumour syndrome associated with a germline nonfunctional p16INK4a allele. *J Natl Cancer Inst.,* **88**, 1489–91.

CHAPTER 19

NON-SMALL CELL LUNG CANCER: SURGICAL MANAGEMENT

Brian C. McCaughan

INTRODUCTION

Patient selection is the key to the appropriate surgical management of patients with lung cancer. The majority (60–70%) of patients present with advanced disease, are inoperable and incurable, and the aim of treatment is effective palliation. On the other hand, in those patients presenting with a localised and often aysmptomatic malignancy, surgical resection affords the most consistent curative results and all such patients must be evaluated for surgery.

Appropriate surgical selection focuses on three basic questions:

1. Is the malignancy non-small cell lung cancer (NSCLC)? — *Tissue Diagnosis*
2. Is the NSCLC resectable and confined to one hemithorax? — *Staging*
3. Is the patient's cardiorespiratory function adequate for the required resection? — *Fitness*

Tissue Diagnosis

Whether established by sputum cytology, percutaneous fine needle biopsy, bronchoscopy or occasionally at thoracoscopy or thoracotomy, a tissue diagnosis of NSCLC is necessary to avoid inappropriate surgery for small cell lung cancer or other malignancies. The histological subtype of NSCLC (squamous, adenocarcinoma, large cell or mixed) does not alter treatment recommendations.

Staging

The staging of lung cancer is undertaken to estimate prognosis and to decide if curative or palliative treatments are indicated. Staging may be clinical, post-surgical or pathological. The American Joint Committee on Cancer utilises the internationally accepted TNM classification where T refers to primary tumour characteristics, N refers to regional lymph nodes and M to the presence or absence of distant metastases. The derived classification is then grouped into Stages 1 to 4 (Table 19.1).

Table 19.1 Summary of the modified (July 1997) American Joint Committee on Cancer (a) TNM staging and (b) grouping system for primary lung cancer

(a) TNM staging for primary lung cancer

Primary Tumour (T)

T1	=< 3 cm in diameter, surrounded by lung without bronchoscopic evidence of invasion more proximal that lobar bronchus
T2	> 3 cm in diameter or visceral pleural invasion or involving main bronchus 2 cms or more distal to carina
T3	Direct invasion of chest wall, diaphragm, mediastinal pleura or parietal pericardium or in main bronchus less than 2 cm distal to carina
T4	Direct invasion of mediastinum, heart or great vessels or adjacent structures (trachea, oesophagus, spine or carina) or malignant effusion

Regional Nodes (N)

N0	No nodal involvement
N1	Involved ipsilateral peribronchial and/or hilar nodes
N2	Involved ipsilateral mediastinal and/or subcarinal nodes
N3	Involved contralateral mediastinal or hilar or scalene or supraclavicular nodes

Distant Metastases (M)

M0	No distant metastases
M1	Distant metastases

(b) Grouping system for primary lung cancer

Stage	Classifications
Stage 1	T1 N0 M0
	T2 N0 M0
Stage 2A	T1 N1 M0
Stage 2B	T2 N1 M0
	T3 N0 M0
Stage 3A	T3 N1 M0
	T1 N2 M0
	T2 N2 M0
	T3 N2 M0
Stage 3B	T4 and/or N3 M0
Stage 4	T any N any M1

Surgery in NSCLC is only indicated with curative intent. There is virtually no role for a palliative thoracotomy in NSCLC. It is therefore essential to exclude:

- direct invasion of non-resectable structures (T4);
- contralateral hilar/mediastinal or scalene/supraclavicular nodal involvement (N3); and
- distant metastases (M1).

Therefore, staging of NSCLC patients should include:

- A detailed history and examination to identify sites of potential metastatic disease.
- Computerized tomography (CT) of chest and upper abdomen to assess the presence and extent of:
  — invasion by primary tumour
  — a pleural effusion
  — mediastinal lymphadenopathy
  — distant metastases (liver, adrenal, bone)
  — multiple lung lesions
- The role of routine CT brain and nuclear bone scan is not clearly defined. Cost-benefit analysis suggest they are not indicated. However, in individual patients a positive bone scan may significantly alter therapy and prognosis.
- Routine mediastinoscopy and biopsy of draining lymph nodes has been replaced by selected targeted mediastinoscopy based on the CT imaging of mediastinal nodes.
- Newer innovative staging investigations such as positive emission tomography (PET) report promising results for identifying N2, N3 and M1 disease not detected by conventional imaging. Further evaluation is required before PET is standard practice prior to thoracotomy for NSCLC.

Thus by staging, a subset of NSCLC patients with Stage 1 (T1–2 N0 M0) or Stage 2A/B (T1–2 N1 M0) is identified, all of whom should be offered surgical resection if they meet fitness criteria (see below). Selected Stage 2B (T3 N0 M0) patients with locally invasive, but resectable tumours (such as direct chest wall invasion by a peripheral tumour) and selected Stage 3A (T1–3 N2 M0) patients are potentially resectable, although recent randomized data indicates that the latter group (so called N2 disease) may be better served by induction chemotherapy followed by surgical resection if there is a response to chemotherapy.

Patients with Stage 3B (T4 and/or N3) or Stage 4 (M1) disease are not surgical candidates.

Fitness for Surgery

Cardiorespiratory assessment is required in all NSCLC patients who fulfill the first two criteria for surgery. Prolonged exposure to tobacco not only induces malignant change but also parenchymal damage and functional impairment of the lung. Coronary artery disease is a frequent comorbidity in these smoking patients.

There is no single test that indicates the patient's ability to tolerate thoracotomy and resection. The surgeon assesses the individual patient's clinical status (particularly their ability to exercise), basic respiratory function tests (FEV 1.0 is the most predictive) and the resection that is required for that particular patient.

A greater cardiorespiratory reserve is required for pneumonectomy and therefore a more detailed assessment is mandatory. Borderline surgical patients may require detailed lung function tests including diffusion capacity, differential V/Q scan and formal exercise testing. Cardiac stress testing and coronary angiography is indicated in patients with symptoms or ECG changes suggestive of ischaemic heart disease.

Operative Strategy

- Pulmonary lobectomy remains the gold standard of surgical management in NSCLC. It offers the same survival advantage as pneumonectomy but with significantly less mortality and morbidity.

- Pneumonectomy is reserved for central tumours or nodal disease involving mainstem bronchus or main pulmonary artery and tumours crossing the major fissure involving upper and lower lobes.

- Lesser resections (segmentectomy or wedge resection) are only performed for patients with peripheral tumours whose cardiorespiratory function precludes lobectomy.

- En bloc resection of adjacent structures (such as chest wall) and involved lung is performed for selected T3 tumours.

- Mediastinal lymph node dissection is routinely performed to accurately stage the patients and provide appropriate prognostic information and to determine the need for adjuvant therapy.

- Modern anaesthetic and perioperative management, including absolute tobacco abstinence for one month prior to surgery, results in acceptably low operative mortality and morbidity.

Surgical Results

Following complete surgical resection, reported 5-year survival rates are illustrated in Figure 19.1 and Table 19.2.

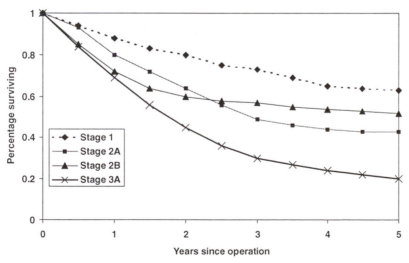

Figure 19.1 Overall survival by stage following surgical resection

Source: Data from The Lung Cancer Surgical Database, University of Sydney, Australia.

Table 19.2 Non-small cell lung cancer: Five-year survival rates following complete surgical resection

Stage 1	T1–2 N0 M0	60–70%
Stage 2A/B	T1–2 N1 M0	45%
Stage 2B	T3 NO MO (selected)	55%
Stage 3B	T1–3 N2 M0 (selected)	20–30%

REFERENCES

1. McCaughan, B. (1997) Recent advances in managing non-small-cell lung cancer: surgery. *Medical Journal of Australia*, **166** (suppl. S7–10), Jun 2.

2. Martini, N., McCaughan, B.C., McCormack, P.M. and Bains, M.S. (1986) Lobectomy for Stage 1 lung cancer. In *Current controversies in Thoracic Surgery*, edited by C.F. Kittle, pp. 171-174. Philadelphia: WB Saunders.

3. Martini, N., Burt, M.E., Bains, M.S., McCormack, P.M., Rusch, V.W., Ginsberg, R.J. (1992) Survival after resection of stage II non-small cell lung cancer. *Annals of Thoracic Surgery*, **54**(3), 460–466.

4. McCaughan, B.C., Martini, N., Bains, M.S. and McCormack, P.M. (1985) Chest wall invasion by carcinoma of the lung: Therapeutic and prognostic implications. *J Thoracic Cardiovas Surg*, **89**, 836–841.

5. Martini N, Flehinger BJ, Zaman, M.B., Beattie, E.R. Jr. (1983) Results of resection in non-oat cell carcinoma of the lung with mediastinal lymph node metastases. *Annals of Surgery*, **198**(3), 386–97.

6. Roth, J.A., Fossella, F., Komaki, R., Ryan, M.B., Putnam, J.B. Jr., Lee, J.S., Dhingra, H., De Caro, L., Chasen, M., McGavran, M. et al. (1994) A randomized trial comparing perioperative chemotherapy and surgery with surgery alone in resectable stage IIIA non-small-cell lung cancer. *Journal of the National Cancer Institute*, **86**(9), 673–80

CHAPTER 20

NON-SMALL CELL LUNG CANCER: RADIATION THERAPY

Graham Stevens

ROLE OF RADIATION THERAPY

Radiation therapy has had a major role in the management of lung cancer throughout its epidemic this century. Historically, this role has been mainly palliative. However, current emphasis is on combined modality treatments with curative intent.

TREATMENT INTENT

Following diagnosis and staging of patients with non-small cell lung cancer (NSCLC) it is possible in most cases to determine the intent of treatment, i.e. whether the patient should be considered for curative or palliative treatment. This assessment is based on:

- Patient factors — performance status, weight loss, comorbidity, respiratory function and age.
- Tumour factors — stage.
- Treatment factors — ability to tolerate the acute and late sequelae of treatment(s).

Curative treatment should not be offered to patients with reduced performance status (ECOG ≥ 2), weight loss >10%, poor respiratory function or Stage IV disease.

CURATIVE RADIOTHERAPY

Stages I/II Non-Small Cell Lung Cancer

Surgery is the most important modality for early lung cancer. High-dose radiation therapy with curative intent is used for patients who:

- refuse surgery; or
- would not tolerate surgery, especially a pneumonectomy, due to respiratory insufficiency.

A dose of 60 Gy in 30 fractions, or equivalent, is used, based on the dose response data generated by the RTOG (Radiation Therapy Oncology Group)[1]. There is no experience of multimodality treatment for Stage I/II tumours. Results expected from high-dose radiation therapy are 5-year survival rates of approximately 30%[2]. These survival rates are less than surgical series, but the groups are not comparable.

Stage III Non-Small Cell Lung Cancer

Operable Tumours

For operable or potentially operable tumours, radiation therapy has been used both preoperatively and postoperatively.

Preoperative irradiation results in tumour down-staging and reduces local recurrence but has no influence on survival rates. Preoperative irradiation has been largely superseded by preoperative, or neoadjuvant, chemotherapy.

Postoperative irradiation to the mediastinum is indicated for:

- positive mediastinal lymph nodes;
- positive margins at the bronchial stump.

A dose of 50 Gy in 25 fractions is generally used. Local control is improved and there is some evidence for a survival benefit. Positive surgical margins on the chest wall are best managed by further surgical resection.

Apical Sulcus, or Pancoast, Tumours

Local control in these tumours is particularly important, because they:

- tend to metastasise late;
- invade into the brachial plexus, causing pain that is difficult to control.

A short course of preoperative radiation therapy has been used. More commonly, postoperative radiation therapy is used for close or positive margins, especially on the medial, vertebral, aspect. A combination of external beam and intraoperative interstitial implantation boost has been used.

Inoperable Tumours

These patients may be offered curative treatment with radiation therapy alone or in combination with chemotherapy if they have good performance status and no significant weight loss. The optimal management of this patient group is uncertain and is the subject of extensive current research. Treatment options being investigated in ongoing randomised clinical trials include the following.

1. Radiation Therapy using Accelerated or Hyperfractionated Schedules

These trials are based on the finding that many tumours proliferate rapidly during treatment, so that higher control rates may be obtained by delivering the radiation in a shorter overall treatment time. Interim analysis of the CHART (Continuous Hyperfractionated Accelerated Radiation Therapy) schedule using 1.5 Gy tds for 12 continuous days to a total dose 54 Gy, has shown an increase in survival compared with conventional daily treatment (30% vs 20% 2-year survival rate respectively)[3].

2. Chemotherapy combined with Radiation using Sequential or Concurrent Treatment

A meta-analysis of randomised trials comparing radiation alone with radiation and chemotherapy showed a small survival advantage for the combined treatments when cisplatin was one of the chemotherapy agents[4]. The optimal combination, scheduling and choice of chemotherapy agents is the subject of much current clinical research. There is clearly a trend towards concurrent treatment.

A Phase II trial of preoperative concurrent chemoradiation using cisplatin and etoposide in Stage III disease yielded a pathological complete response rate of 21%, a median survival time of 15 months and a 3-year survival rate of 29%[5]. These survival rates are typical of the results from the chemoradiation arms of current randomised trials and represent an approximate doubling of 5-year survival rate compared with conventional radiation therapy alone.

TREATMENT PLANNING AND DELIVERY

Radiation therapy delivered with curative intent must be planned carefully to maximise the therapeutic ratio. Essential steps in the planning process include:

- reproducible patient position (usually prone or supine, with arms above head);
- simulation to determine the extent of tumour movement with respiration;
- CT scanning in the treatment position, to identify the tumour volume, normal (critical) structures and the patient body contour;
- computer planning with inhomogeneity corrections, especially for lung;
- multiple treatment fields with wedges and/or compensators;
- three-dimensional (including beam's eye view) imaging of treatment volume and critical structures;
- simulator films to check treatment fields;
- dose delivery prescription to define the total dose, fractionation and overall time of treatment.

During treatment, the following are required:

- weekly review of patient to assess toxicity of treatment (especially with concurrent chemotherapy); and
- weekly portal films or EPI (electronic portal imaging) to check reproducibility of treatment setup.

SIDE EFFECTS AND COMPLICATIONS OF HIGH DOSE (RADICAL) IRRADIATION

Side effects

- pneumonitis (dyspnoea, hypoxia, fever, cough)
- oesophagitis (odynophagia)
- skin reaction (dry, red skin, hair loss)
- tracheitis (cough)
- transient myelitis (Lehmitte's syndrome of shooting pain)
- transient pericarditis (chest pain, tachycardia, dyspnoea)

Complications

- pulmonary fibrosis (onset ~6 months; exertional dyspnoea)
- thoracic spinal cord injury (onset ~6–24 months; leg weakness, paraplegia, sphincter dysfunction)
- coronary artery disease (requires years to decades)
- mediastinal fibrosis (usually asymptomatic)

'Radical irradiation' refers to a dose/fractionation schedule that approaches the accepted tolerance dose of the normal tissues within the treatment volume. This list above represents potential side effects and complications. In practice, the accepted tolerance doses of normal tissues are respected, reducing the possibility of these complications. For example, treatment field sizes and orientations are selected to restrict the volume of normal lung irradiated to a high dose and limit the dose delivered to the thoracic spinal cord. Tolerance doses using combined modality radiation and chemotherapy remain to be defined.

PALLIATIVE RADIOTHERAPY

Radiation therapy is highly effective in the palliation of symptoms caused by lung cancer in both intrathoracic and extrathoracic sites. Approximately two-thirds of patients with NSCLC are incurable at diagnosis, due to either locally advanced or metastatic disease and could benefit from this approach.

Intrathoracic Radiotherapy

Common symptoms and signs in locally advanced NSCLC, are palliated by radiation therapy in 50–80% of patients and include:

- haemoptysis
- cough
- superior vena caval (mediastinal) obstruction
- dyspnoea due to partial or complete major bronchial obstruction
- chest or chest wall pain
- dysphagia due to mediastinal adenopathy compressing oesophagus

Hoarse voice from recurrent laryngeal nerve palsy and pain due to brachial plexus invasion, however, respond poorly to radiation. The optimal dose and schedule have been investigated by the Medical Research Council of the UK[6]. For patients with a poor prognosis, there were no significant differences between a single fraction and a two-week course of fractionated external beam therapy for response rates and duration of response. Haemoptysis and/or partial obstruction of a major bronchus are well-palliated with single fraction endobronchial brachytherapy, particularly as a re-treatment option following previous external beam therapy. Endobronchial brachytherapy is effective also for the treatment of endobronchial metastases from extrathoracic primary sites.

Extrathoracic Radiotherapy

Short courses of radiation therapy are usually effective in the palliative treatment of distant metastases to a range of sites.

1. Cerebral metastases are treated by steroids and fractionated whole brain irradiation to 20–30 Gy in 1–2 weeks. A small solitary metastasis could be considered for resection or stereotactic radiosurgery.

2. Spinal cord compression is manage by high-dose steroids and urgent irradiation to 30 Gy in 2 weeks; the functional outcome depends on the neurological status pre-treatment.

3. Bone metastases causing pain are treated by a fractionated course of 20 Gy in 5 fractions for weight-bearing bones or a single fraction of 8 Gy for non-weight-bearing bones. Severe pain on weight-bearing and cortical destruction are indications for orthopaedic intervention.

REFERENCES

1. Perez, C.A., Stanley, K., Rubin, P., Kramer, S., Brady, L., Perez-Tamayo, R., Brown, G.S., Concannon, J., Rotman, M.and Seydel, H.G. (1980) A prospective randomised study of various radiation doses and fractionation schedules of inoperable non-oat cell carcinoma of the lung: preliminary report by the Radiation Therapy Oncology Group. *Cancer*, 45, 2744–2753.

2. Gauden, S., Ramsay, J. and Tripcony, L. (1995); The curative treatment by radiation therapy alone of stage I non-small-cell carcinoma of the lung. *Chest*, 108, 1278–1282.

3. Saunders, M.I., Dische, S., Barrett A., Parmar, M.K., Harvey, A. and Gibson, D. (1996) Randomised multicentre trials of CHART vs conventional radiation therapy in head and neck and non-small cell lung cancer: an interim report. *Br J Cancer*, 73, 1455–1462.

4. Non-small cell Lung Collaborator's Group (1995) Chemotherapy in non-small cell lung cancer: a met-analysis using updated data on individual patients from 52 randomised clinical trials. *BMJ*, 311, 899–909.

5. Albain, K.S., Rusch, V.W., Crowley, J.J., Rice, T.W., Turrisi, A.T.-3rd, Weick, J.K., Lonchyna, V.A., Presant, C.A., McKenna, R.J. and Gandara, D.R.(1995) Concurrent cisplatin/etoposide plus chest RT followed by surgery for stages IIIA(N2) and IIIB non-small-cell lung cancer: mature results of South West Oncology Group phase II study 8805. *J Clin Oncol*, 13, 1880–1892.

6. Medical Research Council Working Party (1991) Inoperable non small cell lung cancer (NSCLC): a Medical Research Council randomised trial of palliative radiation therapy with two fractions or 10 fractions. *Br J Cancer*, 63, 265–270.

CHAPTER 21

NON-SMALL CELL LUNG CANCER: CHEMOTHERAPY

Michael Boyer

ACTIVE DRUGS AND COMBINATIONS

Although a wide range of anti-cancer drugs have been evaluated for the treatment of non-small cell lung cancer, only a small number of these consistently produce tumour response, with shrinkage by at least 50%, in more than 15% of treated patients. These drugs include cisplatin, carboplatin, ifosfamide, mitomycin and vinblastine. In addition, several newer cytotoxic drugs, such as gemcitabine, vinorelbine, paclitaxel, docetaxel, and irinotecan also possess substantial activity.

In common with many other types of tumour, several drugs are usually combined for the treatment of NSCLC. Most combinations are based on cisplatin or carboplatin. Frequently used combinations include cisplatin (or carboplatin) and etoposide; cisplatin and a vinca alkaloid; cisplatin and gemcitabine; cisplatin and paclitaxel or docetaxel; and carboplatin and paclitaxel. It is not clear which of these combinations has the greatest degree of activity although those including newer agents may possibly be more active. Trials which are underway should assist in answering this question.

USES OF CHEMOTHERAPY IN NSCLC

Adjuvant Therapy

Early trials of adjuvant chemotherapy treatment following surgical resection of early-stage NSCLC failed to demonstrate consistently a survival advantage. Consequently, adjuvant chemotherapy has not become part of the routine management of NSCLC. However, many of the drugs used in the early trials are now known to be relatively inactive. The negative outcome of these studies is therefore not surprising. Also, several of the studies were too small to be likely to detect a difference, even if one existed.

Recently, the introduction of newer drugs with greater levels of activity in advanced NSCLC has led to an increase in interest in the use of chemotherapy in the adjuvant setting. Several randomised

118

clinical trials are in progress for patients with resectable NSCLC. These studies are designed to evaluate the effects on survival of adding chemotherapy to the standard treatments of surgery and radiotherapy.

Combined Modality Therapy for Locally Advanced Disease

Alternate approaches to the incorporation of chemotherapy into the treatment of NSCLC are to administer it prior to or simultaneously with definitive local therapy. These approaches have been used in locally advanced (Stage IIIA and B) NSCLC.

For patients with Stage IIIA disease, initial chemotherapy, sometimes called neo-adjuvant chemotherapy, has been given to reduce the bulk of primary and mediastinal disease prior to attempted surgical resection. The aim of this approach is to make the tumour more easily resectable, and to treat any micrometastatic disease which may be present. Two randomised trials evaluating this type of treatment have been completed, and have demonstrated an improvement in median and long-term survival. Despite this, the approach has remained controversial. It is unclear whether or not surgery is truly necessary and whether similar results be achieved with chemotherapy and radiotherapy. The optimal type and duration of chemotherapy is also unknown.

Stage IIIB disease is not considered to be surgically resectable and the traditional treatment has been with radiotherapy. The relatively poor outcome of patients treated in this manner has led to the evaluation of combined modality treatment with chemotherapy and radiotherapy. Two different approaches have been used, either sequential therapy, where chemotherapy is given prior to the use of radiotherapy, or concurrent therapy where both treatments are given simultaneously.

In randomised trials, both of these approaches have been shown to produce improvements in survival when compared to radiotherapy alone. Furthermore, in a meta-analysis the addition of chemotherapy to radiotherapy has been shown to produce small but significant improvements in the survival rate. Most of the benefit is due to an improvement in local (intrathoracic) control, with little or no impact on the occurrence of metastatic disease. However, the chemotherapy that has been given has usually been of short duration only, and, in the case of concurrent treatment, at relatively low doses. Therefore, an effect on systemic disease is less likely. In the future, it is likely that combined modality treatment programs will incorporate longer periods of chemotherapy which will have a greater likelihood of eradicating micrometastatic disease. Following treatment with currently available regimens, the median survival rate   is around 14 months, with 3- and 5- year survival rates of 25% and 15% respectively.

CHEMOTHERAPY FOR METASTATIC DISEASE

Controversy has surrounded the use of chemotherapy for metastatic NSCLC. While there is clear evidence from a well-performed meta-analysis that the use of chemotherapy results in an improvement in survival for these patients, many doctors do not regard the benefits as being sufficiently great to justify the perceived toxicity of treatment.

Several factors are changing the toxicity associated with chemotherapy for NSCLC. Included amongst these are: better anti-emetics, such as the serotonin antagonists ondansetron and tropisetron; the introduction of newer anti-cancer agents, such as the taxanes and gemcitabine which are generally better tolerated than older drugs; and better selection of patients for treatment, with the recognition that patients of poor performance status benefit less from treatment.

Modern chemotherapeutic regimens produce objective tumour response, with shrinkage of > 50% in 25% to 45% of patients with metastatic NSCLC. Median survival time following treatment is 10–12 months, approximately 2–3 months longer than without treatment. Few studies have addressed directly the impact of chemotherapy on quality of life but in those that have, treatment seems to be associated with an improvement.

REFERENCES

Bonomi, P., Kim, K., Chang, A., and Johnson, D. (1996) Phase III trial comparing etoposide cisplatin versus taxol with cisplatin-G-CSF versus taxol-cisplatin in advanced non-small cell lung cancer. An Eastern Cooperative Oncology Group Trial. *Proc Amer Soc Clin Oncol,* **15**, 382–382 (Abstract).

Dillman, R.O., Herndon, J., Seagren, S.L., Eaton, W.L., and Green, M.R. (1996) Improved survival in stage III non-small-cell lung cancer: seven year follow-up of cancer and leukemia group B (CALGB) 8433 trial. *J. Natl. Cancer Inst.,* **88**(17), 1210–1215.

Non-small Cell Lung Cancer Collaborative Group (1995) Chemotherapy in non-small cell lung cancer: a meta-analysis using updated data on individual patients from 52 randomised clinical trials. *Br. Med. J.,* **311**, 899–909.

Rossell, R., Gomez-Codina, J., Camps, C., Maestre, J., Padille, J., Canto, A., Mate, J.L., Li, S., Roig, J., Olazabal, A., Canela, M., Ariza, A., Skacel, Z., Morera-Prat, J., and Abad, A. (1994) A randomized trial comparing preoperative chemotherapy plus surgery with surgery alone in patients with non small cell lung cancer. *N. Engl. J. Med.,* **330**, 153–158.

Roth, J.A., Fossella, F., Komaki, R., Ryan, M.B., Putnam, J.B., Lee, J.S., Dhingra, H., DeCaro, L., Chasen, M., McGavran, M., Atkinson, E.N., and Hong, W.K. (1994) A randomized trial comparing perioperative chemotherapy and surgery with surgery alone in resectable stage IIIA non-small cell lung cancer. *J. Natl. Cancer Inst.,* **86**(9), 673–680.

CHAPTER 22

SMALL CELL LUNG CANCER

James F. Bishop

INTRODUCTION

Small cell lung cancer (SCLC) comprises about 20% of all lung cancers and is considered separately from non-small cell lung cancer (NSCLC) because the natural history, staging and the treatment are quite different. SCLC is frequently disseminated at presentation, has a short natural history if untreated, with a median survival of 6 weeks for extensive stage patients and 12 weeks for limited disease, is very sensitive initially to chemotherapy and radiotherapy, and has a propensity to metastasise to the CNS.

EPIDEMIOLOGY AND AETIOLOGY

SCLC has an incidence of approximately 12 per 100,000 in males and 4 per 100,000 in females. As with other types of lung cancer, cigarette smoking is the primary cause of this type of lung cancer. It is more common in uranium miners and after radon exposure than other lung cancers.

PATHOLOGY AND BIOLOGY

Small cell lung cancer has been traditionally thought to arise from epithelium, particularly basal neuroendocrine or Kulchitsky cells. However, recently this concept has been challenged. Silver stains are positive in about half and neurosecretory granules are usually present on electron microscopy. The light microscopy appearance is that of small round or ovoid cells with darkly staining nuclei and scanty cytoplasm with characteristic nuclear moulding by adjacent cells. A mixed small cell–large cell variant has been described but is less common.

Small cell lung cancer may have elevated levels of amine precursor uptake and decarboxylation cells (APUD cells), L-dopa decarboxylase, gastric releasing peptide (GRP) and neurone specific enolase. GRP may act as a growth factor, and this and other products may be useful markers.

Molecular analysis has demonstrated that lung cancer cells have a number of genetic lesions which appear to be required for the development of lung cancer. For example, deletions of the short arm of chromosome 3 (3p) is present in over 90% of SCLC suggesting the importance of tumour suppressor genes in this region.

PRESENTATION

Symptoms

Patients frequently present with symptoms consistent with central bronchial obstruction such as dyspnoea, cough, wheeze, haemoptysis, chest pain or post-obstruction pneumonia. Since the features of this disease are rapid growth and early dissemination, patients may also present with superior vena caval (SVC) obstruction, liver or cerebral signs from metastasis, hoarseness from recurrent laryngeal nerve palsy or dysphagia. Approximately half of all SVC obstructions are due to small cell lung cancer.

Signs

Signs depend on the extent of disease in the lung, mediastinum, liver or brain. Pleural effusions or bone tenderness from metastasis may be present. Central bronchial obstruction may cause a pneumonia which is obvious from the history and on chest examination.

Para-neoplastic phenomenon seen with SCLC include inappropriate ADH secretion, ectopic Cushing's syndrome and the Eaton-Lambert or myasthenia-like syndrome. About 4% of small cell carcinoma presents, without an obvious lung primary, in the cervix, oesophagus, oro-pharynx, colon, prostate or paranasal sinuses.

STAGING AND PROGNOSIS

Staging

The staging for SCLC differs from NSCLC since it does not use the TNM surgically based system. SCLC is simply divided into limited disease (33%) or extensive disease (66%). Limited disease is defined as confined to the chest, within one radiation portal, and includes contralateral mediastinal nodes and bilateral supraclavicular nodes. Extensive stage disease includes all disease outside these limits.

Prognosis

This simple system is one of the most powerful prognostic variables in SCLC and is the basis for most therapeutic decisions. Given optimal therapy, the median survival for limited stage SCLC is 18 months, whereas it is only 7–9 months for extensive stage disease.

Other important prognostic factors are performance status (see appendix I) and female sex, the latter associated with long-term survival. LDH, serum sodium, albumin and alkaline phosphatase have all been suggested as providing added prognostic information.

Staging Procedures

The work-up for SCLC is directed towards identifying immediate clinical problems, such as obstruction, and to staging the patient as limited or extensive disease. Suggested staging procedures include histological or cytological proof of SCLC, full blood examination, electrolytes, liver function tests, CT scan of the chest and upper abdomen and bone scan. Brain scan and bone marrow biopsy are usually ordered on clinical suspicion of disease at these sites.

TREATMENT

Limited Stage SCLC

The mainstay of treatment for SCLC is chemotherapy and radiotherapy. Surgery has only a limited role in providing biopsy material and in the occasional patient with a peripheral lung lesion which is either resected prior to the diagnosis or can be resected following other therapy.

Combination chemotherapy has been responsible for the prolonged median survival now seen in limited stage SCLC. The most useful drugs are cisplatin or carboplatin used with etoposide. Alternatively other combinations of drugs use doxorubicin, cyclophosphamide or ifosphamide in addition to etoposide. These combinations will result in a complete response in about 50% of patients with a further 30% achieving a good partial response. Attempts to improve on these results with more intense chemotherapy regimens, such as the CODE program, or the use of cytokines such as G-CSF or GM-CSF, have not improved survival. High-dose chemotherapy with bone marrow transplantation has not been of proven value. However, some newer agents show promise in this disease especially paclitaxel, docetaxel, vinorelbine and topotecan.

Radiotherapy has a proven role in SCLC. Its main effect appears to be to improve the percentage of longer term survivors. Advances have recently been made by giving the radiotherapy concurrently with platinum etoposide chemotherapy and by giving it early in the chemotherapy course. Such therapy has significantly reduced the local relapse rate and improved overall survival.

SCLC presents with CNS metastasis in 12%, with up to 30% relapsing in brain at some time. However, the use of prophylactic radiotherapy to the brain is controversial. Earlier randomised studies of radiotherapy showed a reduction in cerebral metastases but no survival advantage with radiation. There have been concerns that this approach may compromise intellectual function. More recent studies of prophylactic cranial irradiation, only in patients with a complete response, suggest that relapses are less, a small survival difference may be present and that intellectual function may not be compromised.

Extensive Stage SCLC

In contrast to limited stage SCLC, extensive stage patients receive chemotherapy alone using the same drugs and combinations as above. While local control rates and long-term survival have slowly improved in limited disease with radiotherapy and chemotherapy, little progress has been made in outcome in extensive stage SCLC for the last 15 years.

Combination chemotherapy will result in a complete response in 25%, with a further 40% with a partial response. However, these responses are generally worthwhile for the patient with good quality of life. The use of continuous oral etoposide alone has been tried as an alternative to standard intravenous combinations in extensive stage patients or those with poor prognosis. Unfortunately, oral etoposide has been associated with poorer control of the SCLC, more side effects and poorer quality of life than standard IV etoposide regimens.

Second line treatment for relapsed small cell lung cancer is seldom very effective. In general, for patients who have not had radiotherapy and have a progressive, troublesome mass, symptoms can be relieved with a short course of appropriately planned palliative radiotherapy. The use of chemotherapy in this setting must be balanced with the patient's wishes, possible side effects and the likelihood of success.

LONG-TERM SURVIVAL

The long-term survival in patients with limited stage SCLC is only 6–10% at 5 years and 1% with extensive stage disease. Female sex, performance status and stage are the major determinants for long-term survival.

REFERENCES

Carney, D.N. (1992) Biology of small cell lung cancer. *Lancet,* **339**, 843–6.

Idhe, D.C. (1992) Chemotherapy of lung cancer. *N Engl J Med,* **327**, 1434–41.

Minna, J.D., Sekido, Y., Fong, K.W. and Gazdar, A.F. (1997) Molecular biology of lung cancer. In *Cancer: Principles and Practice of Oncology* (5th edn), edited V. DeVita, S. Hellman and S. Rosenberg, pp. 849–858. Philadelphia: Lipponcott-Raven Publ.

Murray, N., Goy, P., Pater, J.L., Hodson, I., Arnold, A., Zee, B.C., Payne, D., Kostashuk, E.C., Evans, W.K., Dixon, P., Sadura, A., Feld, R., Levitt, M., Wierzbicki, R., Ayoub, J., Maroun, J.A. and Wilson, K.S. (1993) Importance of timing for thoracic irradiation in the combined modality treatment of limited stage small cell lung cancer *J Clin Oncol,* **11**(2), 336–44.

Pignon, J.P., Arriagada, R., Ihde, D.C., Johnson, D.H., Perry, M.C., Souhami, R.L., Brodin, O., Joso, R.A., Kies, M.S. and Lebeau, B. (1992). A meta-analysis of thoracic radiotherapy for small cell lung cancers *N Engl J Med,* **327**(23),1618–24.

PART V

BREAST CANCER

FAST FACT SHEET 2

BREAST CANCER

Bruce K. Armstrong and H. L. Nguyen

WORLD IMPACT

In 1985, some 719,000 breast cancers were diagnosed in women worldwide, making it the second most common cancer in women, after nonmelanocytic skin cancer, and the fourth most common cancer in all people, after nonmelanocytic skin cancer and lung and stomach cancers[1]. It was the largest cause of death from cancer in women[2.].

In 1988–92, worldwide incidence rates of breast cancer varied more than five-fold with highest rates in North American and European populations and lowest rates in some Asian populations and African populations. New Zealand also recorded a high incidence rate[3].

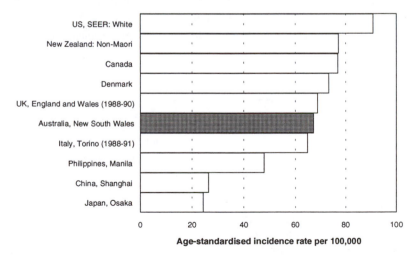

Figure FFS 2.1 Age-standardised incidence rates of breast cancer in females in selected countries, 1988–1992[3]

IMPACT IN AUSTRALIA

In 1992, 7,585 breast cancers were registered in Australian women[4]. In 1990, 75 were registered in Australian men[5]. Based on 1994 figures for New South Wales[6], breast cancer is the second most common cancer in Australian women, after nonmelanocytic skin cancer, and the fourth most common cancer in all Australians, after nonmelanocytic skin cancer and cancers of the prostate and colon and rectum. In 1995, it was the largest cause of death from cancer in Australian women with a total of 2,629 deaths[7].

INCIDENCE BY AGE

Incidence of breast cancer in Australian women is very low before 25 years of age. It increases steeply with age between 30–34 and 45–49 years of age and then more slowly to the oldest age groups[4]. The number of new cases in 1990 was between 600 and 830 in each 5-year age group from 40–44 to 75–79 years of age[5].

INEQUALITIES IN INCIDENCE

Breast cancer incidence varies appreciably by country of birth in Australian women[4]. The age-standardised incidence in Australian born women in New South Wales in 1987–95 was 72 per 100,000 per year. Only New Zealand born women had a higher incidence at 89 per 100,000. The lowest incidence was in women born in China at 39 per 100,000. In Sydney, incidence was 19% higher in women in the highest quintile of socioeconomic status than in the lowest quintile in 1987–91[8]; this differential was highly significant. The mortality from breast cancer in rural women in Australia was 95% of that in urban women in 1991–94; corresponding data were not available for incidence[4].

INCIDENCE AND MORTALITY TRENDS

Breast cancer incidence has been increasing steadily in Australian women since 1982 with a more rapid rate of increase since the mid 1980s[4]. This trend is probably due to increased detection by screening mammography. Mortality was steady from 1982 to 1991 but has fallen a little since.

Table FFS 2.1 Australian breast cancer statistics

Statistics	Females
Crude incidence 1992	86.4 per 100,000
Age adjusted incidence 1992	66.9 per 100,000
Cumulative incidence to 75 years of age 1987–92	7.3%
Crude mortality 1995	29.0 per 100,000
Age adjusted mortality 1995	19.6 per 100,000
Person years of life lost to 75 years of age 1990	26,572 years
Trend in age adjusted incidence 1982 to 1992	+1.5% p.a.
Trend in age adjusted mortality 1982 to 1994	Minimal
Five year relative survival 1986–94 in South Australia	78.0%

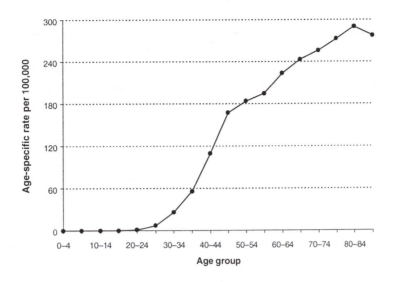

Figure FFS 2.2 Age-specific incidence rates of breast cancer in Australian females, 1987–1992[4]

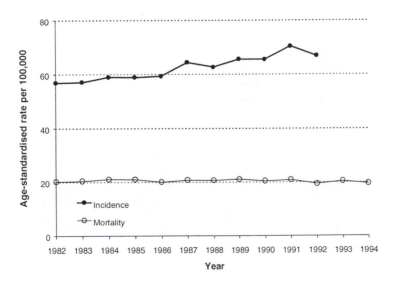

Figure FFS 2.3 Trends in annual age-standardised incidence and mortality rates of breast cancer in Australian females, 1982–1994[4]

SURVIVAL RATE

The five-year relative survival rate from breast cancer in women in South Australia increased from 72.8% in those diagnosed in 1977–85 to 78.0% in those diagnosed in 1986–94[9]. Relative survival in 1977–94 was highest in those under 55 years of age (77.9%) and least in those 75 years of age and over (68.0%). Among 2,101 breast cancers recorded in hospital-based cancer registries in South Australia from 1987–95 (one-third of all breast cancers diagnosed in South Australia during this period), 5-year relative survival fell from 90% in TNM Stage I cancers to 20% in TNM Stage IV cancers[10]. The 5-year relative survival rate for all these cancers was 74% compared with 78% for all breast cancers in South Australia in 1986–94.

RISK FACTORS

Risk of breast cancer increases with early menarche and late menopause and increases at its highest rate with age during menstrual life. These and other observations suggest that risk is substantially determined by the number of ovulatory cycles a woman has and probably, therefore, her total accumulated exposure to ovarian oestrogen[11]. Nulliparous women have about a 40% higher risk of breast cancer than parous women and the earlier a woman's first childbirth the lower is her risk of breast cancer. However, women who have their first childbirth later than about 30 years of age, have a higher risk of breast cancer even than nulliparous women. There is about a 2.5-fold difference in risk between women who have their first childbirth under 20 years of age and women who have it at 30 years of age or older. Risk of breast cancer falls with increasing parity, independently of age at first birth.

After the menopause, risk of breast cancer increases with body weight at a rate of up to about 80%

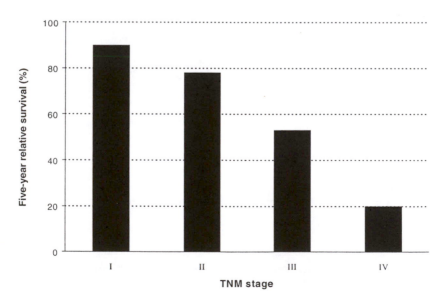

Figure FFS 2.4 Five-year relative survival by TNM stage at diagnosis of breast cancer in females in South Australia, 1987–1995[10]

for each 10-kg increase in weight[11]. This effect is probably due to conversion of adrenal androgen to oestrogen in adipose tissue.

Oestrogen containing medications also increase risk of breast cancer. Risk is increased by an average of 24% while a woman is taking the oral contraceptive pill[12]. The effect of the pill on lifetime risk of breast cancer is small, however, because the underlying risk of breast cancer is low when women commonly take it. Oestrogen replacement therapy after the menopause also appears to increases risk by about 30%[13]. The excess risk increases with increasing duration of use, but disappears within about 2 years of cessation of use of oestrogen.

Breast cancer risk is increased by about 68% in women who drink alcohol at harmful levels (more than 4 standard drinks a day)[14]. However, hazardous (2–4 standard drinks a day) and harmful drinking of alcohol explain only about 3% of breast cancer in Australia. Other dietary factors are thought to explain much of the international variation in breast cancer incidence, but those responsible have not been shown with any certainty. Risk may be increased by high-energy intake and growth rate in childhood and adolescence and reduced by a high intake of fruit and vegetables at any age[15].

History of a benign epithelial proliferative lesion of the breast, such as fibrocystic disease, is associated with an increased risk of breast cancer[11]. This association probably also explains the association between a 'DY' (dysplastic) mammographic pattern and breast cancer.

On average, risk of breast cancer is increased two- to three-fold in women who have one or more first-degree relatives with breast cancer[11]. An inherited mutation of any one of several major genes, BRCA1, BRCA2 and TP53, confers about an 80% lifetime risk of breast cancer, compared with about 7% for women in general. These inherited mutations, however, probably explain only about 1% to 2% of all breast cancers.

REFERENCES

1. Parkin, D.M., Pisani, P. and Ferlay, J. (1993) Estimates of the worldwide incidence of eighteen major cancers in 1985. *Int J Cancer,* 54, 594–606.
2. Pisani, P., Parkin, D.M. and Ferlay, J. (1993) Estimates of the worldwide mortality from eighteen major cancers in 1985. Implications for prevention and projections of future burden. *Int J Cancer,* 55, 891–903.
3. Parkin, D.M., Whelan, S.L., Ferlay, J., Raymond, L. and Young, J. (1997) *Cancer Incidence in Five Continents Volume VII,* Lyon, International Agency for Research on Cancer.
4. Kricker, A. and Jelfs, P. (1996) *Breast cancer in Australian women 1921–1994.* Canberra: Australian Institute of Health and Welfare.
5. Jelfs, P., Coates, M., Giles, G., Shugg, D., Threlfall, T., Roder, D., Ring, I., Shadbolt, B. and Condon, J. (1996) *Cancer in Australia 1989–1990 (with projections to 1995).* Canberra: Australian Institute of Health and Welfare.
6. Coates, M. and Armstrong, B. (1997) *Cancer in New South Wales Incidence and Mortality 1994.* Sydney: NSW Cancer Council.
7. Australian Bureau of Statistics (1996) *Causes of Death Australia 1995*, Canberra, Australian Government Publishing Service.
8. Smith, D., Taylor, R. and Coates, M. (1996) Socioeconomic differentials in cancer incidence and mortality in urban New South Wales, 1987–1991. *Australian & New Zealand Journal of Public Health,* 20, 129–137.

9. South Australian Cancer Registry (1996) *Epidemiology of Cancer in South Australia. Incidence, mortality and survival 1977 to 1995, incidence and mortality 1995 analysed by type and geographical location - nineteen years of data.* Adelaide: South Australian Health Commission.

10. South Australian Cancer Registry (1997) *Epidemiology of Cancer in South Australia. Incidence, mortality and survival 1977 to 1996, incidence and mortality 1996 analysed by type and geographical location - Twenty years of data.* Adelaide: South Australian Health Commission.

11. Henderson, B.E., Pike, M.C., Bernstein, L. and Ross, R.K. (1996) Breast Cancer. In *Cancer Epidemiology and Prevention*, edited by D. Schottenfeld and J.F. Fraumeni, pp. 1022–1039. New York: Oxford University Press.

12. Collaborative Group on Hormonal Factors in Breast Cancer (1996) Breast cancer and hormonal contraceptives: collaborative reanalysis of individual data on 53 297 women with breast cancer and 100 239 women without breast cancer from 54 epidemiological studies. *Lancet,* **347,** 1713–1727.

13. Colditz, G.A., Hankinson, S.E., Hunter, D.J., Willett, W.C., Manson, J.E., Stampfer, M.J., Hennekens, C., Rosner, B. and Speizer, F.E. (1995) The use of estrogens and progestins and the risk of breast cancer in postmenopausal women. *N Engl J Med,* **332,** 1589–1593.

14. English, D.R., Holman, C.D.J., Milne, E., Winter, M.G., Hulse, G.K., Codde, J.P., Bower, C.I., Corti, B., deKlerk, N., Knuiman, M.W., Kurinczuk, J.J., Lewin, G.F. and Ryan, G.A. (1995) *The quantification of drug caused morbidity and mortality in Australia 1995 edition.* Canberra: Australian Government Publishing Service.

15. Hunter, D.J. and Willett, W.C. (1996);Nutrition and breast cancer. *Cancer Causes Control,* 7, 56–68.

CHAPTER 23

EARLY BREAST CANCER: SURGICAL TREATMENT

David Gillett

Breast cancer is the most common cancer in women and the only curative treatment is surgery with or without adjuvant therapy (see Fast Fact Sheet 2).

DIAGNOSIS

Asymptomatic Women

Twenty per cent of cancers presenting at major centres are screen detected. These are asymptomatic women, over the age of 40, who are being screened in accordance with the guidelines of the screening program or privately screened patients with or without a family history of breast cancer. One of the characteristics of this group is the high incidence of pre-invasive cancer, ductal carcinoma *in situ* (DCIS) which is approximately 20%.

Symptomatic Women

- Eighty per cent of the breast cancers diagnosed in most practices are in women who present with a symptom.

- The most common symptom, in 90% of these patients, is a lump usually noticed by the patient herself either at the time of breast self-examination or when showering or bathing.

- Nipple changes occur in 5% of patients and in half of these it is nipple discharge and in the other half retraction, scaliness or eczema.

- Skin changes, dimpling, discolouration, nodules or oedema (peau d'orange), occurs in 5% to 10% of patients with breast cancer.

- Pain is associated in 10% of patients.

EXAMINATION

Patient Seated

Breast examination requires careful attention to inspection and palpation. Inspection must be done with the patient seated to note:

- inequality of the level of the nipples
- retraction of the nipples
- eczema of the nipple
- contour changes in the breast
- skin tethering or dimpling
- oedema of the skin
- nodules in the skin

Many of these signs are made more obvious when the patient elevates the arms above the head and in particular discrepant levels of the nipples will be exaggerated as will skin dimpling.

The patient should then be examined leaning forward with the breasts hanging away from the body and pushing down on her knees or the hands of the examiner to tense the pectoral muscles. This will again accentuate any tethering or attachment.

Examination of the breast tissue should be done in a systematic manner using the palmar surfaces of the distal two phalanxes and examining.

While the patient is seated, the left breast is examined with the right hand commencing in the lower outer quadrant feeling the four quadrants carefully and the area behind the nipple. If the breasts are pendulous they should be felt bimanually. The right breast is felt with the left hand.

When the breasts have been felt the axillae should be examined feeling carefully for medial, anterior, posterior and lateral node groups.

Patient Lying

The patient should then be examined lying down either flat or with a pillow under the appropriate shoulder if bodily habitus indicates this. The breasts should again be examined in the four quadrants and behind the nipple with the patient's arms by the side, the arms should then be placed above the head to thin the breast tissue on the chest wall and the process repeated. Axillary gland palpation should also be done with the patient lying down although it is more common to feel the significant glands with the patient seated.

Characteristics of the Lump

If a lump is felt the attachments of the lump to the skin and deeper structures should be carefully checked by pinching the skin and by tensing the pectoral muscles to see if the mobility of the lump becomes limited. A carcinoma usually feels hard and tethered within the breast tissue with ill-defined margins. Some variants of carcinoma can however feel quite discrete and mobile, in particular the mucinous cancer occurring in the older age group. In some cases a diffuse difference in breast texture without a localised lump is felt and this occurs particularly in lobular carcinomas.

Having examined the patient's breast and found a lump, the lump should be allocated a score between 1 and 5; 1 being normal, 2 — benign lump, 3 — indeterminate, 4 — suspicious and 5 — clinically malignant.

INVESTIGATION

Following examination of the breast, investigation is necessary to determine the presence of carcinoma.

Mammography

The most sensitive imaging technique is mammography which has a sensitivity of 90% overall and a specificity of 50% and a Positive Predictive Value (PPV) of 53%[1]. These figures are lower in the younger age group (under 40) where sensitivity drops to 80% or 85% and specificity to 40%[2].

The mammographic abnormalities seen are stellate (star shaped) lesions (see Figure 23.1), solid lesions (well defined or ill defined) (see Figure 23.2) microcalcification and parenchymal distortion. The abnormalities seen on mammogram have predictive values of:

- 94% for stellate lesions
- 83% for comedo (casting) microcalcifications
- 54% for ill-defined masses
- 35% non-comedo microcalcification
- 37% for parenchymal distortion

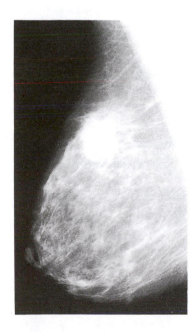

Figure 23.1 (Left) A typical example of a stellate lesion

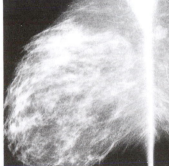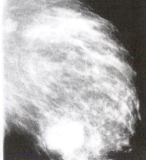

Figure 23.2 A typical example of a well-defined solid lesion

On completion of mammography a diagnostic score should be allocated between 1 and 5 as indicated previously.

Ultrasound

Ultrasound is complimentary to mammography and is commonly done when mammography shows an indeterminate lesion, or as a first line investigation of women under the age of 35. It is a more sensitive diagnostic tool in younger patients than mammography, which is less sensitive. The ultrasound features are:

- An irregular hypoechoic lesion with posterior shadowing (not always present).
- Increased soundwave reflection anterior and lateral to the lesion due to oedema.
- Interruption of tissue planes by the lesion and failure of the tissue planes to curve around the lesion.
- The height of the abnormality is greater than its width.

Ultrasound findings should also be allocated a diagnostic score of 1 to 5.

Cytology

Fine needle aspiration is the most sensitive and specific of the diagnostic modalities for breast cancer with a sensitivity of 95% and a specificity of 99%[3]. This is again allocated a diagnostic score of 1 to 5.

Indication For Biopsy

If suspicion of carcinoma exists, that is there are two 3s or one 4 or 5 scores in the diagnostic work-up of a breast lump, core biopsy or open biopsy must be performed to obtain histology.

Core biopsy, although it provides a cylinder of breast tissue and is subject to histological rather than cytological examination, still has a false negative rate of 5% and a false positive rate of 1%[4].

Open biopsy is the absolute diagnostic test.

STAGING

The staging of breast cancer is undertaken to estimate prognosis and to decide if curative or palliative treatments are indicated. Staging may be on either clinical or pathological grounds. The most commmonly used classifcation, is the TNM classification where T refers to tumour characteristics, N refers to nodes and M to presence or absence of distant metatases. The American Joint Committee on Cancer describes this system[5] and relates it to the 1 to 4 staging system (see Table 23.1).

Clinical staging is used to estimate progress and help decide treatment, and is based on clinical findings. Stages 1 and 2 are considered 'surgical', while Stages 3 and 4 are not usually treated surgically, although selected Stage 3 patients may be amenable to surgery

Pathologic staging is used to estimate prognosis and indicate the need for adjuvant therapy on the basis of complete histopathology of the breast and axillary lymph nodes.

PATHOLOGY

Breast cancer develops from the terminal ductal lobular units. In the vast majority of cases it develops from the ductal cells, less frequently it develops from the lobular cells.

Table 23.1 Summary of American Joint Committe on Cancer (a) TNM staging and (b) grouping system for breast cancer

(a) TNM staging for breast cancer

Primary tumour (T)

TX	Primary tumour can not be assessed
TO	No evidence of primary tumour
TIS	Carcinoma *in situ*: intraductal carcinoma, or lobular carcinoma *in situ*, or Paget's disease of the nipple with no tumour
T1	Tumour 2 cm or less in greatest dimension
T1a	0.5 cm or less in greatest dimension
T1b	0.5 cm to 1 cm in greatest dimension
T1c	1 cm to 2 cm in greatest dimension
T2	Tumour more than 2 cm but not more than 5 cm in greatest dimension
T3	Tumour more than 5 cm in greatest dimension
T4	Tumour of any size with direct extension to chest wall or skin
T4a	Extension to chest wall
T4b	Oedema (including peau d'orange), or ulceration of the skin of the breast, or satellite skin nodules confined to the same breast
T4c	Both 4a and 4b above
T4d	Inflammatory carcinoma

Regional lymph nodes (N)

NX	Regional lymph nodes can not be assessed
N0	No regional lymph nodes metastasis
N1	Metastasis to movable ipsilateral axillary lymph node/s
N2	Metastasis to ipsilateral axillary lymph node/s fixed to one another or to other structures
N3	Metastasis to ipsilateral internal mammary lymph node/s

Distant metastasis (M)

MX	Presence of distant metastasis can not be assessed
M0	No distant metastasis
M1	Distant metastasis (includes metastasis to supraclavicular lymph nodes)

(b) Grouping system for breast cancer

Stage	Classifications
Stage 0	Tis N0 M0
Stage I	T1 N0 M0
Stage IIA	T0 N1 M0
	T1 N1 M0
	T2 N0 M0
Stage IIB	T2 N1 M0
	T3 N0 M0
Stage IIIA	T0 N2 M0
	T1 N2 M0
	T2 N2 M0
	T3 N1 M0
	T3 N2 M0
Stage IIIB	T4 any N M0
	any T N3 M0
Stage IV	any T any N M1

Lobular Carcinoma

Lobular carcinoma insitu (LCIS) is a neoplasm of the lobular cells which is not invasive. It does not usually progress to invasion but it is an indication that the patient has a high likelihood of developing a carcinoma of some type either lobular or ductal in the same or the contralateral breast within the next five years, this occurring in 15% of cases.

Lobular carcinoma develops from the lobular cells of the breast and is characterised by a diffuse infiltration with unclear margins and widespread invasion of surrounding tissues. It makes up 8% of breast cancers.

Ductal Carcinoma

Ductal carcinoma insitu (DCIS) which is pre-invasive may be of a high grade or low grade. It progresses to invasive carcinoma, high grade progressing in 30% of cases within 5 years and low grade 5% of cases within 5 years. They are important because removal of the precancerous lesion should theoretically give 100% cure. This is particularly important as these tumours are becoming more frequently detected by the screening programs.

Invasive ductal carcinoma is divided into the non-specific or invasive ductal carcinoma not otherwise specified (IDCNOS) which constitutes 80% of breast cancers and various special types including medullary, mucinous and tubular. The special types generally have a better prognosis than the IDCNOS and in particular tubular carcinoma is regarded as a very minimally aggressive tumour.

TREATMENT

Treatment needs to be directed towards the breast, the axilla and distant areas. Associated with the treatment may be breast reconstruction.

Breast

The surgical treatment of carcinoma involves removal of all the carcinomatous tissue. If this can be effected by a complete local resection (CLE) and a satisfactory cosmetic result is obtained (as it can in approximately 70% of cases) then that may be the procedure of choice but it must be followed by radiotherapy (RT) to the breast. There is no difference in long-term disease control between mastectomy and CLE plus RT. RT is necessary to reduce the incidence of local recurrence to an acceptable level. Without radiotherapy local recurrence will occur in 20 to 40% of patients in 10 years depending upon the margins of clearance at the original resection[5]. This figure will reduce to approximately one quarter with radiotherapy. If the tumour is large, diffuse or multicentric and complete removal of malignancy would leave an unsatisfactory result, mastectomy is indicated.

The different pathological types vary in their management. LCIS requires excision only because it is not a carcinoma but purely a marker for the deveopment of carcinoma. DCIS (pre-invasive cancer) and invasive cancer should be treated by local excision or mastectomy according to the above criteria. As DCIS is a non-invasive tumour axillary dissection is not indicated.

Axilla

The presence of metastatic disease in the axillary lymph nodes indicates that the tumour is capable of producing metastases and there is thus a likelihood the tumour will be in distant sites such as bone, lungs, liver, brain. Axillary dissection should be performed for all tumours except DCIS. Axillary dissection is important to:

- estimate the likelihood of distant spread
- remove a tumour load from the body
- determine prognosis

The axillary nodes are divided into levels 1, 2 and 3 by the pectoralis minor muscle, level 1 being lateral to the minor, level 2 being behind the pectoralis minor and level 3 being medial to it. It is practice to remove levels 1 and 2 as this gives the optimum prognostic information. Removal of level 1 gives incorrect information in 30% of cases and removal of level 3 will only give information not available with level 1 and 2 dissection in 1% of cases. At least 10 nodes must be removed to give reliable prognostic data[7].

If axillary lymph nodes are extensively involved or there is extra capsular spread then radiotherapy to the area is indicated to prevent local recurrence.

Distant Metastases

Distant metastases should be treated by systemic therapy appropriate to the final histopathology and prognostic factors.

PROGNOSIS

The prognosis of breast cancer varies depending upon many factors, including tumour type, size, stage, lymph node involvement and grade. Other factors, such as receptor levels, CErb2, and epidermal growth factor, ploidy, and Ki67, are also of prognostic significance. The major prognostic factors, however, are size, nodal involvement, grade, receptor status and stage. The prognosis relative to these factors is shown in Figures 23.3, 23.4, 23.5 and 23. 6. The overall 5-year survival in New South Wales is approximately 75%.

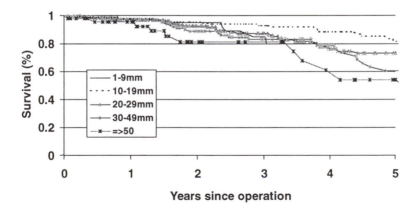

Figure 23.3 Survival by size of lesion

Source: Data from The Strathfield Breast Centre, New South Wales, Australia.

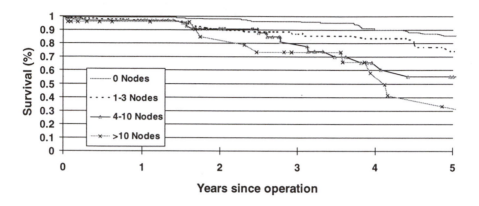

Figure 23.4 Survival by number of positive nodes

Source: Data from The Strathfield Breast Centre, New South Wales, Australia.

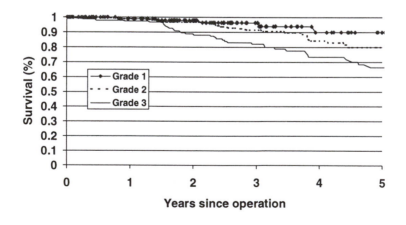

Figure 23.5 Survival by grade of lesion

Source: Data from The Strathfield Breast Centre, New South Wales, Australia.

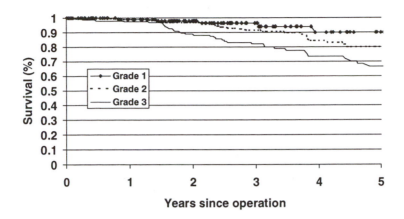

Figure 23.6 Survival by stage

Source: Data from The Strathfield Breast Centre, New South Wales, Australia.

REFERENCES

1. Burrell H.C., Pinder S.E., Wilson A.R.M., Evans, A.J., Yeoman, L.J., Elston, C.W. and Eillis, I.O. (1996) The positive predictive value of mammographic signs: A review of 425 non-palpable breast lesions. *Clin. Radiology*, **51**, 277–281.

2. Chew, S-B., Hughes, M., Kennedy, C., Gillett, D. and Carmalt, H. (1996) Mammographically negative breast cancer at The Strathfield Breast Centre. *Aust N.Z. J. Surg.*, **66**, 134–137.

3. Sterrett, G., Harvey, J., Parsons, R.W., Sterrett, G., Harvey, J., Parsons, R.W., Byrne, M.J., Jamrozik, K., Fitzgerald, C.J., Dewar, J.M., Ingram, D.M., Sheiner, H., Cameron, F. et al. (1994) Breast cancer in Western Australia in 1989: III: Accuracy of FNA cytology in diagnosis. *Aust. N.Z. J. Surg.*, **64**, 745–749.

4. Hirst, C. and Davis, N. (1997) Core biopsy for microcalcifications in the breast. *Aust. N.Z. J. Surg.*, **67**, 320–324.

5. AJCC (1997) AJCC Cancer Staging Manual (5th edn). Philadelphia: Lippencott Raven Publishers.

6. Fisher, B., Redmond, C., Poisson, R., Fisher, B., Redmond, C., Poisson, R., Margolese, R., Wolmark, N., Wickerham, L., Fisher, E., Deutsch, M., Caplan, R., Pilch, Y. et al. (1989) Eight year results of a randomised clinical trial comparing total mastectomy and lumpecteomy with or without radiation in the treatment of breast cancer. *N.Engl. J. Med.,* **320**, 822–828.

7. Veronesi, U., Luini, A., Galimberti, V., Marchini, S., Sacchini, V. and Rilke, F. (1990) Extent of metastatic axillary involvement in 1446 cases of breast cancer. *European J. Surg. Oncology,* **16(2)**, 127–133.

CHAPTER 24

EARLY BREAST CANCER: ADJUVANT SYSTEMIC THERAPY

Alan Coates

INTRODUCTION

Early breast cancer means operable disease, and includes all stages which are neither metastatic nor locally advanced. Management involves both local and systemic treatments.

This chapter is focussed on systemic therapies used in addition to local therapy, including all forms of hormonal manipulation and cytotoxic chemotherapy. The goals of treating undetectable remaining cancer cells are to reduce the risk of metastatic disease and local recurrence and to improve overall survival. Twenty years of carefully conducted randomised controlled trials have yielded irrefutable evidence that these goals can be achieved.

The remaining questions concern the selection of the most appropriate type, intensity and duration of adjuvant therapy for each patient, adapted to her age and general health and to the inherent risk of recurrence of her tumour. Wherever possible, consideration should be given to participation in randomised clinical trials addressing the remaining unsolved questions.

TYPES OF ADJUVANT SYSTEMIC THERAPY

Ovarian Ablation

For more than a century it has been known that altering the hormonal milieu by oophorectomy can alter the behaviour of breast cancer. Trials in the 1940s and 1950s used surgical or radiotherapeutic ovarian ablation as adjuvant therapy for early breast cancer. Although delay of relapse was observed, individual trials were too small to detect improved overall survival, and oophorectomy fell into undeserved disuse.

It was not until the overviews described below that ablation was established as a fully effective adjuvant modality. More recent trials have investigated pharmacological ovarian suppression using LHRH analogues such as goserelin as an alternative to surgery or radiotherapy. Ablation is only used for premenopausal women.

Tamoxifen

This non-steroidal anti-oestrogen is probably the most widely used single drug in the treatment of all stages of breast cancer. It was first shown to be effective in post-menopausal women, but is now recognised as an effective adjuvant at all ages, though likely to be more effective in women whose tumours contain oestrogen receptors. It has the additional benefit of substantially reducing the risk of a new primary breast cancer in the contralateral breast, a property not seen with cytotoxic chemotherapy.

Recent studies suggest that tamoxifen should be given for several years, with most suggesting that five years is best. Tamoxifen has relatively few side effects, but causes menopausal flushing and may increase the risk of endometrial carcinoma.

Cytotoxic Chemotherapy

Many cytotoxic agents are effective against metastatic breast cancer. In general, combinations of drugs are superior to single agent therapy. Although a very wide range of combinations has been used, several standard regimens have emerged, among which cyclophosphamide, methotrexate and 5-fluorouracil (CMF) and combinations of or including doxorubicin (Adriamycin®) and cyclophosphamide (AC) sometimes with 5-fluorouracil (FAC, CAF) are most prominent.

The evidence from the most recent overview and a subsequent publication from the US National Surgical Adjuvant Breast Project (NSABP) confirms that chemotherapy adds to survival at all ages up to 70, even in patients whose axillary nodes were not involved and whose tumours were oestrogen-receptor positive.[1,2] Sequential rather than alternating use of doxorubicin and CMF seems superior.[3]

Outside a clinical trial, AC, CMF or the sequential regimens are reasonable choices for adjuvant cytotoxic therapy. Evidence about adjuvant therapy is changing rapidly, so it is important that those advising women with early breast cancer are up to date. In most settings, referral to a medical oncologist should be considered.

CHOICE OF ADJUVANT THERAPY

Whether in a clinical trial or otherwise, the treatment chosen should be tailored to the degree of risk for an individual patient, to any tumour factors, such as oestrogen receptor positivity, which may predict responsiveness, and to the patient's likely ability to tolerate the treatment (see below). In general, a combination of chemotherapy plus one or both of the endocrine options is likely to be superior to single modalities. Endocrine therapies are less valuable in patients whose tumours are oestrogen-receptor negative, while cytotoxic therapy may be omitted in older patients with low-risk, receptor-positive tumours.

EVIDENCE FOR EFFICACY OF ADJUVANT SYSTEMIC THERAPY

The highest level, most secure evidence derives from a properly conducted overview or meta-analysis of all available randomised controlled trials. Such evidence is available for the major questions of efficacy in adjuvant systemic therapy for early breast cancer.

The Early Breast Cancer Triallists Collaborative Group, led by Richard Peto, conducts regular systematic meta-analyses of all available trial data. Each individual trials group provides individual patient data for statistical re-analysis, so that all available evidence is brought together to answer major questions of efficacy. This series of publications provides the best evidence available to support the fact that all the three main adjuvant therapies work.[1] The overview process will underestimate the magnitude of the benefit, both because it must analyse by 'intention to treat' and because it must group together types of treatment, which maybe more or less effective.

IS DOSE IMPORTANT?

One large randomised trial has shown that it is important not to reduce below standard doses of CAF, but so far has not shown additional benefit of increasing above standard dose intensity.[4] Very high doses of chemotherapy which require autologous stem cell support have not yet been established as beneficial, and should not be used outside randomised clinical trials.

NEW AGENTS

Several new endocrine agents have recently become available, both aromatase inhibitors and pure anti-oestrogens. Their place in adjuvant therapy remains to be determined. Among newer cytotoxic agents the role of the taxanes paclitaxel and docetaxel in sequence or combination with anthracyclines is being investigated.

QUALITY OF LIFE

Only recently have adjuvant therapy trials included self-assessment of patient quality of life. The results were reassuring. Cytotoxic therapy had a measurable but transient and minor effect on quality of life, and there was no substantial interference with the steady improvement in quality of life reported by patients with early breast cancer.[5]

IS ADJUVANT SYSTEMIC THERAPY WORTHWHILE?

Independent of the statistical evidence for efficacy, and even the quality of life scores, the fundamental question to be answered by women and their advising clinicians is whether the benefits likely to accrue in any particular case make the likely adverse effects worthwhile.

One direct approach to this balance involved asking patients who had experienced chemotherapy just what increase in survival duration or probability would justify the use of six months of CMF chemotherapy. As is commonly seen in such surveys, relatively minor advantages were considered sufficient to justify treatment. The minimum increment at which the *majority* of patients would accept treatment was a trade-off of one extra year of survival (5 to 6 or 15 to 16 years), or a 2% improvement in 5-year survival probability (65% to 67% or 85% to 87%)[6]. Such benefits are well within the projected benefits of therapy, even among patients with high or intermediate risk node-negative disease. It seems reasonable therefore to offer cytotoxic treatment to most women at above minimal risk, and tamoxifen to an even wider group.

SUMMARY

Adjuvant systemic therapy works. It saves lives, at an acceptable cost. Apart from very old patients, and those with extremely low risk tumours, adjuvant systemic therapy should be considered in the management of most patients with early breast cancer.

REFERENCES

1. Early Breast Cancer Triallists' Collaborative Group (1992) Systemic treatment of early breast cancer by hormonal, cytotoxic or immune therapy. 133 randomised trials involving 31,000 recurrences and 24,000 deaths among 75,000 women. *Lancet*, **339**, 1–15, 71–85.

2. Fisher, B., Dignam, J., DeCillis, A., Wickerham, D.L., Wolmark, N., Emir, B., Dimitrov, N., Abraham, N., Atkins, J.N., Shibata, H. and Deschenes, L. (1997) The worth of chemotherapy and tamoxifen (TAM) over TAM alone in node-negative patients with estrogen-receptor positive invasive breast cancer: first results from NSABP B-20. *Proc Amer Soc Clin Oncol*, **16**:1a (Abstract #1).

3. Bonadonna, G., Zambetti, M. and Valagussa, P. (1995) Sequential or alternating doxorubicin and CMF regimens in breast cancer with more than three positive nodes: ten-year results. *JAMA*, **273**, 542–547.

4. Wood, W.C., Budman, D.R., Korzun, A.H., Cooper, M.R., Younger, J., Hart, R.D., Moore, Al, Ellerton, J.A., Norton, L. and Ferree, C.R. (1994) Dose and dose intensity of adjuvant chemotherapy for stage II, node-positive breast carcinoma. *N Engl J Med*, **330**, 1253–1259.

5. Hürny, C., Bernhard, J., Coates, A.S., Castiglione-Gertoch, M., Peteson, H.F., Gelber, R.D., Forbes, J.F., Rudenstam, C.M., Simoncini, E., Crivellari, D., Goldhursch, A. and Senn, H.J. (1996) Impact of adjuvant therapy on quality of life in women with node-positive operable breast cancer. *Lancet*, **347**, 1279–1284.

6. Coates, A.S. and Simes, R.J. (1993) Patient assessment of adjuvant treatment in operable breast cancer. In *Introducing New Treatments for Cancer: Practical, Ethical and Legal Problems*, edited by C.J. Williams, pp. 447–458. Chichester: John Wiley & Sons Ltd.

CHAPTER 25

RADIOTHERAPY IN BREAST CANCER

Susan C. Pendlebury

INTRODUCTION

Radiotherapy plays an established role in the treatment of all stages of breast cancer.

In early stage disease, defined in the previous chapter as operable disease, the aim of treatment is curative and the role of radiotherapy is to maximise local control in the conserved breast.

In more locally advanced disease, characterised by large tumours or heavy nodal involvement, radiotherapy has been shown to reduce local recurrence on the chest wall after mastectomy.

In metastatic breast cancer, the aim of treatment is palliative with the goal of all treatment modalities including radiotherapy being to reduce symptoms and improve quality of life for patients.

EARLY STAGE BREAST CANCER

Rationale and Outcome

Clinical trials have demonstrated the equivalence of conservative surgery plus radiotherapy with mastectomy for loco-regional control and survival. The most important determinant in the treatment choice is patient preference.

For patients who choose to retain their breast rather than undergo mastectomy, radiotherapy is delivered after breast conserving surgery (lympectomy) to reduce the rate of local recurrence in the conserved breast. The recurrence rate after lympectomy is reduced from around 30% to 8% at 10 years by the addition of radiotherapy. A good cosmetic result is also achieved in 75–80% of patients.

Precautions

- Contraindications to breast irradiation are pregnancy and prior radiotherapy to the breast.
- Patients who have a large tumour in a small breast may have a reduced cosmetic outcome and so may prefer to be treated by mastectomy.

- If the surgical margins are positive, a re-excision of the tumour bed or a mastectomy should be considered because conservative surgery plus radiotherapy in the presence of positive resection margins carries up to 50% risk of local recurrence in the breast.

What Does Radiotherapy Involve?

The conserved breast following lympectomy for breast cancer, should receive whole-breast irradiation. The recommended dose is 45 to 50 Gy in 25 daily fractions plus a boost of 10 to 16 Gy in five to eight fractions. This provides optimal cosmetic outcomes and cancer control rates in the breast. The boost allows for a higher dose to be delivered to the primary site which is the site of 50–80% of local recurrences.

The regional lymph nodes both axillary and supraclavicular are not routinely included in the treatment volume if an axillary dissection has been performed. Thus, the risk of lymphoedema is not increased above the 6% incidence seen with surgical axillary dissection.

Can Radiotherapy be Omitted in Any Patients?

Tumours less than 1 cm arising in older patients, excised with clear margins, carry a reduced risk of local recurrence. However, these risks are further reduced with radiotherapy. Thus, this technique will maximise the outcome from breast conservation.

Most recurrences in the breast can not be salvaged by further breast conserving therapy and must be managed with mastectomy. Thus, a higher local recurrence rate will mean a higher mastectomy rate.

The improvement in local control achieved with radiotherapy, must be balanced against the toxicity of treatment. The common side effects of radiotherapy are shown in Table 25.1.

Role of Radiotherapy in Ductal Carcinoma *in situ*

Ductal carcinoma *in situ* is a non-invasive, pre-malignant, breast lesion which has become more frequently diagnosed with the increased use of mamography. Whilst it does not carry the metastatic potential of invasive breast cancer, DCIS can progress to invasive malignancy.

There is a spectrum of available treatment ranging from wide local excision to mastectomy. The increasing use of breast conserving treatment for invasive breast cancer is making it harder to justify mastectomy for many cases of DCIS.

Following a wide local excision the risk of recurrence of the DCIS is about 10%, with half of the recurrences being invasive cancers. The addition of radiotherapy following local excision of these lesions reduces the invasive recurrences to around 2%.

LOCALLY ADVANCED BREAST CANCER

Patients with locally advanced breast cancer are at high risk of both local relapse and metastatic spread. The risks of progressive local or metastatic disease increase with increasing tumour size and numbers of lymph nodes involved. The traditional management of these patients with mastectomy alone resulted in unacceptably high rates of local relapse. The addition of chemotherapy, while increasing survival in this group of patients, did not improve local control rates.

- Currently, the optimal management is with a combination of all three modalities of treatment, surgery, radiotherapy and chemotherapy.

- The criteria for offering patients combined modality treatment varies, but evidence suggests a benefit for patients who have tumours greater than 5 cm and in whom 4 or more axillary lymph nodes are involved.

- Some benefit may exist for patients with smaller tumours or fewer nodes but these benefits must be weighed against the side effects of treatment.

- In operable cases, with a small breast primary, but advanced, due to the number of involved lymph nodes at operation, both chemotherapy and radiotherapy are sequenced postoperatively.

Table 25.1 Side effects of radiotherapy

• **Tiredness**

Tiredness affects most patients, but most of those who work continue to do so.

• **Redness of the breast**

This usually begins in the third week and is worst seven to ten days after treatment is completed. The redness is more intense and lasts about seven days longer if chemotherapy is also given. There is frequently some skin desquamation (resembling sunburn) at the peak of the reaction.

• **Symptomatic pneumonitis**

This is rare and occurs in only 1% of patients receiving radiotherapy alone and 3% of those receiving chemotherapy as well. It commences three weeks to three months after completing radiotherapy and presents as a cough or mild shortness of breath. Management is with combined antibiotic and corticosteroid use. The differential diagnosis rests with pulmonary emboli and infection.

Radiological changes of pneumonitis seen on chest X-ray or CT scans at any time after radiotherapy to the breast are common but usually involve a small anterior sliver of the lung, are asymptomatic and require no treatment. The X-ray changes correspond to the radiotherapy fields and should not be mistaken for metastatic disease in the lungs.

• **Rib fracture**

Fracture of the ribs beneath the treated breast is an uncommon long-term side effect occurring in 1% of patients receiving radiotherapy alone and up to 6% in those also receiving chemotherapy. Treatment is with simple analgesics for pain control.

• **Lymphoedema**

The risk of arm lymphoedema after a surgical axillary lymph node dissection is about 6%. Radiotherapy to the breast alone does not increase this risk. When the axilla is treated by radiotherapy alone without surgery, the risk is similar to that of surgery alone, at about 6%. The risk of lymphoedema increases to 25–30% when radiotherapy is given to the axilla in addition to surgery. Recurrent cancer in the axilla frequently presents as lymphoedema of the arm. Radiotherapy is indicated for this presentation provided it has not already been given.

• **Second malignancy**

The most common second malignancy following radiotherapy to the breast is a recurrence of the original breast cancer (8% at 10 years). The risk of a new malignancy arising as a result of the radiotherapy is extremely rare, occurring in only 0.2% of patients alive at 10 years.

• **Heart disease**

A number of old studies showed that heart disease is a risk in patients receiving radiotherapy for breast cancer. Modern techniques minimise radiation dose to the heart and it appears that this risk is now extremely low.

- Where the primary is clinically large or inoperable, or the lymph nodes are fixed at presentation, neoadjuvant or preoperative chemotherapy and radiotherapy are frequently employed.
- Preoperative treatment reduces the size of the tumour and may then allow conservative surgery to be performed.
- Response to initial chemotherapy is a recognised prognostic sign in locally advanced disease.

Where is the Radiotherapy Directed?

The region at greatest risk in locally advanced disease is the chest wall, where at least 50% of all local recurrences occur. This area is always included in the treatment volume. The other areas at risk are the regional lymph nodes particularly the supraclavicular fossa and axilla.

The internal mammary lymph nodes, whilst the site of lymphatic drainage of some breast cancers, particularly those medially placed, are rarely the site of isolated local relapse. The disadvantage of irradiating this group of lymph nodes is the necessary inclusion of part of the heart in the treatment field. The overall benefit of internal mammary irradiation is being studied in ongoing clinical trials.

The dose to these regions is generally 50 Gy in 25 daily fractions. For locally advanced disease radiotherapy is often 'sandwiched' between doses of chemotherapy. It is not given concurrently with doxorubicin. When the axilla is included in the treatment field after axillary dissection the risk of arm lymphoedema is increased to around 25–30%.

METASTATIC BREAST CANCER

Effective palliation is achieved by the judicious sequential use of observation, surgery, radiotherapy, endocrine therapy and chemotherapy. The choice of therapy at any one time is governed by the patients symptoms, age, previous treatment and response to it. If two treatment options are equally effective, the less toxic is recommended.

Situations where Radiotherapy is Used

- Brain or retinal metastases. A high rate of response has consistently been achieved with radiotherapy in these sites.
- Chest wall recurrence may be controlled by radiotherapy alone in 40–50% of cases.
- Bone metastases. Radiotherapy gives rapid pain relief, even after the patient has failed to respond to systemic therapy. Judicious use of node therapy in metastatic breast cancer involving weight bearing bones can prevent pathological fractures.
- Spinal cord compression. Immediate radiotherapy is used for metastases anywhere in the spine that are compressing the spinal canal. This is an emergency because the patients long-term mobility and continence are threatened.

Radiotherapy Dose in Metastatic Bone Disease

The optimal dose of radiotherapy for bone palliation differs in each clinical situation. In patients with multiple sites of visceral metastases and rapidly progressive disease, good palliation may be achieved with a single fraction of 8 Gy. Patients in better general condition who have only bony disease and a longer anticipated survival may be better served by up to 10 fractions. In the palliative setting, treatment over four to six weeks is not usually appropriate.

REFERENCES

Fisher B., Redmond C., Poisson R., Margolese, R., Wolmark, N., Wickerham, L., Fisher, E., Deutsch, M., Caplan, R. and Pilch, Y. (1989) Eight year results of a randomized clinical trial comparing total mastectomy with or without radiation in the treatment of breast cancer. *N.Engl.J.Med.,* **320**, 822–828.

Fowble B., Gray R., Gilchrist K., Goodman R., Taylor S., Tormey D. (1988) Identification of a subset of patients with breast cancer and histologically positive axillary lymph nodes who may benefit from postoperative radiotherapy. *J. Clin Oncol,* **6**, 1107–1117.

Schnitt S., Hayman J., Gelman R., Eberlein T. and Love S.A (1996) Prospective study of conservative surgery alone in the treatment of selected patients with Stage 1 breast cancer. *Cancer,* **77**, 1094–1100.

Pierce S., Recht A., Lingos T., Abner A., Vincini F., Silver B., Harris J. (1992).Long-term radiation complications following conservative surgery and radiation therapy in patients with early stage breast cancer. *Int J Radiat Oncol Biol Phys.,* **23**, 915–922.

Henderson I.,Garber J., Breitmeyer J., Hayes, D. and Harris J.(1990) Comprehensive management of disseminated breast cancer. *Cancer,* **66**, 1439–1448.

Pendlebury S.,Bilous M.,Langlands AO. (1995) Sarcomas following radiation therapy for breast cancer. *Int J Radiat Oncol Biol Phys.,* **31**, 405–410.

CHAPTER 26

LOCALLY ADVANCED AND METASTATIC BREAST CANCER

Stephen P. Ackland and John F. Stewart

METASTATIC BREAST CANCER

Background

Metastases beyond the breast and regional lymph nodes are almost always incurable with a survival time from diagnosis of metastases of only about 3 years. Cure is rarely possible with current therapies.

Breast cancer is a slow growing tumour with a low growth fraction. Thus, doses of effective cytotoxic agents kill only a modest proportion of the tumour. The growth kinetics are Gompertzian with the relative growth decreasing as the tumour becomes larger and so as a tumour is reduced in size by a toxic agent, it reverts to a faster growth rate.

In addition, drug resistance, either intrinsic or acquired through exposure to cytotoxic treatments, is the reason for ultimate failure of therapy to control the disease. Strategies to minimise or overcome drug resistance are needed.

The general aim of treatment is palliation of symptoms and lengthening of survival, with acceptable toxicity of the treatment, so that quality of life is maintained or enhanced.

Work-Up

- The initial assessment of a patient with metastatic breast cancer must include a careful history and physical examination, to assess the biological aggressiveness of the disease and its extent. Breast cancer can metastasise to many organs, but the most common are bones, lung, liver, skin, and soft tissues (chest wall, regional lymph nodes).

- A full blood cell count, liver function tests, alkaline phosphatase, chest X-ray and bone scan are useful staging tests, and if clinically indicated liver ultrasound and/or CT scans can define the extent of disease. Tumour markers such as CEA and CA15.3 are of uncertain value and should not be routinely ordered outside of clinical trials.

- An evaluation of the hormone receptor status is worthwhile as it may determine the choice of

151

therapy. Hormone receptors are usually estimated on the primary tumour specimen, but metastases can be biopsied for this purpose if appropriate.

• The likelihood of benefit from systemic treatment depends to some extent on prior adjuvant therapy. Patients previously treated with adjuvant agents are less likely to respond to such agents when used in the advanced setting.

Management

Management should be individualised, because breast cancer is heterogeneous. Options include no treatment, surgery, radiation and systemic chemotherapy (including hormone therapy). Therefore a multidisciplinary approach to management is necessary[1].

No active treatment may be considered where the risks of treatment outweigh the potential benefits, such as advanced disease in the very elderly or infirm, or asymptomatic disease. Local therapy (e.g. surgery or radiation) can be used for local problems, such as isolated chest wall disease, CNS or choroidal metastases, spinal cord compression, impending fractures, pericardial or pleural effusions. Conventional treatments usually show benefit for limited periods, so future treatments should be anticipated so as not to eliminate them.

Personal preference including quality of life issues should guide therapy. Time to response may be an issue since endocrine treatments usually take 6–12 weeks to take effect whereas cytotoxic chemotherapy works more quickly.

Hormonal Therapy of Metastatic Breast Cancer

Hormonal therapy is generally the treatment of choice for patients who have metastatic but non-life-threatening breast cancer. Factors that are associated with a greater chance of response to hormonal

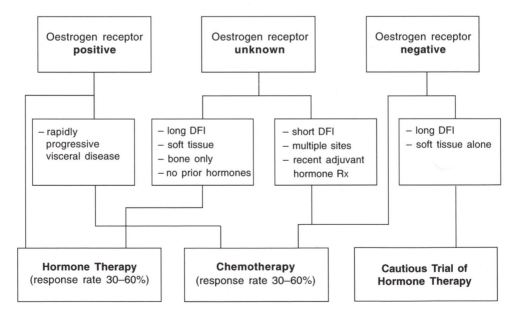

Figure 26.1 Decision tree for systemic therapy of metastatic breast cancer (DFI = disease-free interval)

agents include having a tumour that contains oestrogen (ER) and progesterone (PR) receptors, long disease-free interval, having soft tissue and bone lesions rather than visceral metastases, a previous regression on prior endocrine therapy, and an older age for additive hormonal therapies.

The exact mechanism by which hormonal therapy induces tumour regression is not defined. It could possibly be interference with transcription of oestrogen regulated genes or possibly an effect on growth factors.

Appropriately selected patients have a response rate of 30–60% (see Table 26.1). ER negative tumours rarely respond. The choice of agent depends on the menopausal status and toxicity profile, but the response rate is similar for all agents. Combinations of hormonal agents may be no better than single agents. The median duration of response is 1–2 years, and eventually almost all tumours become refractory.

Tamoxifen

Tamoxifen is the most popular additive endocrine therapy for advanced breast cancer. Although other hormonal therapies have similar efficacy, in general tamoxifen is better tolerated. Some 30% of unselected patients and 50% of patients with hormone receptor positive tumours will respond (see Table 26.1). Other anti-oestrogens with less oestrogenic activity than tamoxifen have only undergone limited clinical testing.

Aromatase Inhibitors

The primary source of oestrogen production in post-menopausal women is the peripheral conversion of adrenal androstenedione to oestrone via the aromatase enzyme. Aminoglutethimide blocks aromatase, but also the conversion of cholesterol to pregnenolone leading to a medical adrenalectomy. It is an effective second-line hormonal therapy in post-menopausal patients with a 30% response rate. Side effects are a problem in over one-third of patients and include lethargy, transient rash, dizziness, nausea and vomiting. Doses over 250 mg twice daily generally require steroid supplementation.

More recently, specific inhibitors of the aromatase enzyme have been available. These include formestane (lentaron), letrozole, anastrozole (arimidex), and vorozole. Preliminary data suggests that responses to these agents are at least as good as those to aminoglutethimide and with less toxicity.

Progestagens

Randomised studies indicate that progestational agents such as medroxyprogesterone and megestrol have similar response rates as tamoxifen and other hormonal agents. Toxicity is apparently similar to

Table 26.1 Results of systemic treatment for metastatic breast cancer

Intervention	Response Rate (%)	Median Time to Progression
Endocrine Therapy		
first line	30–60	~ 10 months
second line	15–25	~ 6 months
Chemotherapy		
first line	40–60	~ 8 months
second line	20–40	~ 4 months

tamoxifen although weight gain is much more common with progestagens and thromboembolic events are also more common. It is not clear whether there is a dose-response relationship for progestagens.

Ablative Hormonal Therapies

Pre-menopausal patients may respond to surgical, radiation, or chemically-induced menopause. Gonadotrophin-releasing hormone analogue such as goserelin and leuprolide induce reduction in gonadotrophin and prolactin levels and a subsequent fall in plasma sex steroids. Fifty percent of pre-menopausal patients with hormone receptor positive tumours will respond to chemical castration whereas only 5% of similar patients with oestrogen poor tumours will respond.

Bisphosphonates

Seventy percent of patients with disseminated breast cancer have metastatic bone disease. This is a major cause of morbidity. Tumour osteolysis is produced by activation of osteoclasts which resorb bone. Bisphosphonates are potent inhibitors of osteoclast-mediated bone resorption. Early studies suggest that regular use of these agents may delay or prevent skeletal complications in patients with osteolytic bone metastases.

Chemotherapy

Almost all patients need to be considered for chemotherapy during their disease.

Candidates for chemotherapy include patients with rapidly progressive disease, with a short disease-free interval, who are refractory to hormonal therapy, with negative hormone receptors, or predominantly visceral metastases.

Overall response rates to first-line chemotherapy are in the range of 40–70% with complete responses of 5–15%, and a median duration of response of 6–12 months (see Table 26.1). Factors that predict for a good outcome include good performance status, one or two sites of metastases especially in soft tissue, and prior hormonal therapy. Poor prognostic factors include prior chemotherapy and/or radiation therapy, bone and visceral metastases (especially liver) and large numbers of metastases. Menopausal status, hormone receptors and age have no effect on outcome from chemotherapy.

The most frequently used drugs include anthracyclines (doxorubicin, epirubicin), cyclophosphamide, fluorouracil and methotrexate (see Table 26.2). Combinations of cytotoxic agents have consistently demonstrated a higher response rate than single agents in almost all trials. However, the overall benefit of combinations compared to the same drugs given sequentially is still debatable.

Doxorubicin combinations may be more active than CMF but are also more toxic with alopecia and cardiotoxicity[2].

Patients with aggressive disease may be better served by the rapid reduction in tumour mass by a combination therapy, whereas patients with indolent cancer may benefit more from the potentially lower toxicity of a single agent. The optimal use of some highly active new drugs, such as the taxanes (paclitaxel and docetaxel), vinorelbine and gemcitabine have not yet been established. Continuous infusions of drugs (e.g. fluorouracil, doxorubicin) have been described as active and less toxic but are not in common use.

The optimal duration of therapy is not clear. There is no evidence that treatment beyond the achievement of maximal response (complete response or stable partial response) is beneficial. However, a shorter duration of standard dose treatment is less ideal in terms of quality of life[4]. In general treatment should be continued until the maximum response is achieved plus 1–2 cycles.

Second-line Chemotherapy

Second-line chemotherapy is often useful for palliation after first-line treatment has failed. Disease responsiveness tends to decline with second-line and subsequent treatment, both in response rate and time to progression (see Table 26.1).

Generally drugs with different mechanisms of action are preferred. Mitomycin C, taxanes, vinorelbine, continuous infusion fluorouracil and the combination of cisplatin and etoposide all have significant efficacy in providing palliation in this setting. For example, docetaxel has shown a 41% response rate after anthracycline failure.

High Dose Chemotherapy

High dose chemotherapy, in which reinfusion of autologous peripheral blood progenitor cells is used to rescue from lethal myelosuppression, has not yet been proven to be more effective than standard chemotherapy in the management of advanced breast cancer[3]. One randomised controlled study showed a significantly better survival for high dose therapy compared to standard treatment, but the response rate for standard therapy was lower than usually seen[6]. The results of confirmatory studies are awaited. Similarly, moderately high doses, requiring G-CSF support but not autologous progenitor cell reinfusion, are of uncertain value and are the subject of clinical trials.

Table 26.2 Chemotherapeutic agents in breast cancer

Agent	Response Rate
Very active	
Doxorubicin (A)	43–54
Docetaxel	38–70
Epirubicin (E)	45–55
Paclitaxel	30–60
Vinorelbine	35–60
Moderately Active	
Cyclophosphamide (C)	36
Fluorouracil (F)	28
Gemcitabine	18–40
Melphalan	25
Methotrexate (M)	26
Mitoxantrone	21
Mitomycin C	22
Vincristine	19
Vinblastine	21
Combinations	
CMF (P)	30–62
CAF	43–82
CEF	50

CMF(P), cyclophosphamide, methotrexate, fluorouracil with or without prednisolone.

LOCALLY ADVANCED BREAST CANCER

Locally advanced breast cancer (UICC Stage III) accounts for 5–20% of breast cancer in developing countries but is less common in developed countries.

Presentation

- Locally advanced breast cancer is characterised by a large breast tumour (T3 is > 5 cm), involvement of the overlying breast skin, satellite skin nodules, peau d'orange, attachment to deep structures (T4 is direct extension to the skin or chest wall for a cancer of any size), palpable matting or fixation of axillary lymph nodes.
- Generally these features indicate inoperability.
- The spectrum of locally advanced disease ranges from slowly growing, neglected T4N0 tumours to aggressive T1N3 disease with nodal involvement and the high probability of micrometastases. The natural history, response to treatment and survival of patients varies considerably, which is reflected in the results of studies.

Treatment

Historical results with surgery and/or radiation alone are uniformly poor. Treatment with radiotherapy alone resulted in local recurrence rates of between 31% and 72% depending on the dose of radiotherapy given[7,8,9]. Surgery following or preceding radiation has not resulted in improvements in survival or local control.

Combined Modality Therapy

- The introduction of combined modality approaches with the early use of chemotherapy has had a dramatic impact on the outcome.
- Preoperative chemotherapy has a number of advantages:
  — The response rates are generally high, possibly because of an intact blood supply.
  — It may convert an inoperable primary tumour into one which is resectable.
  — It allows direct observation of response to treatment so that treatment can be better individualised. Response to initial chemotherapy is a recognised prognostic factor in this disease.
  — The early introduction of systemic therapy in a disease with a high probability of systemic micrometastases.
- Initial therapy with chemotherapy followed by radiotherapy and/or surgery has been adopted as standard therapy with higher response rates longer survival and improved local-regional control compared to historical controls.
- Doxorubicin containing regimens have resulted in a 60–70% response rate, with pathologic complete response in 10–15% of cases.

Current evidence for this approach remains sparse. The role of surgery in addition to local radiotherapy remains ill defined. In a four-arm study the EORTC Breast Group randomised 410 patients with locally advanced breast cancer to either radiotherapy alone, or radiotherapy followed by systemic therapy which was either endocrine therapy, chemotherapy or both[1]. The patients receiving radiotherapy alone had a shorter time to treatment failure compared to the other three groups with a survival benefit in the group receiving radiotherapy plus combined chemotherapy and endocrine therapy.

Inflammatory Breast Cancer

Inflammatory carcinoma is a distinct clinico-pathologic entity. Although frequently grouped with other locally advanced disease, its prognosis is worse. It is characterised by such features as diffuse erythema, oedema, peau d'orange, tenderness, diffuse enlargement and infiltration in the affected breast. There is often associated pathological evidence of invasion of dermal lymphatics.

With local therapy alone, (i.e. radiotherapy, surgery or both modalities), no more than 15% of patients will be alive at 5 years. Combination chemotherapy including an anthracycline can achieve response in 60–80% of patients and is usually followed by radiotherapy or mastectomy and radiotherapy. Outcome in patients being treated in this fashion is better than historical controls, with local control in 70% of patients and survival in the range of 50% at 5 years and 35% at 10 years[5]. These results may now be similar to treatment results for some other forms of locally advanced breast cancer. It is unclear whether mastectomy offers any additional benefit following combined chemotherapy and radiotherapy.

REFERENCES

1. Bartelink, H., Rubens, R.D., van der Schueren, E. and Sylvester, R. (1997) Hormone therapy prolongs survival in irradiated locally advanced breast cancer: a European Organisation for Research and Treatment of Cancer randomised phase II trial. *J Clin Oncol*, **15**, 207–215.

2. Tomiak, E., Piccart, M., Mignolet, F. et. al. (1996) Characterisation of complete responders to combination chemotherapy for advanced breast cancer: a retrospective EORTC Breast Group Study. *Eur. J Cancer*, **32A**, 1876–1887.

3. Basser, R.L., To, L.B., Begley, G.C., Juttner, C.A., Maher, D.W., Szer, J., Cebon, J., Collins, J.P., Russell, I, Olver, I., Grantly Gill, Fox, R.M., Sheridan, W.P. and Green, M.D. (1995) Adjuvant treatment of high-risk breast cancer using multicycle high-dose chemotherapy and filgrastim-mobilised peripheral blood progenitor cells. *Clin Cancer Res*, **1**, 715–721.

4. Coates, A., Gebski, V., Bishop, J.F., Jeal, P.N., Woods, R.L., Snyder, R., Med., M., Tattersall, M.H.N., Byrne, M., Harvey, V., Grantley Gill, M.D., Simpson, J., Drummond, R., Browne, J. and van Cooten, R. (1987) Improving the quality of life during chemotherapy for advanced breast cancer: a comparison of intermittent and continuous treatment strategies. *New Engl J Med*, **317**, 1490–1495.

5. Perez, C.A., Graham, M.L., Taylor, M.E., Levy, J.F., Mortimer, J.E., Philpott, G.W. and Kucik, N.A. (1994) Management of locally advanced carcinoma of the breast. *Cancer*, **74**, 453–465.

6. Bezwoda, W.R., Seymour, L. and Dansey, R.D. (1995) High-dose chemotherapy with hemopoietic rescue as primary treatment for metastatic breast cancer: a randomised trial. *J Clin Oncol*, **13**, 2483–2489.

7. Ackland, S.P., Bitran, J.D. and Dowlatshahi, K. (1985) Management of locally advanced and inflammatory carcinoma of the breast. *Surg Gynecol Obstet*, **161**, 399–408.

8. Booser, D.J. and Hortobagyi GN. (1992) The treatment of locally advanced breast cancer. *Semin Oncol*, **19**(3), 278–285.

9. Wong, K. and Henderson, I.C. (1994) Management of metastatic breast cancer. *World J Surg.*, **18**, 98–111.

PART VI

GASTROINTESTINAL CANCERS

CHAPTER 27

UPPER GASTROINTESTINAL MALIGNANCY: SURGICAL MANAGEMENT

David W. Storey

INTRODUCTION

Upper gastrointestinal cancers include those of the oesophagus, stomach, duodenum, pancreas and biliary tree. Patients with malignant disease of the upper gastrointestinal tract are particularly unfortunate because these cancers are often diagnosed late and cure is uncommon. The operations required for excision of the cancers can cause major disruption to the function of the GI tract and to the enjoyment of eating.

Apart from squamous carcinoma of the oesophagus, nearly all cancers of these organs are adenocarcinoma. Lymphoma, sarcoma and neuroendocrine cancers make up the remainder.

There are large regional variations in the incidence of these cancers. In a region with a low incidence of gastric and oesophageal cancer like the State of New South Wales in Australia, cancers of the upper gastrointestinal tract as a group make up 7% of all malignancies (excluding non-melanoma skin cancer) and cause 12% of all cancer deaths. Adenocarcinoma of the oesophagogastric junction and lower oesophagus is increasing in frequency, but the total incidence of gastric carcinoma is steadily decreasing. The incidence of the others is steady or increasing slowly.

There have been improvements in management over the last two decades; these relate to earlier detection, better staging and selection, improved surgery and perioperative care and better palliation of patients with incurable disease. There has been little change in cure rates.

There are some features which are common to these cancers.

- They may present with vague malaise, anorexia or weight loss without any distinctive features, and it is the appearance and progression of these symptoms over months which should raise suspicion. Physical signs are rare except in disseminated disease.
- Clinical examination may reveal supraclavicular lymphadenopathy, hepatic metastases, ascites or a shelf of carcinoma in the pelvic peritoneum felt by rectal examination, and these findings exclude the patient from any consideration of curative treatment.

- Computerised axial tomography (CAT) of the chest, abdomen and pelvis will detect pulmonary and hepatic metastases accurately, but lymphadenopathy is not reliably detected and may be misleading, and radiological proximity to vital structures should not be overinterpreted as inoperable malignant involvement.

- For carcinoma from the lower oesophagus to the pancreas, laparoscopy can detect peritoneal disease and small hepatic lesions undetected by CT.

- Endoultrasonography can accurately stage local disease, but the technique is difficult and time consuming.

- Positron emission tomography (PET) can identify metastatic disease undetected by other methods, but expense and availability are limiting factors.

Outcomes

Cure rates are dismal when all patients are included (oesophagus 3%, stomach 15%, pancreas 2%, bile ducts and gallbladder 5%). This is partly because many present with disseminated disease, but the majority of the patients who present with localised disease will still die of cancer, even after operative resection or other treatment undertaken with the aim of cure.

The five-year survival rates for patients who undergo complete resection with curative intent are, oesophagus 20%, stomach 35%, pancreas 5–10%, gallbladder 5–10%, and extrahepatic bile ducts 10–40%. For most patients, recurrence is early, less than 3 years, and survival to five years can be equated with cure. Patients with superficial carcinoma of the oesophagus, stomach or gallbladder diagnosed serendipitously, or as a result of active screening or surveillance endoscopy, have an excellent prognosis but are uncommon.

Effective adjuvant therapies are needed, but so far these have established a place only in oesophageal cancer, and for all other sites the only treatment capable of effecting cure remains surgical resection.

OESOPHAGEAL CANCER

Incidence

There are wide variations in the incidence and histological type of cancer of the oesophagus. In most Eastern countries, squamous cell carcinoma is predominant, with an incidence which varies from 3/100,000 in low risk areas to thirty times that in some regions of Iran, Africa and China. The disease can occur in patients from their mid twenties, but with most over 50 years of age.

Histology

- Adenocarcinomas account for 50% of malignant lesions in most of Europe and the US, and the incidence of this histology is rising, especially in males.

- Most of these arise at or near the lower end of the oesophagus and are associated with metaplastic columnar epithelium which arises in response to prolonged gastric reflux (Barrett's esophagus).

- Anaplastic (small cell) carcinoma, adenosquamous neoplasms and carcinosarcomas are uncommon variants.

Mode of Spread

Spread is by local infiltration, lymphatic spread and haematogenous metastasis. The anatomical location of the oesophagus makes early spread into vital structures likely. Longitudinal spread along submucosal lymphatics is common and extensive, and is an important consideration when surgical resection or radiotherapy is planned.

Symptoms

Most patients present with dysphagia. The dysphagia can be preceded over many months by episodes of bolus impaction, but once constant dysphagia for solids is present, there is inexorable progression to absolute dysphagia over 6–12 weeks. Dysphagia of such a degree that the patient cannot take fluids or swallow their own saliva is usually regarded as such a distressing problem that major treatment is warranted in all but the terminally ill.

Occasional patients will present with pain, haemorrhage or the manifestations of disseminated disease as the predominant problem. Patients with advanced carcinoma of the upper third of the oesophagus can additionally present with persistent cough or pneumonia due to oesophagotracheal or oesophagobronchial fistula, or with hoarseness secondary to involvement of the left recurrent laryngeal nerve.

Diagnosis

Diagnosis will nearly always be made by endoscopy and biopsy. Barium examination can detect early lesions, and can give important information about the position, length and conformation of malignant strictures which can be important for therapy, but should not normally be relied upon alone for diagnosis.

Pre-existing achalasia and caustic stricture, predisposes patients to the development of squamous carcinoma. Clinically, such patients present special problems because the symptoms may change little and biopsy may be difficult.

Routine screening endoscopies with multiple biopsies are indicated in patients found to have Barrett's metaplasia. In such patients, of the risk of development of adenocarcinoma is 1–3% per patient per year.

Staging

In addition to the staging measures outlined above, for cancers in the upper half of the oesophagus, laryngoscopy and bronchoscopy will detect recurrent nerve involvement and invasion of the trachea or bronchus.

Treatment

For most patients, the question is not one of possible cure, but of providing relief from dysphagia with minimal morbidity. Nonetheless, it is important that those with localised and potentially curable disease are recognised and treated appropriately.

Surgery and Adjuvant Therapy

Surgical resection is standard treatment for the patient with early disease (Stage I or IIA) and can result in 5% survival of 30–50%. Proximal resection margins of 10 cm are needed to ensure that the resection is clear of submucosal extension. Uncontrolled experience indicates that inclusion of perioesophageal tissues and lymph nodes improves survival.

Randomised controlled trials indicate that there is a survival benefit in patients treated with preoperative chemoradiation versus operation alone for patients with adenocarcinoma (Hennessy). In patients with squamous cell carcinoma (Bosset) preoperative chemoradiation was shown to increase the incidence of resections with curative intent, increase disease-free survival and increase the time free of local recurrence, but it made no difference to the time to metastasis or to the overall survival. The lack of overall survival benefit may reflect increased postoperative mortality with chemoradiation.

In both of these studies, chemoradiation achieved a complete pathological response in 20–40%. More intensive combined treatment can achieve complete endoscopic response in up to 80%, but endoscopic change correlates poorly with histological CR or survival.

Palliative Treatment

For patients with locally advanced disease or known dissemination, surgical resection still has the important advantage of providing prompt relief of dysphagia, but resection of the oesophagus is a major procedure involving both removal of the oesophagus and formation of a conduit to replace it—either stomach (usually), jejunum or colon. Patients with more advanced disease tend also to have higher postoperative morbidity and mortality, and have less to gain, so increasingly alternatives are sought to resection for those with locally advanced disease or metastases.

These alternatives are passage of an endoprosthesis, palliative radiation or chemoradiation, brachytherapy and laser disobliteration. Intubation is unsatisfactory for cancers of the upper third, and for asymetrical lesions near the lower end. Laser has advantages for bulky asymmetric tumours near the COJ, but the need for repeated treatment is a disadvantage.

New Developments

The high incidence of complete endoscopic response that has been achieved with chemoradiation suggests that the role for surgical resection will diminish.

GASTRIC CARCINOMA

Risk factors for gastric cancer include a family history of cancer, a history of partial gastric resection for benign disease more than 10 years before, pernicious anaemia and Helicobacter pylori infection. Chronic gastritis, hypoacidity and consequent bacterial production of carcinogens all appear to play a role in carcinogenesis.

Diagnosis

- Gastric cancer is diagnosed at an early stage in 10% of patients in most Western countries; in Japan, however, it is diagnosed in 30% or more patients, where the high local incidence has led to screening programmes.

- Early gastric cancer, by definition, which involves mucosa or submucosa, even if local nodes are involved. The cure rate is only 80–90 % because nodes may be involved.

- Early gastric cancer is a surprisingly symptomatic disease, with epigastric pain, anorexia and nausea being reported in up to 30% of patients. Usually these symptoms are not distinguishable from those of patients with benign ulceration.

- Patients with advanced gastric cancer (cancer penetrating beyond the submucosa) present with weight loss, epigastric pain and anorexia as the most frequent symptoms.

- Iron deficiency anaemia is an important but less common feature.

- Growths near the oesophagogastric junction may cause dysphagia, and those near the pylorus may present a picture of gastric outlet obstruction with projectile vomiting and a succussion splash.

Investigations

Barium meal does not distinguish between benign and malignant gastric lesions with sufficient accuracy, so endoscopy with multiple, carefully directed biopsies is mandatory for any patient with known gastric ulceration, and for most patients with persisting upper gastrointestinal symptoms.

Staging

Staging should be according to the TNM system, as defined by the International Union Against Cancer (UICC) and the American Joint Commission on Cancer (AJCC) in 1987. Involvement of local lymph nodes and extension to the serosal surface are the most important features which predict a poor prognosis.

The role of clinical assessment and CT scanning are as outlined above. Laparoscopy is particularly important, since 25% of patients who would be considered for curative resection will be excluded by laparoscopic detection of peritoneal or hepatic dissemination.

Surgical Treatment

- Laparotomy should be avoided in patients with disease spread beyond the stomach and local draining nodes unless there is a specific problem, such as haemorrhage or gastric outlet obstruction which requires an operation for palliation.

- Patients who do not have identifiable disease beyond the stomach and the adjacent lymph nodes should be treated by radical gastrectomy.

- Distal subtotal radical gastrectomy is appropriate for antral and pyloric cancers but radical total gastrectomy is indicated for other sites.

- Partial proximal gastrectomy for proximal lesions gives worse functional results than total gastrectomy and should be avoided.

- Restoration of continuity after total gastrectomy is best performed using a Roux-en-Y oesophagojejunostomy, with the jejunojejunostomy component of the 'Y' placed 50 cm further distal to prevent bile reflux.

- Postprandial fullness and vitamin B_{12} deficiency are universal after total gastrectomy. Other potential sequelae of total or subtotal gastrectomy are dumping, diarrhoea, malabsorption and accelerated osteoporosis.

- The extent of regional lymphadenectomy remains controversial. Randomised controlled trials of resection with involves adjacent nodes only (D1 resection) versus removal of node bearing tissue in groups along the left gastric and common hepatic arteries (and other groups according to the site) (D2 resection) have made it clear that routine removal of the spleen and pancreatic tail is harmful, but the optimal extent of nodal resection is unclear.

- Direct invasion of local organs such the liver, transverse colon, spleen or pancreas usually occurs in patients with extensive lymph node involvement, but when lymph nodes are clear, en bloc resection of the involved organ is indicated and can be curative.

- Cancer of the most proximal stomach and the oesophagogastric junction requires resection of the distal oesophagus. This will often involve the addition of a thoracotomy, with attendant increased morbidity for a cancer which has a lower chance of cure than those in more distal parts of the stomach.

- Diffuse carcinoma of the linitis plastica ('leather bottle stomach') pattern is rarely curable and resection is usually followed within 12 months by local peritoneal recurrence which produces symptoms which are very similar to the original cancer. Chemotherapy may produce better palliation than resection.

Outcome

The five-year survival rates after resection with curative intent varies from 90% for early cancer through 50% for cancers involving muscularis propria only with clear nodes, to under 15% for cancers which involve both the serosa of the stomach and local lymph nodes in the resection specimen.

Palliative Therapy

- Surgical resection or bypass has a role in relieving obstruction or controlling haemorrhage even in patients with disseminated disease, but gradually these palliative operations are being replaced by chemotherapy, radiotherapy and/or endoscopic or radiological interventions.
- Chemotherapy in advanced disease has been associated with improved survival and quality of life, but the proportion of patients who benefit from treatment is low.
- Histamine-2 receptor antagonists or proton pump inhibitors can reduce the pain from malignant ulceration, but narcotic analgesics are often required.
- Blood transfusion can relieve the symptoms of dyspnoea and exhaustion caused by anaemia, but should be used with discretion in the terminal phases of the disease for fear of simply prolonging the suffering.

New Developments

Gastric adenocarcinoma is the most chemosensitive of all the common upper GI malignancies. Postoperative adjuvant chemotherapy has not been supported by many RCTs, but the most recent and effective regimens were not used. Preoperative chemotherapy is currently under investigation. Resection of early gastric cancer using minimally invasive techniques is being studied, especially in Japan.

OTHER GASTRIC NEOPLASMS

Lymphoma

- Non-Hodgkins lymphoma can arise in the stomach.
- Some early lesions (MALT) lymphomas appear to be a response to the presence of Helicobacter pylori, and will resolve with eradication of the organism.
- More advanced lesions can be treated locally with resection and/or radiotherapy with 5-year survival of over 50%, but the trend is to use conventional systemic chemotherapy as for other non-Hodgkins lymphoma (see Chapter 39).
- When the primary treatment is chemotherapy, gastric resection is reserved for those patients who have residual disease after systemic treatment. It may also be required in the patients whose lymphoma or its treatment results in deep ulceration which can threaten massive haemorrhage or perforation.

Carcinoid Tumours

The stomach is one site for midgut carcinoid, a form of neuroendocrine tumour characterised by grey or yellow colour and a histological pattern of small uniform cells. These may be increasing in incidence, but are still less than 1% of all gastric malignancies. The clinical course is characteristically indolent, and aggressive resection is justified. The overall five-year survival rate is just under 50%. As with other GI carcinoids, there is a notable incidence of other synchronous cancers (5–10%).

CARCINOMA OF THE PANCREAS

Adenocarcinoma arising from the exocrine pancreas remains one of the most lethal forms of cancer. Median survival from diagnosis is about nine months. Since there is effective treatment only for a small minority of patients with this disease, the role of the clinician is largely to establish the diagnosis, to exclude more favourable pathologies such as periampullary carcinoma or islet cell tumour, and to provide whatever palliation is possible.

Symptoms

- Patients present with vague malaise, anorexia and weight loss, eventually accompanied by epigastric discomfort and persistent low thoracic back pain.
- Depression may be evident even before the diagnosis is made.
- Half of the patients manifest glucose intolerance, and a third are diagnosed as being diabetic around the time of the diagnosis being made.
- Cancers in the head of the pancreas may present with obstructive jaundice. A palpable mass may be present, and in those who are jaundiced the combination of dark urine, pale stools, pruritus and a palpable gallbladder can make the diagnosis obvious.
- Advanced lesions may cause obstruction of the second part of the duodenum.

Investigations

The Jaundiced Patient

Once the diagnosis of obstructive jaundice is established by the clinical picture, liver function tests and imaging (U/S or CT) showing a dilated biliary system, definitive diagnosis of the site and type of obstruction is sought.

- Serum CA19-9 tumour marker is raised in many patients. Moderate elevation can result from jaundice from any cause, but a level over 2000 usually indicates unresectable malignancy.
- Upper GI endoscopy may show invasion of the mucosa of the duodenum, and will indicate if there is a possibly favourable periampullary tumour.
- Endoscopic retrograde cholangiopancreatography or percutaneous transhepatic cholangiography will distinguish cancer from calculous obstruction, and will allow stenting to be performed.

The Patient with a Pancreatic Mass

The ready availability of ultrasound and CT scanning results in many patients presenting with the radiological finding of a mass in the pancreas.

- Differentiating between chronic pancreatitis and cancer can be problematic; the radiological and ultrasound findings can be similar and percutaneous fine needle cytology can easily miss the actual malignant element in a mass which is partly due to local obstructive pancreatitis. Markedly elevated CA19-9 supports the diagnosis of cancer. Positron emission tomography using F^{18}deoxyglucose may resolve this problem, but is not readily available. Some patients will come to resection without a preoperative diagnosis of cancer.

Staging

- As well as the investigations outlined above to exclude disseminated disease, it is important to try to determine preoperatively if resection is possible.
- Modern helical CT with generous, well-timed intravenous contrast allows excellent definition of the extent of local disease, including whether major mesenteric and portal vessels are involved.
- Arteriography is now rarely indicated.

Treatment

- Surgical resection of adenocarcinoma of the head of the pancreas rarely results in cure, and is appropriate only for small lesions (< 2 cm) (5-year survival 20%) or if there is a possibility that the patient has one of the other more favourable types of neoplasm.
- Masses near the papilla which cause biliary obstruction at an early stage can be small adenocarcinomas of pancreatic origin, but they can also be primary bile duct carcinoma, duodenal carcinoma or carcinoma arising at the papilla itself. Resection may be warranted in this setting because these lesions have a 30–40% 5-year survival after resection.
- Cystadenoma and cystadenocarcinoma may also be cured by resection.
- For most patients, the best that can be aimed at is effective palliation.
- Obstructive jaundice should usually be treated so that the patient can be at least relieved of the associated anorexia, malaise and pruritus.
- Good risk patients, and those with impending duodenal obstruction are usually palliated by a surgical biliary bypass and a gastroenterostomy if needed. Poor risk patients and those with disseminated disease are best treated by the use of biliary stents placed by the endoscopic or percutaneous route.
- Early management of pain is important; this often requires narcotic analgesics, but coeliac blockade can be very useful.
- Adenocarcinoma of the body and tail remain essentially incurable conditions, with only occasional long-term survival after resection.
- Adjuvant treatment has been used to try to improve the dismal cure rates after resection for adenocarcinoma. These methods include systemic chemotherapy, regional chemotherapy and both external beam and intraoperative radiotherapy. The combination of 5-fluorouracil and radiotherapy after resection has produced a significant prolongation of survival, but the benefit is small and affects a minority of patients.

PANCREATIC CARCINOMAS OF ENDOCRINE ORIGIN

Hormone producing tumours which arise from the cells which constitute the pancreatic islets are rare. Insulinomas are usually benign (90%), but the other functioning tumours (glucagonoma, VIPoma, somatostatinoma) are usually malignant. (These cancers are discussed in Chapter 48.) Non-functioning islet cell carcinomas also occur and these share with the functioning tumours the feature that they tend to run an indolent course which makes extensive locoregional excision and even metastasectomy worthy of consideration (Lo).

GALLBLADDER CANCER

- Adenocarcinoma of the gallbladder accounts for only around 1% of all cancers, but is nevertheless the most common malignancy of the biliary tree.

- It is mostly a disease of the elderly, is more common in females than males and is associated in 70% of patients with the presence of gallstones.

- Those patients whose carcinoma was found incidentally after cholecystectomy have an 80% 5-year survival rate if the cancer is confined to the mucosa or muscularis. Reoperation and more radical resection is not indicated in this group. If more advanced disease is found in this setting, radical reoperation is advised, but the cure rate is low.

- Less than 5% of those with symptomatic cancer are cured, because in these the cancer has usually invaded into the liver, the draining lymph nodes, the hepatoduodenal ligament or the hepatic hilum.

- With improved imaging techniques, the disease will be correctly diagnosed before laparotomy with greater frequency, offering some chance of treatment aimed at cure.

- The extent of resection which is appropriate is controversial with some advocating excision of the gallbladder and bile duct with surrounding lymphatics and others major hepatic resection.

- Adjuvant therapies including systemic and regional chemotherapy (Lai) and both external and intraoperative radiotherapy have been used, with individual success and uncertain applicability.

- Palliation principally consists of relief of obstructive jaundice using endoscopic or percutaneous stenting and pain relief, with chemotherapy or radiation holding an uncertain role because of low response rates.

CANCER OF THE EXTRAHEPATIC BILE DUCTS

- Cancer arising in the extrahepatic bile duct is an uncommon disease, curable by surgery in fewer than 10% of all cases.

- Bile duct cancer may occur more frequently in patients with a history of sclerosing cholangitis, choledochal cysts, or recurrent pyogenic cholangitis.

- The most common symptoms caused by bile duct cancer are jaundice, pain, fever, and pruritus.

Surgical Resection

Total resection is possible in 25–30% of lesions that originate in the distal bile duct. This, however, drops to 10% for cancers arising near the confluence of the right and left hepatic ducts; resection here involves major hepatic resection in continuity with resection of the confluence of the hepatic ducts. Inclusion of the caudate lobe in the resection may improve the results.

Other Treatment

In most patients, the tumour cannot be completely removed by surgery and is incurable. Palliative resections or other palliative measures such as irradiation (e.g. brachytherapy or external-beam radiotherapy) or stenting procedures may maintain adequate biliary drainage and allow for often long-term survival. The tumours can be chemosensitive in a small proportion of patients. The patients often succumb when proximal involvement of second order ducts prevents successful stent replacement.

REFERENCES

American Joint Committee on Cancer (1992) *Manual for Staging of Cancer* (4th edn). Philadelphia: JB Lippincott Company.

Bonenkamp, J.J., Songun I, Hermans J., Sasako, M. Welvaart, K., Plukker, J.T., van Elk, P., Overtop, H., Gouma, D.J. and Taat, C.W. (1995) Randomised comparison of morbidity after D1 and D2 resections for gastric cancer in 996 Dutch patients. *Lancet*, **345**, 745–8.

Bosset, J-F, Gignoux M, Triboulet J-P, Tuet, E., Mantion, G., Elias, D. Lozach, P., Ollier, J.C., Pavy, J.J., Mercier, M. and Sahmoud, T. (1997) Chemoradiotherapy followed by surgery compared with surgery alone in squamous cell cancer of the oesophagus. *NEJ Med*, **337**, 161–167.

Cuschieri, A., Fayers, P., Fielding, J., Carven, J., Bancewicz, J., Joypaul, V. and Cook, P. (1996) Postoperative morbidity and mortality after D1 and D2 resections for gastric cancer: preliminary results of the MRC randomised controlled surgical trial. *Lancet*, **347**, 995–9.

Frontiers in Bioscience; Tumors of the Gastrointestinal Tract; Information and Resources. URL: http://vega.crbm.cnrs-mop.fr/bioscience/atlases/tumpath/gitract/resource.htm

Hennessy, T.P. (1996) Cancer of the oesophagus. *Postgraduate Med J.*, **72**, 458–63.

Henson, D.E., Albores-Saavedra, J. and Corle, D. (1992) Carcinoma of the extrahepatic bile ducts: histologic types, stage of disease, grade, and survival rates. *Cancer*, **70**(6), 1498–1501.

Jamieson, G.G. (ed) (1988) *Surgery of the Oesophagus*. Churchill Livingstone.

Lok Tio, T. (1995) Gastrointestinal TNM Cancer Staging by Endosonography. New York: Igaku-Shoin.

Maruyama K. National Cancer Center (1985) *Surgical Treatment and End Results of Gastric Cancer*. Maruyama K. National Cancer Center Press, 5-1-1 Tsukiji, Chuo-ku Tokyo, 104, Japan.

National Cancer Institute (NCI), CancerNet, URL: http://cancernet.nci.nih.gov/canlit/canlit.htm

Rothmund, M. (ed.) (1996) World Progress in Surgery—Carcinoid Tumours. *World Journal of Surgery*, **20**, 125–208.

Terblanche, J. (ed) (1994) *Hepatobiliary Malignancy: Its Multidisciplinary Management*. London: Edward Arnold.

Walsh, N.W. Noonan, N., Hollywood, D., Kelly, A., Keeling, N. and Hennessy, T.P.J. (1996) A comparison of multimodal therapy and surgery for esophageal adenocarcinoma. *NEJM*, **335**, 462–467.

Wanebo H.J., Kennedy B.J., Winchester D.P., Stewart A.K., Fremgen A.M. (1997) Role of Splenectomy in Gastric Cancer Surgery: Adverse Effect of Elective Splenectomy on Longterm Survival. *J. Am Coll. Surgeons*, **195**, 177–184.

CHAPTER 28

UPPER GASTROINTESTINAL MALIGNANCY: SYSTEMIC THERAPY

Michael P. N. Findlay

INTRODUCTION

Upper gastrointestinal malignancies represent a significant proportion of the global cancer burden with stomach, esophageal, liver and pancreas all ranking in the top ten in terms of incidence.

OESOPHAGEAL CANCER

In the last 50 years, there has been a change in the type of esophageal cancer, with a relatively constant incidence and an increase in the proportion of adenocarcinomas, particularly of the distal esophagus. The reason for this observation is unclear but many distal esophageal adenocarcinomas are associated with Barrett's epithelium suggesting it may be related to reflux-induced susceptibility.

Local Therapy

- Surgery of esophageal cancer is associated with a poor overall outcome, with a 5-year survival rate of less than 10%. Some series suggest that with careful selection of patients, better results could be produced.
- Radiation therapy has usually been used in patients with disease that has been unresectable. The outcome in these patients appears to be no worse than the overall results for patients with resectable disease having surgery.
- The pattern of failure after both of these modalities suggests that both local control and systemic relapse are a problem independent of pathology.

Combined Modality Therapy

Chemotherapy has been used in an attempt to enhance local control and to reduce distant metastasis, both in resectable and unresectable disease. A randomised trial initiated by the Radiation Therapy Oncology Group in the United States compared concurrent chemoradiation followed by maintenance chemotherapy with radiotherapy alone, in patients with unresectable esophageal cancer. The

171

chemoradiation consisted of radiotherapy (50 Gy) with cisplatin and 5-fluorouracil (5-FU) during radiation and every 3 weeks afterwards for 2 cycles. The control arm was radiation alone to 64 Gy. A total of 123 patients were randomised, 90% of whom had squamous tumours. The results were better in the combined chemoradiation arm, with a 5-year survival rate of 27%, with no survivors in the radiation alone arm.

Further randomised trials have examined the use of chemoradiation prior to surgery in potentially resectable esophageal cancer. While some of these studies have yielded negative results, they may be criticised on the basis of suboptimal chemoradiation schedules, inadequate duration of follow-up and small study size.

A recent randomised trial in Ireland of 113 patients with resectable esophageal adenocarcinoma had patients assigned to surgery alone or chemoradiation followed by surgery. Radiation, 40 Gy, began concurrently with 5-fluorouracil as a 16-hour infusion on days 1–5, then cisplatin on day 7, of weeks 1 and 6. The patients having preoperative chemoradiation had a lower rate of positive nodes in the resected specimen (42 vs 82%; $p < 0.001$) with 25% on this arm achieving a complete histological response. The 3-year survival rates were significantly better on the preoperative chemoradiation arm (32 vs 6%; $p = 0.001$). While this study is encouraging confirmation in other studies is required.

GASTRIC CANCER

Background

Over the last century gastric or stomach cancer has reduced in incidence, although in the last two decades this fall may have plateaued, possibly because of the rapidly increasing incidence of adenocarcinoma of the proximal stomach and gastro-esophageal junction.

The outcome for patients with adenocarcinoma of the stomach is poor overall, because a large proportion present with unresectable, metastatic, or resectable but advanced disease. Outcome is directly related to stage at presentation with relatively high rates of success in early tumours treated with surgery alone. The increasing number of proximal tumours appear to have a much less favourable outcome with 5-year survival rates of 5% or less.

The patterns of treatment failure after surgery were studied by Gunderson and Sosin in 1992. They found that of 107 patients, 86 relapsed with 62 (72%) showing evidence of systemic or peritoneal disease and 24 (22%) evidence of isolated local recurrence.

Postoperative Chemotherapy

- In an attempt to improve on these results, postoperative chemotherapy has been studied extensively worldwide, but with generally disappointing results.

- A recent meta-analysis of the results of postoperative chemotherapy reported no survival advantage with this approach although it was inadequately powered to detect a survival advantage of less than 7%—a magnitude of questionable clinical importance.

- If postoperative adjuvant chemotherapy is genuinely inactive, it is not possible to know whether the treatments were intrinsically inactive or that they were commenced too late in the natural history of the disease.

Preoperative Chemotherapy

Based on these results there has been an increased interest in the use of chemotherapy in the preoperative setting. The biological basis of the preoperative approach is that the undetectable micrometastases may be exposed to the cytotoxics at a much earlier stage than if the patient had surgery initially and chemotherapy on recovery. An added advantage of this approach is that a more immediate indicator of anti-tumour activity is available when the resected specimen is examined.

The Optimal Chemotherapy Combination

Establishing a suitable chemotherapy regimen for use in the preoperative setting usually draws from the experience in treating patients with advanced and metastatic gastric cancer. Since the development of the FAM (5-FU, adriamycin, Mitomycin C) regimen in the late 1970s there has been more enthusiasm for treating patients with advanced gastric cancer.

FAM and FAMTX Regimens

There have been several randomised trials in this context that are of interest. An EORTC study found the FAM regimen inferior to FAMTX (5-FU, adriamycin, methotrexate) for survival, while a three-arm study, also from Europe, showed no survival difference between 5-FU/cisplatin, etoposide/leucovorin/5-FU (ELF) and FAMTX. An American study compared FAMTX to a newer German regimen containing etoposide, adriamycin and cisplatin (EAP), but found the EAP regimen too toxic, particularly from neutropenic sepsis, requiring early study closure with four toxic deaths.

ECF Regimen

In the United Kingdom a regimen containing epirubicin, cisplatin and protracted venous infusion 5-FU (ECF) was developed in this disease and has just recently completed evaluation in a multicentre UK-based randomised trial. In this study ECF was found to be superior to FAMTX for response, survival, quality of life and cost effectiveness.

Chemotherapy versus No Treatment in Advanced Disease

Chemotherapy has been compared to best supportive care, or no chemotherapy, in advanced disease. There are now four randomised trials comparing best supportive care to chemotherapy plus best supportive care. These studies demonstrate an increase in median survival from about 3 months to 10 months. Although the magnitude of the survival benefit is modest, there have been quality of life benefits demonstrated with chemotherapy in this setting. These results suggest that chemotherapy has some biological activity in this disease, and when given in the optimum sequence with surgery in earlier stage patients may yield improved outcomes.

PANCREATIC CANCER

Background

- The most common form of pancreatic cancer is ductal adenocarcinoma.
- The incidence of this tumour has remained relatively static in recent years. The dismal outcome has also changed little.
- The most important predictors of outcome are the ability to resect the tumour and the stage of the disease.

- Only 10% of patients will present with resectable disease and even their 5-year survival rate will range from only 3% to 25%, but will most often be below 10%.

Postoperative Chemoradiation

Strategies to improve these results have included the use of postoperative chemoradiation. One study from the Gastro-Intestinal Tumour Study Group (GITSG) in the US randomised 43 patients to receive no postoperative therapy or postoperative radiation 20 Gy over 2 weeks repeated after a 2-week break, with 5-FU, days 1–3 of each radiotherapy course, followed by 5-FU weekly for 2 years. The results showed a 2 year survival advantage favouring the chemoradiation (43 vs 18%; p = 0.05). However, this study should be interpreted with caution due to the small numbers and the short duration of follow-up. The results of a recent, larger European study of similar design are awaited.

The role of chemoradiation in unresectable pancreatic cancer has also been examined in an earlier randomised trial performed by the Gastrointestinal Study Group (GITSG). One hundred and ninety-four patients were randomised to receive either radiation alone (60 Gy), radiation (40 Gy) with 5-FU, or radiation (60 Gy) with 5-FU. The results showed that while there was no advantage of radiation at 60 Gy vs 40 Gy in the combined modality arm, chemoradiation gave a better one-year survival compared to radiation alone (40% vs 10%). These results suggest there may be some impact on tumour outcome with chemoradiation, that this is modest and further developments are required to improve outcome.

Advanced Pancreatic Cancer

- The palliation of patients with advanced and metastatic pancreatic cancer has been investigated in randomised trials comparing various chemotherapy combinations with best supportive care.
- Three studies have now shown that chemotherapy improves the median survival of patients from 2–3 months to 6–11 months. One of these studies examined quality of life and found it improved with chemotherapy.
- Preliminary evidence from a randomised trial suggests that gemcitabine has greater impact on patient quality of life than 5-FU given as an IV bolus, although the absolute survival benefit over 5-FU is only about 1 month.

BILIARY CANCER

- Tumours of the biliary tract comprise tumours of the gall bladder, intra-hepatic, and those of the extra-hepatic biliary tract.
- Gall bladder tumours often present at an advanced stage but may be an incidental finding at cholecystectomy.
- Biliary tumours may present earlier than gall bladder tumours. However their location make them often difficult to remove.
- Peri-ampullary tumours may be resected with a comparatively good outcome but the majority will present at an advanced stage.

- A randomised trial in advanced, unresectable disease has shown chemotherapy can improve survival from a median of 2 to 6 months while increasing quality of life, compared to best-supportive care alone.
- Phase II studies suggest combinations such as FAM and ECF (see above) have some anti-tumour activity.

REFERENCES

Ahlgren and Macdonald (eds) (1992) *Gastrointestinal Oncology*. Philadelphia: JB Lippincott.

Al-Sarraf, M., Martz, K., Herskovic, A., Leichman, L., Brindle, J.S., Vaitkevicius, V.K., Cooper, J., Byhardt, R., Davis, L. and Emami, B. (1997) Progress report of combined chemoradiotherapy versus radiotherapy alone in patients with esophageal cancer: an Intergroup study. *J Clin Oncol*, **15**, 277–284.

Findlay, M. and Cunningham, D. (1993) Chemotherapy of carcinoma of the stomach. *Cancer Treatment Reviews*, **19**, 29–44

Findlay, M., Cunningham, D., Norman, A., Mansi, J., Nicolson, M., Hickish, T., Nicolson, V., Nash, A., Sacks, N., Ford, H., Carter, R. and Hill, A. (1994) A new regimen for the treatment of gastric cancer: epirubicin, cisplatin and infusional 5 fluorouracil (ECF). *Ann Oncol*, **5**, 609–616

Glimelius, B., Hoffman, K., Sjoden, P.O., Jacobsson, G., Sellstrom, H., Enander, L.K., Linne, T. and Svensson, C. (1996) Chemotherapy improves survival and quality of life in advanced pancreatic and biliary cancer. *Ann Oncol*, **7**, 593–600.

Hermans, J., Bonenkamp, J.J., Boon, M.C., Bunt, A.M.G., Ohyama, S., Sasako, M. and van de Velde, C.J.H. (1993) Adjuvant therapy after curative resection for gastric cancer: meta-analysis of randomised trials. *J Clin Oncol*, **11**, 1441–7.

The Gastrointestinal Tumour Study Group (1981) Therapy of locally unresectable pancreatic carcinoma: a randomised comparison of high dose (6000 rads) radiation alone, moderate dose radiation (4000 rads + 5-fluorouracil) and high dose radiation + 5-fluorouracil). *Cancer*, **48**, 1705–1710.

The Gastrointestinal Tumour Study Group (1987) Further evidence of effective adjuvant combined radiation and chemotherapy following curative resection of pancreatic cancer. *Cancer*, **59**, 2006–2010.

Walsh, T.N., Noonan, N., Hollywood, D., Kelly, A., Keeling, N., Hennessy, T.P.J. (1996) A comparison of multimodal therapy and surgery for esophageal adenocarcinoma. *N Engl J Med*, **335**, 462–7

Webb, A., Cunningham, D., Scarffe, J.H., Harper, P., Norman, A., Joffe, J.K., Hughes, M., Mansi, J., Findlay, M., Hill, A., Nicolson, M., Hickish, T., OBrien, M., Iveson, T., Watson, M., Underhill, C., Wardley, A. and Meehan, M. (1997) A randomised trial comparing ECF with FAMTX in advanced oesophago-gastric gastric. *J Clin Oncol*, **15**, 261–267.

FAST FACT SHEET 3

COLORECTAL CANCER

H. L. Nguyen And Bruce K. Armstrong

WORLD IMPACT

In 1985, there were an estimated 678, 000 new cases of colorectal cancer diagnosed worldwide, accounting for 9% of all cancers[1]. More than two-thirds of these cases occurred in developed countries, making it the third most common cancer of both sexes in developed countries, after non-melanocytic skin cancer and lung cancer in males and after non-melanocytic skin cancer and breast cancer in females. It was the third largest cause of death from cancer with an estimated total of 394,000 deaths in 1995[2].

The incidence of colorectal cancer varies some 10-fold among different countries. The highest incidence rates in 1988–92 were recorded in New Zealand, Australia, and North America (particularly the black population). Rates in some African and Asian populations (except Japan and Singapore) were low[3].

IMPACT IN AUSTRALIA

In 1990, 8,726 new cases of colorectal cancer were registered in Australia, accounting for 15% of all registered cancers[4]. In 1994 in New South Wales[5], colorectal cancer was the fourth most common cancer, after non-melanocytic skin cancer and cancers of the prostate and breast. In 1995, 4,495 people died from colorectal cancer in Australia, making it the third most frequent cancer causing death in males after lung and prostate cancers, and the second most frequent in females after breast cancer[6].

INCIDENCE BY SEX AND AGE

In 1990–94, incidence of colorectal cancer in New South Wales increased steadily in males and females from 25–29 to 45–49 years of age. Thereafter, rates increased more steeply with age,

176

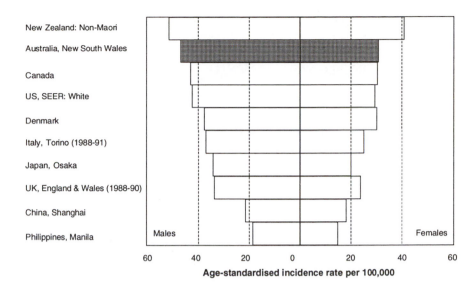

New Zealand: Non-Maori

Australia, New South Wales

Canada

US, SEER: White

Denmark

Italy, Torino (1988-91)

Japan, Osaka

UK, England & Wales (1988-90)

China, Shanghai

Philippines, Manila

Males   Females

60   40   20   0   20   40   60

Age-standardised incidence rate per 100,000

Figure FFS 3.1 Sex specific, age-standardised incidence rates of colorectal cancer in selected countries, 1988–1992[4]

Table FFS 3.1 Australian colorectal cancer statistics

Statistics	Males	Females
Crude incidence 1990	55.3 per 100,000	46.8 per 100,000
Age adjusted incidence 1990	44.8 per 100,000	31.4 per 100,000
Cumulative incidence to 75 years of age 1990	5.3%	3.7%
Crude mortality 1995	26.8 per 100,000	23.0 per 100,000
Age adjusted mortality 1995	19.7 per 100,000	13.0 per 100,000
Person years of life lost to 75 years of age 1990	14,624 years	12,154 years
Trend in age adjusted incidence 1973 to 1994 in New South Wales	+1.7% p.a.	+1.4% p.a.
Trend in age adjusted mortality 1973 to 1994 in New South Wales	Very minimal	−0.8% p.a.
Five year relative survival for colon cancer 1977–94 in South Australia	51.9%	53.8%,
Five year relative survival for rectal cancer 1977–94 in South Australia	52.5%	56.0%

particularly in males. Incidence was more than 50% higher in males than in females over 60 years of age[5,7].

INEQUALITIES IN INCIDENCE

Incidence of cancer of the colon increased with increasing socioeconomic status in both males and females in urban New South Wales in 1987–91[8]. In contrast, cancer of the rectum fell with increasing socioeconomic status in males and showed no net trend either way in females.

Mortality from colorectal cancer in 1979–88 was significantly higher in people born in Australia and New Zealand than in Australian residents born in most other countries. The lowest rates were in people born in Asia and the Middle East[9].

INCIDENCE AND MORTALITY TRENDS

Incidence of colorectal cancer in New South Wales increased steadily from 1973 to 1983 at rates of 2.7% and 2.8% a year in males and females respectively. The rates were then stable in both sexes from 1984 to 1994. This stability, however, belies a continuing flat or upward trend in people over 45 years of age and a downward trend in people under 45 years of age.

Mortality from colorectal cancer in males was fairly stable from 1973 to 1994. In females, the mortality rate fell by an average of 0.8% a year from 1972 to 1994; the rate of decrease from 1984 to 1994 was twice the rate of decrease from 1973 to 1983[5,7].

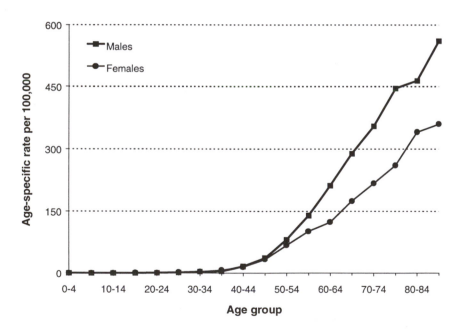

Figure FFS 3.2 Age-specific incidence rates of colorectal cancer by sex and age in New South Wales, 1990–1994[5,7]

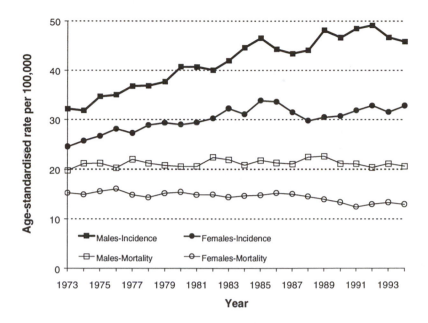

Figure FFS 3.3 Trends in annual age-standardised incidence and mortality rates of colorectal cancer in New South Wales, 1973–1994[5,7]

SURVIVAL RATE

The five-year relative survival rate from colon cancer in people in South Australia increased from 48.3% in those diagnosed in 1977–85 to 56.6% in those diagnosed in 1986–94[9]. In the same periods, the survival rate from rectal cancer increased from 51.8% to 55.2%. Females diagnosed in 1977–94 had a slightly higher five-year relative survival than males for both cancers of the colon and the rectum. In the same period, five-year relative survival from rectal cancer was highest in those under 55 years of age (58.5%) and least in those 75 years of age and over (50.7%). For colon cancer, relative survival was highest in those 55–64 years of age (55.9%) and least in those 75 years of age and over (50.8%). Among 1,902 colonic cancers and 1,184 rectal cancers recorded in hospital-based cancer registries in South Australia from 1980–95, the five-year relative survival rate fell from 87–88% in ACPS Stage A cancers to only 7–8% in ACPS Stage D cancers[11]. The five-year relative survival rate for all these colorectal cancers was around 50% compared with around 56% for all people diagnosed with cancers of the colon and rectum in South Australia in 1986–94.

RISK FACTORS

Diets high in meat and fat and low in fruit and vegetables are associated, probably causally, with an increased risk of colorectal cancer[12,13]. People in sedentary jobs have about a 60% higher risk of colorectal cancer than people in active jobs. This difference does not appear to be explained by confounding with dietary or other possibly causal factors[13]. Non-occupational as well as occupational physical activity is associated with a reduced risk. Smokers have an increased risk of colorectal adenoma,

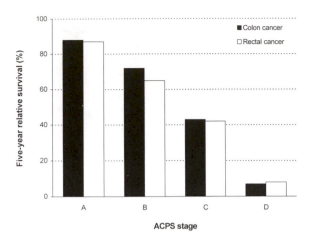

Figure FFS 3.4 Five-year relative survival by ACPS stage of cancers of the colon and rectum in South Australia, 1980–1995[11]

but the evidence for an association with carcinoma is inconclusive. Regular use of nonsteroidal anti-inflammatory drugs may reduce the risk of colorectal cancer.

Adenomatous polyps of the colon and rectum are precursors of colorectal cancer and, therefore, associated with an increased risk[13]. The malignant potential of an adenoma is related to its size, a predominance of villous features and the presence of dysplasia. Patients with inflammatory bowel disease affecting the colon are at increased risk of colorectal cancer with risk proportional to the extent of disease and the severity of associated dysplasia.

There is significant familial aggregation of colorectal cancer, and major gene mutations, such as those in the APC gene (responsible for familial adenomatous polyposis coli) and in the mismatch repair family of genes (probably responsible for the majority of what has been called hereditary non-polyposis colorectal cancer), are responsible for up to 5% of these cancers[13]. The lifetime risk of colorectal cancer is 100% (by 55 years of age) in people with a mutated APC gene and about 80% in people with mutations of the relevant mismatch repair genes. APC gene mutations are also associated with an increase in risk of cancers of the stomach and proximal small intestine, and mismatch repair gene mutations with an increase in risk of endometrial, ovarian and other gastrointestinal, biliary and urinary tract cancers.

REFERENCES

1. Parkin, D.M., Pisani, P. and Ferlay, J. (1993) Estimates of the worldwide incidence of eighteen major cancers in 1985. *Int J Cancer,* **54,** 594–606.
2. Pisani, P., Parkin, D.M. and Ferlay, J. (1993) Estimates of the worldwide mortality from eighteen major cancers in 1985. Implications for prevention and projections of future burden. *Int J Cancer,* **55,** 891–903.
3. Parkin, D.M., Whelan, S.L., Ferlay, J, Raymond, L. and Young, J. (1997) *Cancer Incidence in Five Continents Volume VII.* Lyon: International Agency for Research on Cancer.

4. Jelfs, P., Coates, M., Giles, G., Shugg, D., Threlfall, T., Roder, D., Ring, I., Shadbolt, B. and Condon, J. (1996) *Cancer in Australia 1989–1990 (with projections to 1995)*. Canberra: Australian Institute of Health and Welfare.

5. Coates, M. and Armstrong, B. (1997) *Cancer in New South Wales Incidence and Mortality 1994*. Sydney: NSW Cancer Council.

6. Australian Bureau of Statistics (1996) *Causes of Death Australia 1995*. Canberra: Australian Government Publishing Service.

7. Bell, J., Coates, M., Day, P. and Armstrong, B. (1996) *Colorectal Cancer in NSW in 1972 to 1993*. Sydney: NSW Cancer Council.

8. Smith, D., Taylor, R. and Coates, M. (1996) Socioeconomic differentials in cancer incidence and mortality in urban New South Wales, 1987–1991. *Australian & New Zealand Journal of Public Health,* **20**, 129–37.

9. Giles, G., Jelfs, P. and Kliewer, E. (1995) *Cancer Mortality in Migrants to Australia 1979–1988*. Canberra: Australian Institute of Health and Welfare.

10. South Australian Cancer Registry (1996) *Epidemiology of Cancer in South Australia. Incidence, mortality and survival 1977 to 1995, incidence and mortality 1995 analysed by type and geographical location - nineteen years of data*. Adelaide: South Australian Health Commission.

11. South Australian Cancer Registry (1997) *Epidemiology of Cancer in South Australia. Incidence, mortality and survival 1977 to 1996, incidence and mortality 1996 analysed by type and geographical location - Twenty years of data*. Adelaide: South Australian Health Commission.

12. Willett, W.C. and Trichopoulos, D. (1996) Nutrition and cancer: a summary of the evidence. *Cancer Causes Control,* 7, 178–80.

13. Schottenfeld, D. and Winawer, S.J. (1996) Cancers of the large intestine. In *Cancer Epidemiology and Prevention,* edited by D. Schottenfeld and J.F. Fraumeni, pp. 813-40. New York: Oxford University Press.

CHAPTER 29

COLORECTAL CANCER: SURGICAL MANAGEMENT

E. L. Bokey and Brian D. Draganic

INTRODUCTION

Colorectal cancer (CRC) is one of the most common internal malignancy amongst men and women in Australia. The incidence of this common tumour is increasing and its aetiology is basically unknown.

There are several predisposing factors including adenomoteus polyps, Familial Adenomoteus Polyposis (FAP), Hereditary Nonployposis Colorectal Cancer (HNCC), ulcerative colitis and to a lesser extent Chrohn's colitis. Whereas in the past, most CRCs were considered to be sporadic, there is growing evidence that many have a hereditary basis and a first-degree family history is considered an important predisposing factor.

PRESENTATION

- Approximately 50% of CRCs arise in the rectum with the right side of the colon as the next most common site (40–45%).

- The symptoms are often subtle and include rectal bleeding, a change in bowel habits and mucus per rectum.

- Abdominal pain, distension and relative or absolute constipation denote luminal obstruction.

- The tumour spreads locally through the bowel wall, thence to lymph nodes and eventually haematogenous spread to the liver, lungs and beyond.

MANAGEMENT

Whereas the primary treatment for CRC is surgical, it is essential that the management approach is multidisciplinary. Several disciplines are involved, including nursing, enterostomal therapy, gastroenterology, medical and radiation oncology, psychology, medical genetics, pathology and family medicine. Frequent, precise and meaningful communication is required to ensure the best outcome for the patient.

Management starts with a history and physical examination. Amongst other issues, the history should identify whether there is a family history of CRC, and if there is any comorbidity. Physical examination should include a rectal examination and abdominal examination to detect the presence of hepatomegaly, abdominal masses or ascites.

INVESTIGATION

Most CRCs are diagnosed either at sigmoidoscopy, colonoscopy or barium enema. Biopsies usually confirm the diagnosis. A chest X-ray, abdominal ultrasound or abdominal and pelvic CT scan may be useful in identifying the presence of distant metastases. Although the latter two investigations are not universally accepted as essential.

INFORMED CONSENT

Once the diagnosis is confirmed, informed consent is obtained. A careful explanation of the operative procedure and its potential complications is given. Alternative procedures are explained. It is often useful to draw a diagram to explain the operation. Whenever possible this should be done in the presence of a spouse, relative or friend. The practitioner needs to demonstrate sensitivity and kindness, especially at this time when patients maybe particularly frightened and vulnerable.

ADMISSION

Admission to hospital usually occurs the day before surgery. Any preoperative, cardiovascular or respiratory assessment should be done before surgery. Preparation for surgery includes a full blood count, serum electrolyses, renal and liver function tests, chest X-ray and ECG.

ENTEROSTOMAL THERAPY CONSULTATION

An enterostomal therapy muse consultation may be necessary if temporary or permanent stoma are contemplated. Enough time should be allowed to inform the patient, carefully explain what stoma is, discuss stomal management and if necessary introduce the patient to another patient with a stoma. The stoma is sited a position which is visible and accessible to the patient, clear of scars and bony prominence, and not between fat folds.

PERIOPERATIVE ANTIBIOTICS

A high blood level of antibiotics is necessary in the preoperative period. Intravenous gentamycin and metronidazole may be given at the induction of anaesthesia and for 24 hours postoperatively.

PERIOPERATIVE THROMBOEMBOLIC PROPHYLAXIS

Subcutaneous heparin and T.E.D. stocking should be used to prevent deep vein thrombosis and pulmonary emboli.

BOWEL PREPARATION

An othrograde osmotic agent is used to cleanse the colon. Many preparations are available. GLYCOPREP is one of the most common in use. These preparations should only be given to patients undergoing elective surgery, and not patients with impending or established bowel obstruction. Care should also be exercised with elderly patients and those with cardiac failure.

ELECTIVE SURGICAL TREATMENT OF COLON CANCER

In the operating room, after general anaesthesia, a urinary catheter and nasogastric tube are introduced. The general principles underpinning surgical treatment is to resect that segment of bowel bearing the cancer together with its blood supply, and accompanying lymphatic drainage, as close to its origin as possible.

Thus for a cancer of the right colon, the right colic, ileocolic and right branch of the middle colic vessels are ligated and divided close to their origins and the right side of the colon resected.

For cancers in the left colon, the inferior mesenteric and ascending left colic vessels are ligated and divided close to their origin. Having resected the colon, intestinal continuity is restored by anastomosis using either sutures or staples.

SURGICAL MANAGEMENT OF RECTAL CANCER

The past 15 years have seen major advances in the management of rectal cancer. Whereas in the past most cancers of the rectum were treated by complete excision of the rectum with a permanent abdominal wall colostomy, new techniques have been developed to obviate the necessity of permanent colostomy.

It is now possible to resect most of the rectum and anastomose the proximal colon to the distal rectum or even to the anal canal. This procedure is called an anterior resection, and when the anastomosis is low in the pelvic, it is usual to divert the faeces away from it temporarily by constructing a synchronous proximal loop ileostomy which is closed within 12 weeks after the initial surgery.

SURGICAL TREATMENT OF OBSTRUCTED CRC

Obstructed Right-sided CRC

The usual procedure is an immediate right hemicolectomy with an ileotransverse anastomosis.

Obstructed Left-sided CRC

The colon proximal to the cancer is very distended and the cecum bears the brunt of the distension. Because of distension and poor preparation of the proximal colon it is not possible to resect and immediately anastomose: a bowel anastomosis under these circumstances would be at great risk of leaking leading to faecal peritonitis and significant sepsis. It is therefore usual to resect the obstructing tumour and exteriorise the proximal colon as a colostomy whilst oversewing the distal end. This is called a Hartmann's procedure. Several months later, the colon and rectum can be re-anastomosed at a subsequent operation. A simple, diverting loop colostomy can relieve the obstruction with resection performed later.

LAPAROSCOPIC SURGERY

There is little doubt that laparoscopic resection of cancer in all segments of the colon can and has been performed with similar lymphatic clearance and peri-operative morbidity and mortality as open colectomy. Whether there is any significant benefit to the patient's resumption of mobility and resolution of ileus, or to the hospital in shortened bed stay and cost savings remains an area of controversy. More importantly, there is justifiable concern whether cancer clearance and survival is compromised by laparoscopic resection. There are reports of port site wound recurrences in several series, a complication which is exceedingly rare in open surgery. Until these issues are resolved and the true longer term survival rate and complication rates following laparoscopic colectomy for cancer are known, this technique should remain confined to randomised prospective trials.

HISTOPATHOLOGY

Traditionally, CRC has been staged to determine the degree of spread of tumour in order to discuss prognosis with the patient, and to determine whether adjuvant chemotherapy or radiation therapy may be useful. There are two principle methods of staging bowel cancer: a purely pathological and a histopathological method.

The Dukes staging system is purely pathological, and describes the spread of tumour in the specimen; Stage A is cancer confined to the bowel wall, Stage B is beyond the bowel wall and Stage C is spread to regional lymph nodes.

The problem with Dukes staging system is it does not cater for those 20% of patients who at the time of surgery have distant metastases or cancer remaining locally. It is for this reason that Clinical Pathological Staging (CPS) has been developed. This system includes a CP Stage D, which accounts for patients with distant metastases and local residual tumour.

PROGNOSIS

Using CP Stage, long-term survival is directly related to stage. Patients with CP Stages A and B have a survival rate equivalent to a matched group of the general population. Patients with CP Stage C have a significantly reduced survival and 90% of patients with CP Stage D, do not survive longer than twelve months.

ADJUVANT THERAPY FOR COLON CANCER

Until recently, there was little indication that adjuvant therapy was useful in CRC. In the past decade however, there has been evidence to suggest that certain combinations of chemotherapeutic agents may improve survival in patients with lymph node metastases.

This is not universally accepted and one has to consider the potential side effects of chemotherapy. A close working relationship with medical oncology is essential in order to give the patient the best possible chances of survival (see Chapter 30).

ADJUVANT THERAPY FOR RECTAL CANCER

There is an added incentive to consider adjuvant therapy for patients with rectal cancer. Not only is survival an issue, but also attempts to prevent local recurrence of the cancer. There is evidence to suggest that combination chemoradiotherapy diminishes the incidence of local recurrence as well as improving survival. This is by no means a universally accepted practice but it should at least be considered, and patients with locally advanced disease or those with lymph node metastases should be given the benefit of a consultation with a radiation oncologist.

PALLIATIVE CARE

Approximately 20% of patients have distant metastases at the time of surgery and many others subsequently develop local and distant spread. It is essential to have a close working relationship with a palliative care team who will keep patients free of pain and permit death with dignity.

FAMILY CANCER GENETICS

First-degree relatives of patients with CRC are at higher risk of developing CRC themselves. They should be screened by colonoscopy at regular intervals.

REFERENCES

Bokey, E.L., Chapuis, P.H., Debt, O.F., Newland, R.C., Koorey, S.G., Zelas, P.J. and Stewart, P.J. (1997) Factors affecting survival after excision of the rectum for cancer. *Dis. Colon Rectum*, **40**, 3–9.

Bokey, E.L., Moore, J.W.E. and Chapuis, P.H. (1996) Morbidity and mortality following laparoscopic assisted-colectomy for cancer. *Dis. Colon. Rectum*, **39**(Suppl), S24–8.

Davis, N., Evans, E. and Cohen, J. 1984Staging of colorectal cancer. The Australian Clinico-Pathological Staging (ACPS) system compared with Dukes system. *Dis. Colon Rectum*, **27**, 707–14.

Moertl, C.G., Fleming, T.R., Macdonald, J.S., Haller, D.J., Laurie, J.A., Tangen, C.M., Ungerleider, J.S., Emerson, W.A., Tormey, D.C. and Glick, J.H. (1995) Fluorouracil plus Levamisole as effective adjuvant therapy after resection of stage III colon carcinoma: A final report. *Annals of Internal Medicine*, **122**, 321–6.

Williams, N.S. (1993) Results of elective surgical treatment of colonic carcinoma. In *Surgery of the Anus, Rectum and Colon*, edited by M.R.B. Keighley and N.S. Willams, pp. 924–38. Philadelphia: W.B. Saunders Company Ltd.

CHAPTER 30

COLORECTAL CANCER: SYSTEMIC THERAPY

Stephen J. Clarke

INTRODUCTION

Colorectal cancer affects 1 in 20 people in the Western world (see Fast Fact Sheet 3). While surgery remains the principal treatment for bowel cancer, 30% of patients will present with inoperable advanced or metastatic disease, while another 25% will recur after apparently curative surgery. Thus, over 50% of patients with colorectal cancer could benefit from effective systemic therapies, either in the adjuvant setting to prevent relapse, or as palliation for metastatic disease.

SYSTEMIC THERAPY FOR ADVANCED COLORECTAL CANCER

5-Fluorouracil (5-FU)

5-fluorouracil has been the mainstay of chemotherapy for advanced colorectal cancer for over 2 decades. This drug has multiple putative sites of cytotoxic activity including competitive inhibition of thymidylate synthase (TS) via the derivative FdUMP, and through disruption of RNA and DNA synthesis.

When used as single agent bolus therapy there is wide variation in response rates. It appears necessary for regimens to induce consistent levels of severe myelosuppression, with about 20% Common Toxicity Criteria (CTC) Grades III and IV, to produce response rates of between 25% and 35% in advanced disease. Other common toxicities include mucositis (which is lessened by sucking ice), rash and diarrhoea. The accepted response rate with tolerable doses of 5-FU alone in metastatic colorectal cancer is 10–15%. The median survival for patients treated with 5-FU is approximately 6–8 months with no proven impact on overall survival, although responding patients may survive a median of 12–18 months.

Modulation of 5-FU

Colon cancers have a low proliferative index and 5-FU has a short plasma half-life of approximately 10–15 minutes, which means only a small percentage of colon cancer cells will be exposed to the drug after bolus administration. In addition, intracellularly, increasing concentrations of dUMP behind the block at thymidylate synthase (TS) can compete out the inhibitory effect of FdUMP, while rapid increases in TS levels may also result in 5-FU resistance. In order to overcome potential drug resistance mechanisms and increase anti-tumour activity, a wide range of studies have been undertaken aimed at modulating the schedule of administration and biochemical pharmacology of 5-FU.

Chronic infusions of 5-FU overcome the short half-life of the compound and alter the spectrum of toxicities. Response rates of 30–40% have been reported using continuous infusions with the principal toxicities being plantar/palmar erythroderma and complications associated with the central venous catheters required to deliver the drug. Although these treatments are well tolerated there are no proven survival benefits over bolus administration.

Chronomodulation, or alteration of the timing of administration of drug through a 24-hour period of 5-FU, has demonstrated that increased doses of drug are able to be delivered and response rates appear higher than in conventional dosing schedules.

Alteration of the biochemical pharmacology of 5-FU has been explored through the co-administration of a number of agents including methotrexate (an inhibitor of purine and pyrimidine synthesis), phosphonacetyl-L-aspartate (PALA; an inhibitor of pyrimidine synthesis), α-interferon and folinic acid (leucovorin).

α-interferon has been suggested to prevent up-regulation of TS, increase formation of FdUMP and to alter the pharmacokinetics of 5-FU and initial clinical studies were very encouraging with reported response rates in phase II studies of between 26% and 63% however this promise has not been confirmed in phase III study.

Leucovorin co-administration with 5-FU provides increased amounts of intracellular reduced folates which lead to stability and durability of the ternary complex formed between FdUMP, TS and 5, 10-methylene tetrahydrofolate which results in enhanced inhibition of TS and greater potency compared with 5-FU alone *in vitro* models. The combination of bolus 5-FU and folinic acid has been demonstrated in one study to provide survival advantage over 5-FU alone. A recent meta-analysis has reported the response rate for the combination as 23% compared with 11% for single agent bolus 5-FU, and although the optimal schedule of administration of these two drugs is unclear, this combination is widely regarded as the treatment of choice for patients with metastatic colorectal cancer.

NEW DRUGS IN THE TREATMENT OF METASTATIC COLON CANCER

The following agents are demonstrating activity in patients with colorectal cancer, but their exact place in the management of this condition is as yet uncertain.

CPT-11 (Irinotecan)

CPT-11, a semi-synthetic derivative of the plant alkaloid camptothecin, inhibits the enzyme topoisomerase I, resulting in single-stranded DNA breaks. The active component is 7-ethyl-10-hydroxy-camptothecin (SN-38) which is produced by hepatic metabolism of the parent drug. There are reports that colon cancer cells may have elevated levels of topoisomerase I compared with normal bowel mucosa which may provide relative specificity for CPT-11 in this tumour type.

In the United States and Australia a weekly schedule of administration is being utilised, while in

Europe a higher dose given every 3–4 weeks is favoured. Similar response rates and toxicities have been seen with the different schedules of CPT-11.

The principal side effects of this compound are severe (CTC grades III and IV) delayed diarrhoea which occurs in 36% of patients treated weekly for four consequent weeks with a two week break, and is lessened by high-dose loperamide. Other side effects include neutropenia (22% grades III and IV) and alopecia.

The response rate in patients who have previously received 5-FU is reported at between 13% and 27%, whilst in chemotherapy naïve patients the response rate has ranged between 15% and 32%.

Oxaliplatin

A heavy metal derivative, oxaliplatin has a similar mode of action to cisplatin and carboplatin, but may be non-cross resistant to these agents. The principal toxicities are nausea, vomiting, diarrhoea, and dose-related cumulative and reversible peripheral neuropathy. There has been minimal myelosuppression, nephropathy or ototoxicity reported.

In phase II studies as a single agent in patients with pre-treated colorectal cancer, the response rate was approximately 10%. However when combined with 5-FU and folinic acid in this same setting, the response rate was approximately 28%. In untreated patients the response rate for this combination was between 31% and 53%. When used as a single agent in chemotherapy naive patients the response rate to oxaliplatin is 24%.

Tomudex

Tomudex is a folate-based inhibitor of TS. The principal toxicities associated with its use are myelosuppression, diarrhoea and fatigue.

In phase II studies in patients with previously untreated colorectal cancer the response rate was 26%. Three phase III studies have been performed comparing Tomudex with 5-FU and folinic acid, one of which suggested a modest survival benefit for 5-FU and folinic acid, while the others have demonstrated comparable overall survival.

Phase II and III trials evaulating and comparing these agents and their combinations are in progress and may help to identify the optimal systemic therapy for metatatic colorectal cancer.

SYSTEMIC ADJUVANT THERAPY OF COLON CANCER

Chemotherapy

Early studies of adjuvant chemotherapy in colorectal cancer failed to demonstrate a survival advantage. However, a meta-analysis in 1988 of 25 randomised studies containing approximately 10,000 patients suggested a small benefit for patients receiving 5-FU based regimens.

In 1989, Laurie et al. reported the results of a 3-armed randomised study comparing surgery alone with surgery plus 5-FU and levamisole, or surgery plus levamisole, an anti-helminthic agent with purported immunomodulatory activity. At a median follow-up of 90 months in patients with Dukes C stage cancer, there was a 9% increase in overall survival favouring the 5-FU plus levamisole arm which was statistically significant (p = 0.03).

A subsequent larger intergroup study in Dukes C patients confirmed these results, suggesting an

11% survival advantage at 5 years favouring the chemotherapy arm. This regimen consisted of 12 months of weekly therapy and full compliance was difficult.

Levamisole has no single agent activity in advanced colorectal cancer and it has been difficult to support its use on pharmacologic grounds. Thus, investigators have been keen to investigate the combination of 5-FU and folinic acid in the adjuvant setting.

A number of studies have confirmed that 5-FU and folinic acid following surgery is superior to surgery alone and the advantage appears to apply equally to Dukes' Stage B and C. More recent studies have suggested that 6 months of therapy with 5-FU and folinic acid is as at least comparable to 12 months of treatment. Levamisole does not appear to provide additional benefit to 5-FU and folinic acid.

Panorex

Panorex is a murine monoclonal antibody to a colon cancer antigen. In a small randomised adjuvant study comparing surgery alone to surgery plus postoperative therapy with Panorex, a 30% reduction in mortality was demonstrated favouring the antibody arm. Studies comparing Panorex with conventional therapy are ongoing.

REFERENCES

Haller, D.G. (1995) An overview of adjuvant therapy for colorectal cancer. *Eur J Cancer*, **31A**, 1255–63.

Moertel, C.G. (1994) Chemotherapy for colorectal cancer. *N Eng J Med*, **330**, 1136–1142.

Moertel, C.G., Fleming, T.R., Macdonald, J.S., Haller, D.G., Laurie, J.A., Hoodman, P.J. and Ungerleiden, J.S. (1990) Levamisole and fluorouracil for adjuvant theraphy of resected colon carcinoma. *N Eng J Med*, **332**(6), 352–358.

Wilke, H. (1997) An interventional, multidisciplinary approach to the management of advanced colorectal cancer. International Working Group in Colorectal Cancer. *Anti-cancer Drugs*, 8 (suppl. 2), s27–31.

van Triest, B., van Groeningen, C.J., Pinedo, (1995) Current chemotherapeutic possibilities in the treatment of colorectal cancer. *Eur J Cancer*, **31A**, 1193–1198.

CHAPTER 31

HEPATOCELLULAR CARCINOMA

John E. L. Wong

DIAGNOSIS

Presentation

Patients with hepatocellular carcinoma usually present late with advanced disease. They have right upper quadrant pain and hepatomegaly in the setting of chronic liver disease and known risk factors. Usual risk factors are hepatitis B or C carrier states. Fever and weight loss are common on presentation. Rarely, patients present early, and are detected on an evaluation of an elevated serum alpha-feto protein, or the discovery of a hepatic lesion on radiographic studies.

Investigations

If this diagnosis is suspected, the usual work-up is:

- serum alpha feto protein (AFP)
- serum hepatitis B surface antigen (HBsAg)
- serum antibodies for hepatitis C (anti-HCV)
- CT scan of the liver with intravenous contrast

A firm diagnosis is best made with a histological sample. A CT-guided fine needle aspirate (FNA) by an interventional radiologist is the simplest and least morbid procedure. However, FNA may be accompanied by post-aspiration haemorrhage in this disease and its routine use is controversial.

If a fine needle aspirate is not possible, the triad of positive HBsAg or anti-HCV, elevated AFP to more than 1, 000 U/ml, and characteristic findings on contrast enhanced CT is more than 90% predictive of hepatocellular carcinoma.

Once a diagnosis is made, investigations required to plan treatment options include full blood count, liver function tests, PT, aPTT, renal chemistries, chest X-ray or CT chest and bone scan.

STAGING

There are two common staging systems, the International Union Against Cancer TNM and the Okuda. The Okuda may be preferred because liver function is a key determinant in choosing therapy. The Okuda system uses four simple criteria:

1. tumour size: </> 50% of the liver
2. ascites: present/absent
3. serum albumin: </> 30 g/L
4. serum bilirubin: </> 35 umol/L

Each negative factor is scored with 1 point.

- Stage I: 0 points
- Stage II: 1 – 2 points
- Stage III: 3 – 4 points

TREATMENT

Decisions are made according to the following questions:
- What is the patient's Child's classification?
- Is there evidence of metastasis?
- Is the patient surgically curative?

Operable Patients

Surgery remains the only curative modality. Only 10–20 % of patients are surgical candidates. Most centers prefer patients with Child's A and selected Child's B with unilobar tumours and absence of portal vein invasion. Even with aggressive surgery, up to 50% of patients may relapse. The role of adjuvant therapy is unclear and being evaluated. Such therapy includes retinoids and radioimmunotherapy.

Transplantation is possible in tumours less than 5 cm, but is hampered by the lack of donor organs, cost, significant perioperative morbidity and varying figures for mortality.

Inoperable Patients

For inoperable tumours, there is no standard treatment.

A recent review of randomised controlled trials indicate that current strategies are either ineffective or uncertain to improve survival. Ideally, all patients should be entered onto clinical trials of new agents to improve on this dismal state.

Outside a clinical trial, options depend on the patient's wishes, performance status, co-morbid disease, Child's classification, and portal vein patency.

For patients with a poor performance status, who wish for active therapy in addition to supportive care, tamoxifen is an option given its low toxicity. Cryotherapy and percutaneous alcohol injections have been used with mixed results.

For patients with a good performance status, Child's A or selected Child's B, no evidence of metastasis, and patent portal vein, hepatic artery chemoembolisation has been extensively used. This is limited to centers with trained interventional radiologists, and is complicated by fever, pain, and potential hepatic failure. A randomised study showed that although there was reduced tumour growth, there was no significant survival benefit and considerable morbidity.

Radioimmunotherapy is another option being evaluated for patients with a good performance status and inoperable disease confined to the liver. Agents used include 1^{131} antiferritin antibody, 1^{131} with lipiodol, and 90 Yttrium tagged to resin or glass microspheres. These will have to be tested in a phase III setting, and applicability is limited to centers with access to the above technology.

Systemic therapeutic options for fit patients include interferon and chemotherapy. Interferon may confer a slight advantage, but this is limited by the high dosages needed, with the attendant cost and side effects. Standard chemotherapy has not been shown to offer any significant benefit, and most centers would try to enrol patients in phase I–II trials looking at new agents, e.g. liposomal preparations, or new regimes, such as infusional chemotherapy with novel combinations.

It is hoped that mass vaccination programs against hepatitis B in populations where the disease is endemic will ultimately be the means of impacting on this cancer.

REFERENCES

Farmer, D.G., Rosove, M.H., Shaked., A. and Busuttil, R.W. (1994) Current treatment modalities for hepatocellular carcinoma. *Ann Surg*, **219**(3), 236.

Groupe d'Etude et de Traitement du Carcinome Hepatocellulaire (1995) A comparison of lipiodol chemoembolization and conservative treatment for unresectable hepatocellular carcinoma. *N Engl J Med*, **332**, 1256.

Mazzaferro, V., Regalia, E., Doi, R., Andreola, S., Pulvirenti, A., Bozzetti, F., Montalto, F., Ammatuna, M., Morabit., A. and Gennari, L. (1996) Liver transplantation for the treatment of small hepatocellular carcinomas in patients with cirrhosis. *N Engl J Med*, **334**, 693.

Simonetti, R.G., Rosove, M.H., Shaked, A. and Busuttil, R.W. (1997) Treatment of hepatocellular carcinoma: a systematic review of randomized controlled trials. *Ann Oncol*, **8**, 117.

Venook, A.P. (1994) Treatment of hepatocellular carcinoma: too many options? *J Clin Oncol*, **12**, 1323.

PART VII

UROGENTIAL CANCERS

FAST FACT SHEET 4

PROSTATE CANCER

D. P. Smith and Bruce K. Armstrong

WORLD IMPACT

In 1985, some 291,200 new cases of prostate cancer were diagnosed worldwide[1]. In the same year, prostate cancer caused an estimated 148, 600 deaths[2].

The incidence of prostate cancer varies some 70-fold among different countries. The highest incidence rates of prostate cancer in 1988–92 were recorded in black males in the USA, followed by white males in the USA and Canada. Males in China, Japan and India had the lowest rates of prostate cancer[3].

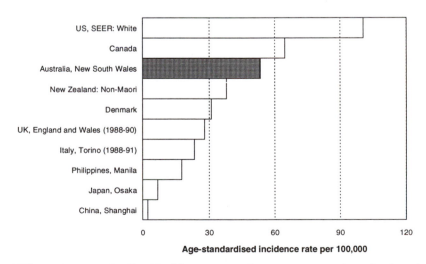

Figure FFS 4.1 Age-standardised incidence rates of prostate cancer in males in selected countries, 1988–1992[3]

Table FFS 4.1 Australian prostate cancer statistics

Statistics	Males
Crude incidence 1990	67.4 per 100 000
Age adjusted incidence 1990	50.4 per 100 000
Cumulative incidence to 75 years of age 1990	5.7%
Crude mortality 1995	28.7 per 100 000
Age adjusted mortality 1995	18.8 per 100 000
Person years of life lost to 75 years of age 1990	4,729 years
Trend in age adjusted incidence 1972 to 1994 in New South Wales	+6.2% p.a.
Trend in age adjusted mortality 1972 to 1994 in New South Wales	+0.7% p.a.
Five-year relative survival 1977–94 in South Australia	65.9%

IMPACT IN AUSTRALIA

In 1990, 5,753 new cases of prostate cancer were recorded in Australian males, accounting for 17.7% of all new cancers in males and 9.6% of all registered cancers in both sexes[4]. In 1994, prostate cancer was the second most common cancer in males in New South Wales after non-melanocytic skin cancer[5]. It was also second only to non-melanocytic skin cancer in both sexes together.

In 1995, 2,575 males died from prostate cancer in Australia, making it the second most common cancer causing death in males after lung cancer[6].

INCIDENCE BY AGE AND SEX

In 1990–94, prostate cancer in New South Wales was rare in males less than 40 years of age[7]. Between the ages of 40 and 69 years, incidence rates more than doubled from each five-year age group to the next and peaked in males aged 80–84.

INEQUALITIES IN INCIDENCE

Prostate cancer incidence increased with increasing socioeconomic status in the Sydney Statistical Division of New South Wales in 1988–94. Incidence in the highest quintile was approximately 23.3% higher than in the lowest quintile. [7]

The death rate from prostate cancer in 1979–1988 in people born in Australia was generally higher than in Australian residents born in other countries. Specifically migrants from England and Wales, Austria, Germany, Poland, Southern Europe, Lebanon, China and Malaysia had lower mortality rates than Australian born residents[8].

INCIDENCE AND MORTALITY TRENDS

Prostate cancer incidence in New South Wales increased by an average of 2.9% per year between 1972 to 1987 and 15.4% per year between 1988 and 1994[7]. Data from South Australia show that incidence peaked in 1994 and 1995 and fell in 1996[9]. Mortality in New South Wales remained stable throughout the entire period 1972 to 1994.

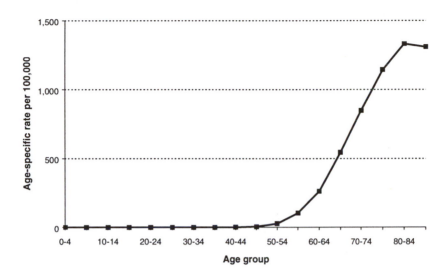

Figure FFS 4.2 Age-specific incidence rates of prostate cancer in males in New South Wales, 1990–1994[7]

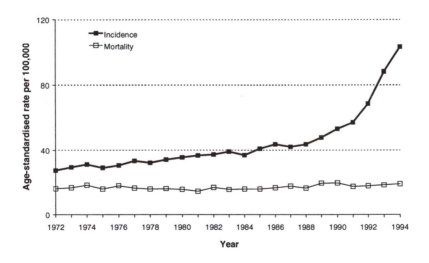

Figure FFS 4.3 Trends in annual age-standardised incidence and mortality rates of prostate cancer in males in New South Wales, 1972–1994.

SURVIVAL RATE

The five-year relative survival rate from prostate cancer in males in South Australia increased from 61.1% in those diagnosed in 1977–85 to 67.8% in those diagnosed in 1986–94[10]. In 1977–94, relative survival was highest in those aged 55 to 64 years at 70.2% and least in those 75 years of age and over at 61.3%. Better survival in the most recent time period is probably due to an increase in the detection of less aggressive lesions due to increasing use, since the late 1980s, of PSA tests for screening.

RISK FACTORS

Little is known with any certainty about risk factors for prostate cancer; dietary, hormonal, and sexual factors are suspected to contribute to risk[11]. A high fat intake probably increases risk, possibly by way of increasing plasma testosterone levels. A high intake of vitamin A has been more often associated with an increase than a decrease in risk. A past history of sexually transmitted disease has been fairly consistently associated with an increased risk and vasectomy has been associated with subsequent prostate cancer in a number of studies.

There is strong evidence of familial aggregation of prostate cancer[11], and strong evidence of linkage to the long arm of chromosome 1 has been found in North American and Swedish families with a high risk of prostate cancer[12]. High frequencies of allelic loss on the short arm of chromosome 8 and the long arm of chromosome 13 in prostate cancers raise the possibility that mutation of tumour suppressor genes at these locations may increase risk[13].

REFERENCES

1. Parkin, D.M., Pisani, P. and Ferlay, J. (1993) Estimates of the worldwide incidence of eighteen major cancers in 1985. *Int J Cancer*, 54, 594–606.
2. Pisani, P., Parkin, D.M. and Ferlay, J. (1993) Estimates of the worldwide mortality from eighteen major cancers in 1985. Implications for prevention and projections of future burden. *Int J Cancer*, 55, 891–903.
3. Parkin DM, Whelan SL, Ferlay J, Raymond L, Young J. (1997) *Cancer Incidence in Five Continents Volume VII*. Lyon: International Agency for Research on Cancer.
4. Jelfs, P., Coates, M., Giles, G., Shugg, D., Threlfall, T., Roder, D., Ring, I., Shadbolt, B. and Condon, J. (1996) *Cancer in Australia 1989–1990 (with projections to 1995)*. Canberra: Australian Institute of Health and Welfare.
5. Coates, M. and Armstrong, B. (1997) *Cancer in New South Wales Incidence and Mortality 1994*. Sydney: NSW Cancer Council.
6. Australian Bureau of Statistics (1996) *Causes of Death Australia 1995*. Canberra: Australian Government Publishing Service.
7. Smith, D.P., Supramaniam, R. and Coates, M.S., Armstrong, B.K. (1998) *Prostate cancer in New South Wales in 1972 to 1994*. Sydney: New South Wales Cancer Council.
8. Giles, G., Jelfs, P. and Kliewer, E. (1995) *Cancer mortality in migrants to Australia 1979–1988*. Canberra: Australian Institute of Health and Welfare.
9. South Australian Cancer Registry (1997) *Epidemiology of Cancer in South Australia. Incidence, mortality and survival 1977 to 1996, incidence and mortality 1996 analysed by type and geographical location - Twenty years of data*. Adelaide: South Australian Health Commission.

10. South Australian Cancer Registry (1996) *Epidemiology of Cancer in South Australia. Incidence, mortality and survival 1977 to 1995, incidence and mortality 1995 analysed by type and geographical location - nineteen years of data*, Adelaide: South Australian Health Commission.

11. Ross, R.K. and Schottenfeld, D. (1996) Prostate cancer. In *Cancer Epidemiology and Prevention*, edited by D. Schottenfeld and J.F. Fraumeni, pp. 1180–1206. New York: Oxford University Press.

12. Smith, J.R., Freije, D. and Carpten, J.D. (1996) Major susceptibility locus for prostate cancer on chromosome 1 suggested by a genome-wide search. *Science,* 274, 1371–4.

13. Bova GS, Isaacs WB. Review of allelic loss and gain in prostate cancer (1996) *World Journal of Urology,* 14, 338–46.

CHAPTER 32

GENITOURINARY MALIGNANCIES: SURGICAL MANAGEMENT

Mohamed H. Khadra

RENAL CELL CARCINOMA (GRAWITZ TUMOUR, HYPERNEPHROMA)

Background

Renal cell carcinoma (RCC) originates from renal tubular epithelium. Cigarette smoking, cadmium exposure, dialysis-induced acquired renal cystic disease, Von Hippel-Lindau Syndrome and some familial syndromes are risk factors. Males are affected twice as commonly as females with most presentations between 50 and 70 years of age.

Diagnosis

- Half are found by chance on ultrasound or abdominal CT scan.
- The classical triad of haematuria, loin pain and loin mass is found in only 10% of patients but each of the component symptoms is found in about 40% of cases.
- When a patient presents with haematuria, loin pain or mass then upper tract imaging should be performed. This may include intravenous pyelogram (IVP), abdominal ultrasound or CT scan.
- Ninety percent of renal masses are benign cysts found in approximately 20% of all patients over 60 years of age.
- An abdominal ultrasound can be useful in differentiating benign cystic lesions from complex cystic lesions or solid tumours. Solid masses of the kidney are malignant in 80% of cases. The main differential diagnosis for such lesions is oncocytoma, angiomyolipoma and inflammatory lesions (e.g. xanthogranulomatous pyelonephritis).
- Fine needle aspiration biopsy is not helpful in differentiating an oncocytoma from a RCC as both contain non-specific oncocytes.
- Imaging is also non specific for diffentiating a benign from a malignant solid mass.
- Patients with a solid renal lesion which does not contain fat and those patients with complex cystic lesions are candidates for surgical exploration.

Important features of a preoperative abdominal CT scan are:

- the size and position of the tumour, the presence of invasion into contiguous structures (hepatic flexure and liver on the right and pancreas, spleen and splenic flexure on the left); and

- the patency of the renal vein and possible involvement of the inferior vena cava, the state and function of the contra lateral kidney, the local lymph nodes and possible hepatic metastases.

Some patients present with a paraneoplastic syndrome. RCC can produce any number of proteins which can mimic intrinsic body hormones. Syndromes produced by these look-alike hormones include polycythaemia (erythropoietin), hypercalcaemia (PTH) hypertension (Renin), Cushing's syndrome (glucocorticiods) and hypoglycemia (insulin).

Treatment

Surgery

There is no known cure for RCC other than surgical excision. This is performed through the flank via a supracostal incision or from an anterior transperitoneal approach. The principles of a radical nephrectomy are to remove the kidney, the proximal ureter, the perinephric fat within the envelope of Gerotas fascia and the hilar lymph nodes. There is no survival advantage to performing a retroperitoneal lymph node dissection. If a tumour is thought to be possibly benign, then frozen sections at the time of surgery can be helpful.

Partial nephrectomies are also used for tumours less than 3 cms in diameter, in patients who have only a single kidney, or who have multiple tumours, or who have progressive renal disease with renal impairment.

Surgery also has a place as a palliative procedure in patients who have metastases but also have severe local symptoms such as haematuria or pain. There are occasional reports of metastasis spontaneously regressing after the nephrectomy. This is not considered sufficient justification for surgery.

Other Treatment

Patients with metastatic disease may benefit from radiotherapy to bone metastases for pain control. Interleukin-2 lymphokine activated killer cells and other immune therapy has been trialed with limited success.

Outcome

The prognosis for RCC for Stage I is a 5-year survival rate of about 80%, Stage II about 60% . If renal vein involvement occurs, the prognosis is still about 50% . However, with lymph nodes metastases the prognosis is poor with 5-year survival of only to 15% . The 5-year survival for Stage IV disease is less than 5% .

TUMOURS OF THE UPPER URETER AND RENAL PELVIS

Background

Tumours of the upper ureter and renal pelvis are transitional cell carcinomas which occur in the renal pelvis, renal calyces and ureter. They are uncommon tumours and account for only about 10% of all genitourinary cancers. Rarely other tumours such as squamous cell carcinomas can occur. The mean age at diagnosis is 65 years with a peak incidence between 60 and 70. Males and females are affected equally. The main predisposing factors are smoking and analgesic abuse.

Diagnosis

- These patients present with haematuria in about 80% of cases as well as with flank pain due to obstruction.
- Ultrasound is poor at detecting ureteric abnormalities.
- CT scan can detect lesions if they are large.
- The diagnosis is usually made on IVP by detecting a filling defect in the urinary tract.
- Cystoscopy and retrograde pyelography with possible ureteroscopy is then performed in order to elucidate the tumour and obtain tissue diagnosis if possible.
  Urine cytology should be performed.

Staging

On diagnosis, clinical staging includes chest X-rays, full blood count, liver function tests and also an abdominal CT scan. The essential features to look for on an abdominal CT scan are the presence of lymph node metastases, the state and function of the contra-lateral kidney, and the presence of lymphatic metastases.

Surgical Management

The surgical approach entails the removal of the kidney, the ureter and the excision of a cuff of normal bladder around the ureter to a diameter of 2 cm. This normally requires 2 separate incisions, a flank incision where the kidney and proximal ureter are removed, and a Pfannensteil incision where the bladder is opened and the distal ureter removed with a cuff of the normal bladder. The main postoperative complications are leakage of urine after bladder opening and the complications of nephrectomy as outlined above.

Five percent of patients present with bilateral TCC of the renal pelvis. This presents management difficulties since bilateral nephrectomies render the patient anephric exposing them to the high morbidity of regular dialysis. Conservative therapy may be required and consists of intrarenal or systemic chemotherapy.

Outcome

The prognosis in patients with early stage disease treated surgically is between 70% and 90% 5-year survival rate. Those with local or distal metastatic disease, have less than a 20% 5-year survival rate.

BLADDER CARCINOMA

Background

Transitional cell carcinomas (TCC) of the bladder account for over 95% of all tumours of the bladder and are 3 times more common in males then females. TCC of the bladder has a peak incidence between 50 and 70 years of age. They are the fourth most common cancer in men and the eighth in females. The main predisposing factors are smoking, analgesic abuse, and occupational exposure to aromatic hydrocarbons. Such compounds include aniline dyes, naphtylamine and benzidine.

Occupations at risk include painters, autoworkers, truck drivers, dental technicians, barbers and beauticians. Other factors increasing risk include chronic cystitis, pelvic irradiation and cyclophosphamide.

Diagnosis

- Patients normally present with haematuria or dysuria but rarely with metastatic disease.
- The initial assessment should include an intravenous pyelogram as long as there is no contraindications, as this allows upper tract tumours to be excluded.
- Cystoscopy is then performed and the urethra, the prostate in males and the bladder are examined visually. The presence of transitional cell carcinoma is detected by the presence of a papillary lesion with fragile fronds. Red velvety patches in the mucosa are associated with carcinoma *in situ*.
- An initial biopsy is performed. This should include some underlying bladder muscle in order to detect the presence of invasion.

Staging

The TNM classification is used for staging. Staging investigations should include a chest X-ray, an abdominal CT scan, liver function tests and a bone scan.

For practical purposes staging can be divided into:

- superficial disease (85% cases)
- carcinoma *in situ*
- invasive disease
- metastatic disease

Treatment

- Superficial disease is treated with a resection biopsy. As long as there is no invasion, check cystoscopies are performed every 3 months initially.
- Carcinoma *in situ* is an aggressive disease which can lead to early metastases. It is treated with intravesical BCG (Bacille Camille Guerin). If the tumour recurs following two courses of BCG then a cystectomy is performed, if the patient is suitable.
- Invasive bladder carcinoma can be treated by either radiotherapy or surgery. Surgery can also be performed to salvage a patient who has failed radiotherapy. However, the complication rate of this surgery being much higher.
- Metastatic disease is treated with chemotherapy.

Surgical Procedures

- When a patient is treated with a cystectomy, urine from the ureters needs to be diverted either into an ileal conduit or neo-bladder.
- An ileal conduit requires patients to catheterise themselves and have a normal renal function.
- Configurations of either ileum or a combination of either ileum and ascending colon are used to construct a spherical organ which is then anastomosed to the urethra. Reconstructions require no tumour in the urethra, so random biopsies from the prostatic urethra are completed prior to selection for diversion.

Complications of Surgery

- Complications of surgery are cardiovascular, respiratory and metabolic derangements because of the long periods of time when patients are nil by mouth.
- Hypochloraemic acidosis is experienced because of the absorption of sodium and secretion of bicarbonate into the intestinal segment used for diversion. The long-term effects of this acidosis are osteoporosis and possible deterioration of renal function.
- Strictures can occur at the ureter ileoanastomosis.

Outcome

The prognosis for patients treated by cystectomy in localised invasive disease is about 80% 5-year survival. If lymph nodes are involved then the survival is reduced to 40% 5-year survival. Metastatic disease has about a 20% 5-year survival.

CARCINOMA OF THE PROSTATE

Background

Ninety-five percent of prostatic malignancies are adenocarcinomas arising from the secretory lining of the ducts or the acini of the glandular tissue of the prostate. Other tumours that can affect the prostate include Transitional cell carcinoma of the prostatic urethra and rhabdomyosarcoma or leiomyosarcoma. See also the Fast Fact Sheet 4: Prostatic Cancer.

Diagnosis

Patients present with clinical symptoms of prostatic obstruction such as a poor stream, hesitancy, intermittancy, frequency and urgency or after screening by digital rectal examination and serum prostate specific antigen (PSA).

Prostate Specific Antigen

- PSA is an enzyme found predominantly in the prostate gland secretions and prevents semen from coagulating.
- It can be detected in blood by antibody immunoassay tests.
- Depending on the test, used normal is set between 2.5 to 4 ng/dl. Age-specific normal levels have been recommended in Australia in order to increase the specificity of PSA in detecting carcinoma in the elderly while increasing the sensitivity in younger patients. The range recommended for the commonly used PSA tests are:
  — 40 to 49 years of age < 2.5 ng/dl,
  — 50 to 59 < 3.5 ng/dl,
  — 60 to 69 < 4.5 ng/dl or less
  — over 70, 6.5 ng/dl or less.
- The presence of an elevated PSA does not necessarily imply carcinoma. Benign prostatic hyperplasia, as well as infection or trauma of the prostate and ejaculation, can all raise the level of PSA above normal in males.
- The total PSA to free PSA ratio appears to increase in patients with carcinoma and can be used to increase the specificity of this test for prostate cancer.

- PSA as a screening tool has not been recommended but is widely used.
- A patient who has a PSA test should be counselled about the relative risks and benefits of discovering carcinoma of the prostate. The natural history is long and little scientific evidence exists to determine the best treatment.

Staging

- Grade, stage, the patient's age and his medical condition are important factors in deciding management strategy.
- The Gleason grade is determined by the architecture under low power microscopy, so that well organised architecture is grade 1 and poorly organised acinar glandular structures are Grade 5. The final score is calculated by adding together the Gleason grade for the most common and second most common area of cancer.
- Gleason scores of 2 to 4 are regarded as well differentiated, 5 to 7 moderately differentiated and 8 to 10 poorly differentiated.
- Staging for a patient involves an abdominal CT scan, bone scan as well as a chest X-ray and liver function tests.
- A PSA of greater than 30 carries a high chance of extra prostatic disease.

Treatment

- A major issue with curative treatment is the significant morbidity associated with these treatments. Surgery carries with it a 5% incidence of incontinence and a 50% to 70% percent of impotence.
- The mortality is about 0.5% to 1%.
- The side effects of radiotherapy include prostatitis and impotence.
- The choice of treatment should be left to the patient. Thus, comprehensive, easily understood information should be provided so that appropriate informed consent can be obtained.
- Disease outside the prostate is treated by androgen deprivation. Bilateral orchiectomy has been the method of choice. Medical orchiectomy can also be performed by LHRH agonists or peripherally acting antiandrogens. Side effects of these medications may include painful gynaecomastia, hot flushes and decreased libido.
- Patients with metastic disease, but localised prostatic symptoms, may benefit from palliative transurethral resection of the prostate. Occasionally pelvic lymphadenectomy is performed in order to exclude lymph node metastases prior to radiation therapy.

Outcome

The prognosis from prostate cancer is good. Localised prostate cancer patients have a 90% disease-free survival rate over 10 years. Patients with metastic disease have a median survival of 2 years after diagnosis.

TESTICULAR CARCINOMA

Diagnosis

- Patients present with a painless testicular mass for investigation. Often there is denial and patients may present late. About 10% of patients will present with pain due to haemorrhage into the tumour.

- A patient with a testicular mass is initially investigated with a scrotal ultrasound. If this mass is confirmed to be a intratesticular lesion then this is assumed to be cancer until otherwise proven as over 97% of such masses are cancer.
- Preoperatively, it is essential to obtain serum for testicular markers. These include serum alphafetoprotein (αFP) and beta human chorionic gonadotropin (βHCG), as well as lacratedehydrogenas (LDH).

Treatment

- Inguinal radical orchiectomy is the safest way of removing the primary cancer.
- This requires an inguinal approach where the cord is clamped prior to manipulation of the testis. The testis is brought up into the wound, biopsied and a frozen section obtained. If this is postive the testis is removed.
- If the markers are positive prior to surgery, the testis is removed without frozen section.
- Surgery may be required for removal of residual retroperitoneal masses following chemotherapy.

Staging

- Staging should include a chest and abdominal CT scan and a repeat set of tumour markers about 3 weeks after the surgery.
- If positive markers return to normal based on half-life (see Chapter 35) and the abdominal CT scan and chest CT are normal, then the patient is presumed to have Stage 1 disease. This is disease is contained within the testis.
- Patients who have positive markers postoperatively or have positive CT scans may have Stage 2 disease (infra diaphragmatic) or Stage 3 disease (supra diaphragmatic).
- Some patients present with metastic disease (Stage 4).

REFERENCES

Hanno, P.M. and Wein, A.J. (1994) *Clinical Manual of Urology* (2nd edn). New York: McGraw-Hill.
Stricker, P. (1996) Prostate Cancer: Issues and Controversies. *Modern Medicine of Australia*, Nov., 16–28.

CHAPTER 33

CANCERS OF THE UROGENITAL TRACT: SYSTEMIC AND RADIATION TREATMENT

Michael Boyer and Michael Jackson

PROSTATE CANCER

Hormonal Therapy

Hormonal therapy is the mainstay of treatment for metastatic prostate cancer, and has an evolving role in the management of locally advanced disease. The basis of hormonal therapy for prostate cancer is the dependence of tumours of the prostate (as well as the normal prostate gland) on androgens (especially testosterone) for continued growth.

Orchidectomy

Suppression of testosterone levels can be achieved by orchidectomy or by agonists of luteinising hormone releasing hormone (LHRH). Orchidectomy has been used for many years to provide a rapid and irreversible decrease in the level of testosterone.

Luteinising Hormone Releasing Hormone Agonists

More recently, LHRH agonists, such as goserelin or leuprorelin, both of which are as effective as orchidectomy, though with slower onset of action, have been used to produce reversible suppression of testosterone levels.

LHRH agonists work by interfering with the pituitary synthesis of LH, which is required for testicular testosterone production. Normal production of LH requires the presence of pulsatile stimulation by LHRH. The continuous stimulation produced by the LHRH agonist drugs results in a suppression of LH production, following a transient rise.

These agents are administered as a depot injection, once a month, with a long acting three monthly injection recently available. The transient rise in LH levels following the commencement of LHRH agonists can be associated with a temporary flare in disease activity.

Maximal Androgen Blockage (MAB)

Prostate cancer can also be treated by the administration of anti-androgens which interfere with the binding of testosterone to its nuclear receptor. Examples of anti-androgens include cyproterone acetate, flutamilde, nilutamide, and bicalutamide. These drugs are usually used together with an LHRH agonist, or following orchidectomy in an approach known as combined or maximal androgen blockade.

The use of MAB is based on the fact that about 5% of androgens are produced by the adrenal gland. Although castration, either surgical or chemical, eradicates testicular androgen synthesis, it does not affect adrenal androgen synthesis. The use of anti-androgens may eliminate the effects of these adrenal androgens.

Although appealing in principle, the use of MAB has not been clearly demonstrated to result in improved outcomes, with contradictory data from randomised trials. A meta-analysis has failed to demonstrate an overall benefit of MAB compared to various, single hormone manipulations.

Outcome

Irrespective of the method used, approximately 70–80% of men with metastatic prostate cancer respond to hormonal manipulation, with a median duration of response of 18–24 months. Response is usually associated with relief of symptoms such as pain.

Treatment is associated with symptoms of androgen deprivation, which include impotence, hot flushes, lethargy, and loss of lean body mass. In contrast to the high response rate seen with initial hormonal therapy, second line hormonal therapy produces responses in less than 25% of patients. Furthermore when second hormonal response occur, they are usually short-lived.

Timing of Hormone Treatment in Prostate Cancer

The timing of treatment for metastatic prostate cancer has been the subject of considerable controversy. Traditionally, men have only received treatment for metastatic disease following the development of symptoms.

There has been an increasing trend towards the treatment of asymptomatic patients with locally advanced or metastatic prostate cancer. This approach is supported by the results of a large randomised trial which showed improved survival in patients with immediate treatment, when compared to those in whom treatment was delayed until they were symptomatic.

Neo-adjuvant therapy

In recent years, there has also been increasing interest in the use of neo-adjuvant hormonal therapy for prostate cancer. This involves the administration of treatment, usually with MAB, to patients with bulky primary disease in an attempt to decrease the tumour volume and make subsequent surgery or radiotherapy easier. It is not yet clear whether or not this approach yields improved survival, though it may decrease the toxicity of treatment.

Chemotherapy

Cytotoxic chemotherapy has only played a small part in the management of advanced prostate cancer. This has been due, in part, to inadequacies in the way in which new treatments have been evaluated. Recently, with the use of palliative endpoints, assessing pain relief, and analgesic requirements, it has been demonstrated that chemotherapy using mitoxantrone produces benefit in men with symptomatic metastatic prostate cancer, following the failure of hormonal therapy.

TRANSITIONAL CELL CARCINOMA OF THE BLADDER

- Transitional cell carcinoma (TCC) of the bladder is treated with systemic chemotherapy when metastatic.
- The disease may metastasise widely, but common sites are lymph nodes, lungs and bone.
- Several drugs have activity in the treatment of TCC. These include cisplatin, adriamycin, vinblastine, methotrexate, and newer agents such as paclitaxel and gemcitabine.
- Usually, multi-agent combination chemotherapy is used, since there is randomised trial evidence that this approach results in higher response rates and longer survival. The major regimens are the MVAC regimen (including methotrexate, vinblastine, adriamycin and cisplatin) and the CMV regimen (containing cisplatin, methotrexate and vinblastine).
- One of the difficulties in the use of these regimens is their toxicity, which may be substantial, especially in the elderly population of patients who typically suffer with TCC. Therefore newer regimens are being evaluated, in an effort to produce equivalent results with less toxicity.

Outcome

Following treatment with chemotherapy, the median survival of patients with metastatic TCC is 12 months. Long-term survival has been reported in small numbers of patients who had metastatic disease confined to the lymph nodes.

Neo-adjuvant Chemotherapy

Chemotherapy has also been advocated as a neo-adjuvant treatment in patients with locally advanced disease. The aims are to decrease the size of the local tumour, and to eradicate micro-metastatic disease. Although this approach results in high response rates with shrinkage, and often disappearance, of the primary tumour, it unfortunately, does not result in an improvement in survival, and is thus not regarded as standard practice.

RADIOTHERAPY IN GENITOURINARY MALIGNANCIES

Radiotherapy has an important role in the curative and palliative treatment of genitourinary malignancies, either alone or in combination with surgery or systemic treatment.

Prostrate Cancer

Localised prostate cancer can be treated with radical radiotherapy and this gives similar results to surgery. Tumour Stage, grade and PSA levels are important prognostic indicators. Surgery tends to be used in patients under 65 but radiotherapy does give good long-term results at all ages.

A four-field arrangement to cover the prostate with a small margin is usually used to a dose of about 66 Gy. Using a large field initially to cover the pelvic nodes increases the side effects and probably is of little benefit. The prostate can be boosted to a higher dose if small, individually shaped fields are used. This does seem to be helpful especially if the initial PSA is over 10 ng/ml. The use of androgen blockade prior to radiotherapy may improve disease control and survival but the results of further trials are awaited.

Ten-year disease-free survivals range from 30–70%.

Acute complications include proctitis, dysuria and skin reaction. Long-term proctitis is a problem in about 5% of patients but less than 0.5% require colostomy. Urinary symptoms usually settle quickly. Impotence may occur in 50% of patients but the contribution of radiotherapy to this is difficult to assess because of the age of the patient.

In an attempt to reduce the side effects and the length of treatment there has been renewed interest in interstitial brachytherapy using Iodine 125. The seeds emit low energy radiation and are implanted through the perineum using ultrasound and fluoroscopic control. Initial results are encouraging with similar disease-free survival to radical prostatectomy in appropriately selected patients. Side effects, particularly impotence, are less than following surgery. Only early tumours can be treated and long-term (> 5 years) data are still awaited. Implants may also be used as a boost following conventional external beam radiotherapy.

Short courses of radiotherapy can be useful in the palliation of bone metastases and pelvic disease. Doses of 20 Gy in 1 week or 30 Gy 2 weeks are usually used. Many patients have widespread bone metastases in which case a single dose to the upper or lower half of the body or an injection of Strontium 89 provides good pain relief, but haematological toxicity can be a problem. Radiotherapy to the breast can prevent gynaecomastia in hormone treated patients.

Bladder Cancer

Radical radiotherapy to a dose of 60–66 Gy with or without chemotherapy can be used as an alternative to cystectomy in localised disease. Five year survival rates are 25–40% but acute complications can be severe and the bladder capacity is reduced after treatment.

Bone and lymph node metastases can be palliated with short courses of radiotherapy.

Renal Cell Carcinoma

Radiotherapy has little role in radical treatment either as a primary modality or post operatively as the tumour is relatively resistant to radiotherapy and is surrounded by sensitive structures.

Bone metastases are common but often respond poorly to radiotherapy.

Testicular Tumours

The role of radiotherapy is covered in Chapter 34.

REFERENCES

Bolla, M., Gonzalez, D., Warde, P., Dubois, J.B., Mirimanoff, R.O., Storme, G., Bernier, J., Kuten, A., Sternberg, C., Gil, T., Collette, L. and Pierart, M. (1997) Improved Survival in Patients with Locally Advanced Prostate Cancer Treated with Radiotherapy and Goserelin. *N. Eng. J. Med.* **337**, 295–300.

Catalona, W.J. (1994) Management of cancer of the prostate. *N.Engl.J.Med.*, **331**(15), 996–1004.

Loehrer, P.J., Einhorn, L.H., Elson, P.J., Crawford, E.D., Kuebler, P., Tannock, I., Raghavan, D., Stuart Harris, R., Sarosdy, M.F.and Lowe, B.A. (1992) A randomized comparison of cisplatin alone or in combination with methotrexate, vinblastine, and doxorubicin in patients with metastatic urothelial carcinoma: a cooperative group study. *J Clin Oncol,* **10**,1066–1073.

Raghavan, D., Shipley, W.U., Garnick, M.B., Russell, P.J. and Richie, J.P. (1990) Biology and management of bladder cancer. *N.Engl.J Med.,* **322**,1129–1138.

The Medical Research Council Prostate Cancer Working Party Investigators Group. (1997) Immediate versus deferred treatment for advanced prostatic cancer: initial results of the Medical Research Council trial. *Br. J. Urol.*, **79**, 235–246.

CHAPTER 34

GERM CELL TUMOURS

Guy C. Toner

INTRODUCTION

- Germ cell tumours comprise > 95% of adult testicular cancers. Germ cell tumours may also arise in midline structures including the mediastinum and retroperitoneum. Germ cell tumours arising in the pineal gland occur predominantly in children.
- Germ cell tumours comprise approximately 2–3% of ovarian cancers in our community and a higher incidence (up to 15%) in Asian countries. The principles of management are similar to testicular germ cell tumours but will not be discussed in detail here.
- Germ cell tumours comprise about 1% of all male malignancy. Approximately 300 new cases of testicular cancer are diagnosed each year in Australia. The incidence is increasing.
- Germ cell tumours are the most common malignancy in 15–35 year age group.
- High proportion of cures possible: approximately 80% of patients with metastatic malignancy achieve long-term disease-free survival with chemotherapy, radiotherapy and surgery.
- These tumours are a model for diagnostic and therapeutic use of serum tumour markers.

AETIOLOGY

- Unknown in the majority of cases.
- Established risk factors are:
  - Age: Median age at diagnosis is 25–30 years.
  - Cryptorchidism: 12% of testicular neoplasms arise in cryptorchid testes. Up to 40 times risk in undescended testis which is improved but not normalised by orchidopexy. Small increased risk in contralateral, normally descended, testis.
  - Race: Most common in Scandinavia and in white males from developed Western countries. Less common in blacks and in Asian races. Intermediate risk in Mediterranean nations. Uncommon in North American blacks suggesting genetic rather than environmental aetiology.

214

- Postulated risk factors include higher socio-economic status, sedentary occupation.
- An isochromosome of the short arm of chromosome 12 is commonly identified in germ cell tumours. Excessive expression of a gene located on 12p is postulated to be an early genetic event in tumourogenesis.

PATHOLOGY

- Distinct management policies for two groups. Each comprises approximately 50% of cases.
  - — Seminoma: comprising pure seminoma only. Median age at presentation approximately 35 years. Highly responsive to radiotherapy treatment (and chemotherapy). Equivalent to dysgerminoma in ovarian germ cell tumours.
  - — Non-Seminomatous Germ Cell Tumours (NSGCT): Often comprising a mixture of histologies including embryonal carcinoma, yolk sac (endodermal sinus) tumour, choriocarcinoma, teratoma and seminoma. Median age at presentation approximately 25 years. Relatively resistant to radiation therapy but highly responsive to chemotherapy.
- Pathological classifications can be confusing. 'Teratoma' as used by the British system can be used in approximately the same way as 'NSGCT', whereas teratoma in the 'World Health Organisation' classification refers to a specific component of NSGCT only.

SERUM TUMOUR MARKERS

- Alphafetoprotein (AFP), human chorionic gonadotropin (HCG), and lactate dehydrogenase (LDH) are useful markers for diagnosis, staging, assessment of prognosis, monitoring response to therapy and monitoring for relapse.
- AFP is elevated in up to 60% of non-seminomatous tumours. AFP is never elevated with pure seminoma. The half-life of AFP decline after complete removal of tumour is approximately 5 days. False positive elevations are possible with hepatoma, gastrointestinal malignancies, and regeneration after hepatic necrosis.
- HCG is elevated in up to 60% of non-seminomatous tumours and approximately 20% of seminomas. The half-life of HCG decline after complete removal of tumour is approximately 2–3 days. False positive elevations are possible with elevation of other hormones sharing a common alpha sub-unit (LH, FSH, TSH), pregnancy and rarely other malignancies.
- LDH is less specific but is an important prognostic factor for outcome of chemotherapy and may be useful in monitoring disease, particularly if HCG and AFP are not elevated.

PRESENTATION

- The most common presentation is with a painless mass in one testicle. Other presenting symptoms include a change in texture or size of the testicle, scrotal pain, back pain due to retroperitoneal metastases or respiratory symptoms due to thoracic metastases, and gynaecomastia and/or galactorrhoea due to HCG secretion.

INITIAL MANAGEMENT

- Initial management of a suspicious testicular mass is testicular ultrasound and measurement of serum tumour markers.
- Inguinal orchidectomy is performed if ultrasound confirms a suspicious testicular lesion. Trans-scrotal approaches for biopsy or orchidectomy must be avoided to prevent disruption of the normal lymphatic drainage, which is important in staging and management.
- Careful pathological examination of the entire testicle is important to assess local extent, the presence or absence of various histological components and lymphatic or vascular invasion. Serum tumour markers should be followed post-operatively until within normal limits.

STAGING

- Staging investigations include a CT scan of chest, abdomen and pelvis.
- The pattern of spread of testicular germ cell tumours is very predictable. The most common site of initial spread is to the retroperitoneal lymph nodes just below the renal vessels. This is the site of origin of the lymphatic and vascular supply of the testes. NSGCT also commonly spread to the lungs via the blood stream either synchronously or separately to retroperitoneal disease.
- Twenty to thirty percent of patients with disease apparently confined to the testis will relapse as a result of occult metastatic disease, most commonly in normal size retroperitoneal lymph nodes.

SUBSEQUENT MANAGEMENT

Non-Seminomatous Germ Cell Tumours

Stage I Disease

- Stage I disease, confined to testis, is most commonly managed with observation following surgery and treatment with chemotherapy for the patients who relapse. Strict compliance with a close observation policy, particularly in the first 2 years after diagnosis, is essential to ensure relapses are diagnosed at an early stage.
- Patients with a high risk of relapse (e.g. those with lymph/vascular invasion in the primary tumour) can be successfully managed with initial chemotherapy. Patients with unexplained elevated markers after surgery should receive chemotherapy for occult metastases.
- In excess of 95% of these patients should be cured with these approaches.

Metastatic Disease

Metastatic disease is managed with chemotherapy and post-chemotherapy resection of any residual masses. Chemotherapy is cisplatin-based and generally consists of cisplatin, etoposide and bleomycin. The short-term toxicities include nausea/vomiting, alopecia, myelosuppression, peripheral neuropathy, tinnitus and high-tone hearing loss, renal impairment, and bleomycin pulmonary disease.

Post-chemotherapy resection of residual masses is an important component of management, particularly to remove mature teratoma, which is present in up to half of the residual masses.

Long-term toxicity includes infertility in approximately 50% due to chemotherapy and retroperitoneal node dissection. Other toxicities include bleomycin lung toxicity, and less commonly second malignancies, Raynaud's phenomenon, hearing loss and tinnitus and renal impairment.

The vast majority of patients return to full employment and normal lifestyles.

Seminoma

Stage I Disease

Stage I disease, confined to testis, is managed post-operatively with radiotherapy to the retroperitoneal nodes to a dose of approximately 25 Gy. This reduces the risk of recurrence from about 20% to 2%. Initial observation with treatment at relapse is an investigational approach that is not in routine practice because of the risk of late relapse and the good results of radiotherapy.

Stage II Disease

Low volume Stage II disease with retroperitoneal lymphadenopathy < 3–5 cm diameter, is managed with radiation therapy to a higher dose, generally 35 Gy. The risk of relapse increases with the size of the lymphadenopathy but is generally < 15%.

More Advanced Disease

More advanced disease is managed with chemotherapy. The chemotherapy used for NSGCT is used in advanced seminoma. Bulky initial tumour often leaves a residual mass after chemotherapy. Generally, this consists of scar tissue only and can be observed. Patients relapsing after radiotherapy are also managed with chemotherapy with excellent results. Approximately 90% of patients remain free of disease and achieve long-term survival after chemotherapy.

REFERENCES

Bosl, G.J., Bajorin, D.F., Sheinfeld, J. and Motzer, R.J. (1997) Cancer of the testis. In *Cancer: Principles and Practice of Oncology* (5th edn), edited by V.T. DeVita, S. Hellman and S.A. Rosenberg, pp. 1397–1425. Philadelphia: Lippincott-Raven.

Boyer, M., Raghavan, D., Harris, P.J., Lietch, J., Bleasel, A., Walsh, J.C., Anderson, S. and Tsang, C.S. (1990) Lack of late toxicity in patients treated with cisplatin-containing combination chemotherapy for metastatic testicular cancer. *Journal of Clinical Oncology*, **8**, 21–26.

Einhorn, L.H. (1981) Testicular cancer as a model for a curable neoplasm: The Richard and Hinda Rosenthal Foundation Award Lecture. *Cancer Research*, **41**, 3275–3280.

PART VIII

GYNAECOLOGICAL CANCERS

CHAPTER 35

GYNAECOLOGICAL CANCERS: SURGICAL MANAGEMENT

Jonathan Carter

INTRODUCTION

All patients with gynaecologic cancers, should have their surgical care undertaken by a certified gynaecologic oncologist (CGO). The ability to perform adequate surgical staging or surgical debulking are improved if performed by a CGO, rather than a general gynecologist or surgeon. These factors have an important impact on survival.

CERVICAL CANCER

Presenting Symptoms

Microinvasive or occult cervical cancers may by asymptomatic, with diagnosis after work-up of an abnormal Pap smear. As lesions progress, for more advanced disease, abnormal vaginal bleeding occurs which may be postcoital or intermenstrual. Occasionally a watery vaginal discharge may be the only symptom. Advanced and metastatic tumours have symptoms and signs related to the site of tumour involvement.

Diagnostic Work-Up

- Once an invasive cervical cancer has been confirmed on biopsy, the work-up is designed to identify tumour spread.
- In the majority of cases, findings of the extent of disease found at an examination under anaesthetic (EUA) allows a stage to be assigned.
- In early cancer, other than a CXR, no other specific work-up is necessary.
- In advanced tumours, a CT scan may give valuable information regarding retroperitoneal nodal involvement, ureteric obstruction and other evidence of spread.

Staging

Cervical cancer is staged clinically.

- Stage I: Carcinoma strictly confined to the cervix.
- Stage II: The carcinoma extends beyond the cervix but has not extended onto the pelvic side wall.
- Stage III: The carcinoma has extended onto the pelvic side wall. On rectal examination, there is no cancer free space between the tumour and the pelvic wall. The tumour involves the lower third of the vagina. All cases with hydronephrosis or non-functioning kidney.
- Stage IV: The carcinoma has extended beyond the true pelvis or has clinically involved the mucosa of the bladder or rectum. Bullous edema of the bladder wall does not permit a case to be allotted to stage IV.

Indications for Surgery

- The overall survival is similar for surgery and radiotherapy. However, most early cervical cancers are treated with radical hysterectomy and pelvic lymph node dissection.
- Surgery allows the accurate delineation of the extent of disease, removal of gross tumour and the option of transposing the ovaries out of any intended pelvic radiation field.
- Irradiation obviates and negates the risks of major surgery. However, therapy takes 5–6 weeks and is complicated by both early and late side effects.
- More advanced stages of cervical cancer, are primarily treated by irradiation. Some centres perform a surgical staging procedure to accurately define the extent of disease prior to this, while others rely on the CT to provide this information.

Type of Surgery

1. Removing primary tumour
   (i) Type II or III hysterectomy (Radical or Wertheim hysterectomy)
2. Defining the extent of disease
   (i) Pelvic lymph node dissection
   (ii) Pelvic washings
3. Debulking
   (i) Debulking grossly positive lymph nodes in advanced or recurrent disease may confer a survival benefit.
   (ii) There is no role however for debulking intraperitoneal disease as is performed in ovarian cancer.

Outcomes

In early stage disease, outcome is related to the presence of lymph node metastasis. Factors significantly associated with microscopic pelvic lymph node metastasis include depth of invasion, parametrial involvement, capillary-lymphatic space invasion, tumour grade and gross versus occult primary tumour.

ENDOMETRIAL CANCER

Presenting Symptoms

The majority of women present with postmenopausal bleeding. Occasionally a watery vaginal discharge may be the only symptom. While uncommon in younger women, if present, will present with abnormal or heavy bleeding.

Diagnostic Work-Up

The diagnosis is usually confirmed on an endometrial biopsy or curettage. Once confirmed, no specific preoperative work-up apart from a CXR is necessary.

Staging

- Stage I: The carcinoma is confined to the corpus of the uterus.
- Stage II: The carcinoma involves corpus and cervix.
- Stage III: Tumour has spread away from the uterus to involve the serosa, adnexa, vagina or retroperitoneal nodes.
- Stage IV: Distant metastasis involving bladder, bowel mucosa, intraabdominal and inguinal metastasis.

Indications for Surgery

- Any patient with postmenopausal bleeding or discharge or abnormal premenopausal bleeding warrants evaluation.
- A diagnosis of endometrial cancer usually is an indication for surgery, as discussed below. Rarely however, with medically unfit patients definitive irradiation may be advised instead of surgery.
- Patients with endometrial cancer treated with primary irradiation have a poorer prognosis than those treated with surgery, unlike cervical cancer.

Type of Surgery

1. Removing the primary tumour
   (i) Type I hysterectomy (extrafascial THBSO)
2. Defining the extent of disease
   (i) Pelvic lymph node dissection
   (ii) Pelvic washings
   (iii) Omental biopsy
3. Debulking
   (i) Removing all gross disease where possible in advanced stage disease.

Outcomes

As most women present in an early stage, the majority of patients are cured with surgery alone or with adjuvant irradiation. Independent prognostic factors for survival in surgical Stage I and II disease include age, depth of myoinvasion, grade and cell type. The outlook for advanced and recurrent tumours is poor.

OVARIAN CANCER

Presenting Symptoms

Ovarian cancer develops insidiously, hence the reason why the majority of cases present in an advanced stage. Patients usually seek medical attention with a variety of nonspecific gastrointestinal symptoms, increasing abdominal girth secondary to accumulating ascites, a feeling of pressure or heaviness secondary to pelvic tumour mass and weight loss and satiety related to the advanced stage of the tumour.

Diagnostic Work-Up

- The presence of a complex pelvic mass and ascites alone are indications for surgical exploration.
- Exclusion of metastatic causes for ovarian enlargement is important.
- Mammography and large bowel studies (barium enema or colonoscopy) are useful.
- Many patients have CT scans performed in their diagnostic work-up. While occasionally helpful, they are not critical when surgical exploration is contemplated.
- Preoperative determination of serum tumour markers (CA-125) are important.

Staging

- Stage I: Tumour limited to the ovaries
- Stage II: Tumour involving one or both ovaries with pelvic extension
- Stage III: Tumour involving one or both ovaries with peritoneal implants outside the .pelvis and/or positive retroperitoneal or inguinal glands; superficial liver metastases; tumour limited to the true pelvis but with histologically proven malignant extension to small bowel or omentum
- Stage IV: Distant metastases including parenchymal liver disease

Indications for Surgery

The presence of a persistent or complex mass associated with an elevated serum CA125 are indications for surgical exploration.

Type of Surgery

1. Removing the primary tumour
   (i) Involves a total hysterectomy and bilateral salpingo-oophorectomy (THBSO). In a young woman with an early tumour, consideration may be given to perform a conservative unilateral salpingo-ophorectomy, assuming a thorough surgical staging has been performed and has failed to document extraovarian disease.
2. Defining the extent of disease
   (i) Pelvic and para-aortic lymph node dissection, most important in apparent early stage disease
   (ii) Pelvic and peritoneal washings
   (iii) Inspecting all peritoneal surfaces
   (iv) Omentectomy

3. Debulking

   (i) For advanced staged ovarian cancer, unlike other solid tumours, survival can be prolonged by aggressive, 'maximal surgical effort'.

   (ii) Patients left with minimal residual disease after primary surgery have a significantly longer survival than those left with bulky or suboptimal disease.

   (iii) An optimal debulking is one where there is no tumour deposit greater than 2 cm in maximum diameter (preferably 1 cm).

   (iv) Such surgery may involve bowel resection to achieve optimal cytoreduction.

Outcomes

Tumour grade is the most powerful predictor of recurrence in early stage disease, followed by dense adherence and large volume ascites. Cell type other than clear cell or mucinous, Taxol-platinoid based treatment, good performance status, younger age, lower stage, clinically nonmeasurable disease, smaller residual tumour volume, and absence of ascites are all favorable characteristics for overall survival in patients with advanced ovarian cancers.

REFERENCES

1. Delgado, G., Bundy, B.N., Fowler, W.C., Stehman, F.B., Sevin, B., Creasman, W.T., Major, F., DiSaia, Zaino, R. (1989) A prospective surgical pathological study of stage I squamous carcinoma of the cervix: a GOG study. *Gynecol Oncol,* **35,** 314–320.

2. Delgado, G., Bundy, B., Zaino, R., Sevin B.U., Creasman, W.T. and Major, F. (1990) Prospective surgical-pathological study of disease-free interval in patients with stage IB squamous cell carcinoma of the cervix: a GOG study. *Gynecol Oncol,* **38**(3), 352–357.

3. Boronow, R.C., Morrow, P.C., Creasman, W.T., DiSaia, P.J. (1984) Surgical staging in endometrial cancer: clinical-pathologic findings of a prospective study. *Obstet Gynecol,* **63,** 825.

4. Orr, J.W., Holimon, J.L. and Orr, P.F. (1997) Stage I corpus cancer: is teletherapy necessary? *Am J Obstet Gynecol,* **176,** 777–789.

5. S. Bush RS, Kjorstad K, Dembo, A.J., Davy, M., Stenwig, A.E., Berle, E.J. (1990) Prognostic factors in patients with stage I epithelial ovarian cancer. *Obstet Gynecol,* **75,** 263–272.

6. Omura, G.A., Brady, M.F., Homesley, H.D., Yordan, E., Major, F.J., Buchsbaum, H.J. and Park, R.C. (1991) Long-term follow-up and prognostic factor analysis in advanced ovarian carcinoma: the GOG experience. *J Clin Oncol,* **9**(7),1138–1150.

CHAPTER 36

GYNAECOLOGICAL CANCERS: SYSTEMIC TREATMENT

Alison Davis and Michael Friedlander

INTRODUCTION

The role of chemotherapy in the management of women with gynaecological cancers has expanded significantly over the past 20 years. Chemotherapy has an important place in the multidisciplinary management in patients with both epithelial and germ cell tumours of the ovary as well as gestational trophoblastic tumours. Furthermore chemotherapy is of value in the palliative management of selected patients with metastatic endometrial cancer, cervical cancer and uterine sarcomas.

EPITHELIAL CARCINOMA OF THE OVARY

Outcomes

- The majority of women with ovarian cancer present with Stage III or IV disease. Most are treated with platinum-based combination chemotherapy, and this has resulted in an improved response rate and a longer median survival period when compared to alkylating agents alone. However, the five-year survival rate is still only approximately 20%.
- There are a number of important prognostic factors that are useful in predicting outcome in advanced ovarian cancer, and these include FIGO Stage, volume of residual disease remaining after initial debulking surgery, performance status, patient age, tumour grade and tumour ploidy.
- Patients with Stage III disease who have had optimal debulking (less than 1 cm of residual tumour) have a 30% five-year survival rate, while those with Stage III or IV disease with suboptimal residual disease have approximately a 10% chance of long-term survival.

Combination Chemotherapy

Cyclophosphamide and Platinum Combinations

Platinum-based combination chemotherapy with either cisplatinum or carboplatin and cyclophosphamide has, until recently, formed the mainstay of treatment for the majority of patients with advanced ovarian cancer. Response rates are in the order of 65–75% with a clinical complete remission rate of approximately 40% to 50% and a complete pathological response of 20% to 30%. The median progression-free survival time is approximately 18 months and the median survival time is 24 months.

There are at least seven randomised trials that have demonstrated that carboplatin and cisplatin have equal efficacy in patients with an advanced ovarian cancer. Cisplatin is associated with significantly more side effects including nausea and vomiting, neurotoxicity and nephrotoxicity, while carboplatin is more myelosuppressive. In view of these data the majority of patients with advanced ovarian cancer are treated with carboplatin-based combinations.

Paclitaxel-Based Chemotherapy

More recently, paclitaxel has been demonstrated to have an important role in the management of women with advanced ovarian cancer. In a recent randomised study which included approximately 400 women with advanced ovarian cancer and suboptimal residual disease, the progression-free survival was significantly longer in the cisplatin/paclitaxel group than in the cisplatin/cyclophosphamide group with a median progression-free survival of 18 versus 13 months. Furthermore, the survival period was also significantly longer in the cisplatin/paclitaxel group with a median of 38 versus 24 months.

These findings have been confirmed in a large co-operative trial from Europe and Canada that also included patients with optimally debulked disease, and it is likely that this combination will be adopted widely. Studies are in progress comparing cisplatin and paclitaxel with carboplatin and paclitaxel as the toxicity and convenience of the carboplatin combination makes it much more attractive.

Other Agents

There are a number of other single agents with documented activity in advanced ovarian cancer and these include the anthracylines, hexamethylmelamine, topotecan, gemcitabine and tamoxifen. At the present time these tend to be used in the setting of recurrent ovarian cancer, although there are ongoing studies addressing their role in first line treatment.

Limited Disease (Stages I and II)

- Patients with Stage IA or B tumours that are well or moderately well differentiated have a five-year survival rate of 91% to 98% which is not improved with adjuvant treatment.
- Patients with either Stage IC (e.g. capsular involvement or positive washings), poorly differentiated tumours or Stage II disease have a higher risk of relapse and these patients are often considered for post-operative adjuvant therapy.
- An improved disease-free survival has been demonstrated with chemotherapy, but the impact on overall survival is less clear.

Recurrent Ovarian Cancer

- Patients who have persistent or recurrent disease after initial chemotherapy are not curable. However, second line treatment can provide useful palliation and improve quality of life.

- Patients with tumours that are intrinsically resistant to platinum-based chemotherapy or who relapse within six months of stopping treatment tend to have a poor prognosis with a low likelihood of responding to second line treatment.
- Patients with a treatment free interval of greater than six months after stopping chemotherapy have a 30% to 50% chance of responding to reintroduction of carboplatin or cisplatin.
- Combination chemotherapy does not appear to be any better than single agents in the salvage setting.

OVARIAN GERM CELL TUMOURS

Ovarian germ cell tumours account for only approximately 5% of all ovarian cancers and almost always occur in young women. The initial treatment approach is surgery for both diagnosis and therapy. If the tumour appears to be confined to one ovary, it is imperative that proper staging biopsies are performed.

The type of primary surgery depends on the findings at laparotomy. Bilateral ovarian involvement is rare, and therefore unilateral salpingo-oophorectomy with preservation of the contralateral ovary and uterus can be performed in most patients with malignant ovarian germ cell tumours thus preserving the potential for fertility.

Dysgerminoma

- Dysgerminoma is the female equivalent of seminoma.
- Approximately two-thirds of patients will have Stage I disease and well-staged patients with Stage IA dysgerminomas are carefully followed up after unilateral salpingo-oophorectomy.
- Careful follow-up is required as 15% to 25% will recur, but because of the sensitivity of this tumour to chemotherapy virtually all patients will be successfully salvaged at the time of recurrence.
- Patients with more advanced dysgerminomas should be treated with cisplatin based chemotherapy along the same lines as non-dysgerminomatous ovarian germ cell tumours.

Immature Teratomas

- Most patients with Grade I Stage I immature teratoma will survive progression free, but the failure rate of less well-differentiated immature teratomas is appreciable.
- As many as 75% of patients with Stage I Grade III immature teratomas will recur after initial surgery as well as similar numbers of patients with a resected endodermal sinus tumour, embryonal carcinoma or mixed germ cell tumours.
- Adjuvant chemotherapy is indicated for all patients except those with Grade I Stage I immature teratoma. These patients are treated with three cycles of cisplatin, etoposide and bleomycin and the vast majority will be cured.
- A similar approach to treatment is used in patients with more advanced disease and 80% to 90% will be cured with chemotherapy.

GESTATIONAL TROPHOBLASTIC TUMOURS

Gestational trophoblastic disease are tumours that arise from the placental trophoblastic tissue following a pregnancy and includes hydatidiform mole, invasive mole and choriocarcinoma.

Although pathology is useful in determining treatment, management decisions are usually based on the clinical course as determined by β HCG measurements.

The WHO staging system is in common usage in Australia and is based on a number of prognostic factors, including age, nature of antecedent pregnancy, interval between pregnancy and at the start of chemotherapy, β HCG level, tumour size and site as well as the number of metastases and prior chemotherapy. These are all used to classify patients as being of low risk, intermediate risk or high risk.

Treatment

- Following diagnosis of a molar pregnancy, patients have a suction curettage (or hysterectomy if no future pregnancy is desired). Approximately 10% of patients with a molar pregnancy will require chemotherapy.
- For those patients with low risk disease, single agent chemotherapy with Methotrexate and Folinic acid is commonly used although Actinomycin D may also be used in this setting. Most patients will go into complete remission and will not require a change of treatment.
- Patients with medium to high risk disease should receive combination chemotherapy. The most widely employed regimen in this country is EMA-CO (etoposide, methotrexate, actinomycin D, cyclophosphamide and vincristine).
- The majority of patients will be cured with this approach although salvage regimens including cisplatinum are sometimes required. The management of patients with gestational trophoblastic tumours can be complex and they are best treated by experienced clinicians in a trophoblastic disease centre.

ENDOMETRIAL CARCINOMA

The role for chemotherapy in endometrial cancer is essentially limited to patients with Stage IV disease at presentation or recurrent disease not amenable to treatment with radiotherapy or hormonal therapy. Active agents, with a response rate 20%, include hormonal agents such as progestins and tamoxifen as well as chemotherapy with doxorubicin, carboplatin and paclitaxel.

Hormonal therapy with progestins or tamoxifen should be considered for those patients with oestrogen or progesterone receptor positive tumours, or in the absence of receptors, with Grade I to II disease.

Chemotherapy may be considered in selected patients with Grade 3, negative receptor status or those no longer responsive to hormones.

Chemotherapy with doxorubicin and cisplatin has been shown to be superior to either agent alone. Paclitaxel has also been recently shown to have significant activity. However responses are usually only partial and the duration is measured in months.

UTERINE SARCOMAS

Uterine sarcomas are rare heterogeneous tumours that account for less than 5% of uterine tumours. Approximately 60% are mixed mesodermal tumours, 30% are leiomyosarcomas, and 10% other types including endometrial stromal sarcomas. Chemotherapy is generally reserved for patients with disseminated or recurrent disease, but is also used in the adjuvant setting in investigational studies. Recommendations for treatment vary according to histological subtype.

For patients with advanced or recurrent mixed mesodermal sarcomas, ifosfamide and cisplatin are associated with response rates of 32% and 19% respectively. Combination regimens have not resulted in higher responses compared with single agents. Doxorubicin has a reported response rate of 25% in leiomyosarcomas. Addition of other agents does not appear to improve response rates or survival, but may increase toxicity.

CERVICAL CANCER

Surgery and radiotherapy form the mainstay of treatment of cervical cancer (see Chapter 36). However, chemotherapy, 5-flurouracil (5-FU), may have a role as a radiosensitiser in conjunction with radiotherapy in the management of patients with locally advanced or locally recurrent tumours.

There are a number of drugs that have activity in cervical cancer and these include cisplatin, ifosfamide, bleomycin and anthracyclines. Although combination chemotherapy is associated with higher response rates than single agents, there is increased toxicity and no improvement in survival.

Recent studies have demonstrated no advantage, and indeed possibly a disadvantage, for neoadjuvant chemotherapy prior to radiotherapy for patients with locally advanced cervical cancer. Chemotherapy has a limited place in the palliative management of patients with metastatic cervical cancer.

REFERENCES

1. McGuire, W.P., Hoskins, W., Brady, M., Kucera, P.R., Partridge, E.E., Look, K.Y., Clark-Pearson, D.L. and Davidson, M. (1996) Cyclophosphamide and cisplatin compared with paclitaxel and cisplatin in patients with Stage III and IV ovarian cancer. *N Eng J Med*, **334**, 1–6,
2. Gershenson, D.M. (1993) Update on Malignant ovarian germ cell tumours. *Cancer*, **71**, 1581–1590.
3. O'Mura, G. (1994) Chemotherapy for cervix cancer. *Semin Oncol*, **21**, 54–62.
4. Ozols, R.F. and Vermorken, J. (1997) Chemotherapy of advanced ovarian cancer: current status and future directions. *Semin Oncol*, **24** (Suppl 2), 1–9.
5. Berkowitz, R.S. and Goldstein, D.P. (1995) Gestational trophoblastic disease. *Cancer*, **76** (10-suppl.), 2079–85.

PART IX

HEAD AND NECK CANCER

CHAPTER 37

HEAD AND NECK CANCER: SURGICAL MANAGEMENT

Christopher J. O'Brien

INTRODUCTION

The term 'head and neck cancer' is a general one which refers to malignant tumours involving the skin, soft tissues or bones of the head and neck region.

These cancers include:

- mucosal squamous cell carcinomas (SCC) of the upper aerodigestive tract
- metastatic cancer involving the lymph nodes of the neck
- salivary gland tumours
- thyroid cancers
- cancers of the skin of the head and neck
- bone tumours, particularly those involving the jaw

Brain tumours are not usually included among cancers of the head and neck. This chapter deals with primary and metastatic mucosal SCC.

Anatomically, the head and neck region is complex and both the malignant process and its treatment can significantly affect appearance and the important functions of speaking and eating. Early diagnosis facilitates best treatment results and is also more likely to lead to preservation of function.

Most head and neck tumours are treated by surgical excision, with appropriate reconstruction where necessary. Radiotherapy is mainly given after surgery to destroy cancer cells which may remain at the edge, or beyond the margins, of excision.

MUCOSAL SQUAMOUS CELL CARCINOMA

Mucosal squamous cell carcinoma is the most common form of head and neck cancer. The typical patient is male, aged between 50 and 70 years, a heavy user of tobacco and alcohol, with poor oral hygiene. These tumours account for 5% of all new cancers in Australia and the United States and approximately 3% of cancer deaths. The incidence among females has risen in recent years due to smoking.

Oral Cavity

The oral cavity extends from the lips to the anterior tonsillar pillars. The most common sites of cancer are the floor of mouth and lateral borders of tongue. Invasion of the mandible readily occurs when cancer involves the mucosa of the gum. Cervical lymph nodes are involved in approximately 30% of cases.

Surgical Management

- Oral cavity cancers can usually be resected through the open mouth.
- Small defects of the tongue can be primarily closed by direct suture.
- Defects of the floor of mouth and larger defects of the tongue require reconstruction. This is best achieved by the use of thin, pliable tissue usually a microvascular radial forearm free flap.
- Skin grafts may also be used but they tend to take poorly and contract.
- Where the tumour encroaches onto the jaw a marginal resection of bone is frequently required to give an adequate surgical margin. This involves taking a sliver of jaw while maintaining the continuity of the mandible.
- A segmental resection, which interrupts the continuity of the jaw, should only be carried out when there is gross bone invasion. Ideally, segmental jaw defects should be reconstructed using vascularised autologous bone.

Oropharynx

The oropharynx lies posterior to the oral cavity and includes posterior third of tongue, tonsillar fossae, soft palate and posterior pharyngeal wall. Oropharyngeal tumours tend to present later than oral cancers. The tongue base and tonsils are the most common sites and these tumours tend to be more poorly differentiated than oral cavity cancers. The incidence of neck node involvement is 50% to 70%.

Surgical Management

- Surgical treatment of oropharyngeal cancers is made difficult because access to the oropharynx is difficult.
- This can be improved by a mandibulotomy, a cut in the mandible, either in the midline or to one side of the midline, allowing the mandible to be retracted laterally to give access to the oropharynx. This is called 'mandibular swing'.
- Resection of oropharyngeal cancers is more likely to affect swallowing than oral cancers and postoperative swallowing rehabilitation is important.
- Primary closure of surgical defects is difficult in the oropharaynx and free flap reconstruction is usually necessary. The radial forearm flap is most frequently used but its lack of bulk is sometimes a limitation.

- Large base of tongue cancers are best treated with radiotherapy because surgery leads to significant morbidity.

Larynx

The larynx is subdivided into supraglottic larynx, glottis (true vocal cords) and subglottis. About 60% of cancers affect the true cord and 35% affect the supraglottic larynx. Hoarseness is the common early symptom for vocal cord cancers and so these patients tend to present with early disease. True vocal cord cancers rarely spread to neck nodes unless very advanced. Supraglottic cancers involve neck nodes in 50% to 60% of cases.

Treatment

- Early laryngeal cancers, where the vocal cord is still mobile, can be effectively treated with radiotherapy. Sometimes, however, these tumours are bulky and conservative surgery, or partial laryngectomy, can be carried out and give better results than radiotherapy.
- Surgery is reserved for advanced laryngeal cancers, that is when the vocal cord is fixed by the tumour.
- A total laryngectomy is usually carried out, removing the entire voicebox and restoring the continuity of the pharynx by suturing the pharyngeal mucosa.
- Reconstruction with new tissue is usually not necessary unless there is insufficient pharyngeal mucosa to form a satisfactory gullet.
- Removal of the larynx leaves the patient unable to phonate, that is, to make a noise. Speech can be restored by a number of mechanisms which allow the patient to make a noise by forming a vibrating column of air in the throat which can then be articulated into words by the lips, teeth and tongue.
- The involvement of a trained speech pathologist in vocal rehabilitation of laryngectomy patients is of great importance.

Organ Preservation

More recently, there has been a trend towards 'organ preservation' in patients with laryngeal cancers. Evidence suggests that if patients are given initial chemotherapy and respond to this treatment they can have radiotherapy to treat their advanced laryngeal cancer rather than surgery.

Approximately 50% of patients treated in the way retain their voicebox and the cure rates are similar to those achieved by laryngectomy. Patients who do not respond to initial chemotherapy or who have persistence of cancer after the radiotherapy need to be treated by laryngectomy.

Hypopharynx

The hypopharynx lies behind the larynx and is the uppermost part of the gullet. Cancers in the hypopharynx are often 'silent' and may present late. Neck node involvement is very common (60–80%).

Treatment

- Cancers of the hypopharynx have been regarded as being more resistant to radiotherapy than laryngeal cancers and even early stage cancers of the hypopharynx are usually treated by surgery.

- Surgery often involves total laryngectomy as well as resection of the involved mucosa of the hypopharynx. Sometimes the larynx can be spared.
- Primary closure of the remaining pharynx can sometimes be achieved but if the entire hypopharynx is resected, total laryngopharyngectomy, it is necessary to reconstitute this circumferential defect in the gullet. A segment of small bowel, usually the jejunum, can be transferred from the abdomen to the pharyngeal defect as a microvascular-free tissue graft.
- As with larynx, however, recent evidence suggests that an organ preservation strategy using chemotherapy and radiotherapy can provide good rates of laryngeal preservation.
- The survival rates are lower than those for larynx with about 25% alive at 5 years rather than 50% at 5 years seen for patients with laryngeal cancer.

Paranasal Sinuses

The paranasal sinuses include the maxillary and ethmoid sinuses and nasal passages. The most common site of cancer is the maxillary sinus. These cancers present late and frequently involve bone while neck metastases are rare.

Treatment

- The best treatment is with combined surgery and radiotherapy.
- Treatment of these tumours usually involves a maxillectomy and resection may include exenteration of the orbit if the orbital contents are involved. The maxillectomy cavity can either be skin grafted and left open for inspection or obliterated with a free flap.
- An open maxillectomy cavity needs to be sealed with an upper dental plate and an obturator to allow normal speaking and eating.

Nasopharynx

The nasopharynx lies above the oropharynx and behind the nasal cavity and cancers occur mainly among Asian patients. The presentation is often late and may include bone and cranial nerve involvement. Neck node involvement occurs in 70–90%. Nasopharyngeal cancer is usually treated with radiotherapy but chemotherapy is sometimes used in addition.

METASTATIC CANCER IN THE NECK

There are approximately 40–60 lymph nodes on each side of the neck. These are frequently involved by metastatic cancer from primary tumours of the skin of the head and neck, the mucosa of the upper aerodigestive tract, the thyroid and salivary glands and also by lymphoma.

The most common cause of lymph node enlargement in the neck in an adult is metastatic cancer, most frequently from a primary tumour above the clavicles, particularly mucosal SCC. Involvement of lymph nodes by cancer seriously worsens prognosis in virtually all disease, except differentiated thyroid cancer. The prognosis of patients with mucosal SCC is halved when lymph nodes are involved.

Surgical removal of the lymph nodes in the neck is called a neck dissection. The extent of neck dissection is specified using the following terminology:

- Elective neck dissection: removal of lymph nodes not clinically palpable.
- Therapeutic neck dissection: removal of clinically palpable lymph nodes.

- Comprehensive neck dissection: indicates that the entire neck is dissected.
- Radical neck dissection: a comprehensive neck dissection including resection of the sternomastoid muscle, internal jugular vein and spinal accessory nerve.
- Modified radical neck dissection: a comprehensive neck dissection but preserving one or more of the sternomastoid muscle, internal jugular vein and spinal accessory nerve.
- Selective neck dissection: removal of only certain lymph node levels.

An elective neck dissection is an integral part of the overall management of patients with mucosal SCC. This procedure can provide important pathological information about possible microscopic involvement of lymph nodes, can improve the control rate of disease in the neck since disease is treated at an earlier stage, can save patients from returning with advanced disease in the neck at a later time and can assist in microvascular free tissue transfer by removing tissue from around recipient blood vessels. Elective neck dissections are usually selective operations aiming to remove only the lymph node groups which are most at risk for metastatic involvement.

A therapeutic neck dissection is used when clinical disease is present in the neck. The safest form of therapeutic procedure is a comprehensive neck dissection. Most frequently this can be a modified radical dissection, preserving especially the spinal accessory nerve in order to avoid a painful, sagging shoulder. Radical neck dissection should only be carried out when massive neck disease is present.

PROGNOSTIC FACTORS AND POSTOPERATIVE RADIOTHERAPY

Some features may worsen prognosis in mucosal SCC and are indications for postoperative radiotherapy. These include:

- Clinicopathological features
    — Advanced disease at presentation (T3, T4).
    — Positive surgical margins.
    — Perineural invasion.
    — Irregular or disordered invasive pattern on tumour histology.
- Other features
    — Involvement of multiple lymph nodes.
    — Involvement of lymph nodes at multiple neck levels.
    — Spread of metastatic disease beyond the lymph node capsule into the surrounding soft tissue, i.e. extracapsular spread.

MULTIDISCIPLINARY TREATMENT

Patients with head and neck cancer should be treated by head and neck surgeons in collaboration with radiation and medical oncologists. Frequently, plastic surgical reconstruction is needed to restore appearance and function. Preoperative evaluation and postoperative treatment by speech pathologists, physiotherapists, dietitians, social workers and nursing staff are most important in this patient group.

REFERENCES

O'Brien, C.J. (1994) A Selective Approach to Neck Dissection for Mucosal Squamous Cell Carcinoma. *Aust N Z J Surg*, **64**, 236–241.

O'Brien, C.J., Lee, K.K., Castle, G.K. and Hughes, C.J. (1992) Comprehensive Treatment Strategy for Oral and Oropharyngeal Cancer. *Am J Surg*, **164**, 582–586.

The Department of Veterans Affairs Laryngeal Cancer Study Group (1991) Induction Chemotherapy plus Radiation Compared with Surgery plus Radiation in Patients with Advanced Laryngeal Cancer. *New Eng J Med*, **120**, 589–601.

Theile, D.R., Robinson, D.W., Theile, D.E. and Coman, W.B. (1995) Free Jejunal Interposition Reconstruction after Pharyngolaryngectomy: 201 Consecutive Cases. *Head Neck*, 83–88.

Urken, M.L., Moscoso, J.F., Lawson, W. and Biller, H.F. (1994) A Systematic Approach to Functional Reconstruction of the Oral Cavity Following Partial and Total Glossectomy. *Arch Otolaryngol Head Neck Surg*, **120**, 589–601.

CHAPTER 38

HEAD AND NECK CANCER: RADIATION THERAPY

Michael Jackson

INTRODUCTION

The head and neck region is the site of origin of many different cancers. The majority, or about 85%, are squamous cell carcinomas of the upper aerodigestive tract. This chapter covers squamous cell carcinomas and tumours of the parotid gland and skin, but carcinomas of the nasopharynx and thyroid, melanoma, lymphoma, sarcoma, and metastatic tumours are discussed elsewhere.

As squamous cell carcinomas of the head and neck are strongly associated with heavy smoking and drinking, these patients often have other significant medical problems, particularly of the respiratory and cardiovascular systems. They may also have social and intellectual problems which cause late presentation and difficulty coping with a prolonged course of treatment.

PRESENTATION

Presentation is usually in a patient with a clear history of cigarette and alcohol abuse, but can occur rarely in young and otherwise fit patients, and the diagnosis is sometimes delayed in this group. Symptoms include:

- sore throat, often unilateral
- no associated signs of infection and no resolution with antibiotics
- difficulty swallowing
- hoarse voice
- weight loss
- problems with teeth and dentures
- halitosis
- lumps in the neck

DIAGNOSIS

The primary site is often visible at clinical examination. Malignant lymph nodes are usually hard and non-tender, and may be unilateral or markedly asymmetric with no general signs of infection. Referral should not be delayed if symptoms persist despite antibiotics.

The lesion is often accessible to biopsy and fine needle aspiration (FNA) of neck nodes can be performed. In some cases, examination may be difficult and may require a laryngeal mirror or a fibre-optic nasopharyngoscope. Examination under anaesthetic is often required to fully stage the tumour and to exclude the presence of other head and neck primary tumours.

STAGING

These tumours usually have a logical spread from primary site to cervical lymph nodes, before metastasising to the lungs and then to other sites. This makes the TNM staging system particularly important in determining therapy and prognosis.

The T stage varies with site but generally T1 and T2 are small tumours with limited local spread and T3 and T4 are larger or involve adjacent structures. The N stage is common for most sites: N0 — no regional nodes, N1— ipsilateral single node ≤ 3 cms, N2a — ipsilateral single node 3–6 cms, N2b — ipsilateral multiple nodes ≤ 6 cms, N2c — bilateral or contralateral nodes > 6 cms, N3 — nodes ≤ 6 cms.

A problem with this system is that Stage III and IV include small primary tumours with nodal spread as well as large primaries with no nodal spread. These have different natural histories and prognosis and treatment may also be different.

TREATMENT

It is important to decide initially if there is a reasonable chance of curing the tumour. Relevant factors include:

- Patient factors
    - general health and performance status
    - willingness to stop smoking and heavy drinking
    - desire for aggressive treatment
    - intellectual ability
    - ability to cope with acute and chronic side effects
    - family and social support

- Tumour factors
    - site, size and degree of differentiation
    - rate of growth
    - nodal involvement
    - distant metastases

Radiotherapy and surgery often produce similar cure rates but with differing toxicities. The choice of treatment depends on patient preference and local availability of resources or expertise. If cure cannot reasonably be attempted palliative radiotherapy is rarely useful.

RADIATION TECHNIQUES

In most cases radiotherapy is given in 1.8 to 2.0 Gy/fraction to a total dose of 60 to 70 Gy over 6–7 weeks. Techniques vary according to site and tumour extent but in many cases lateral fields are used to cover the known tumour, likely microscopic extension and nodal areas.

An anterior field may be used to cover the lower neck nodes, in which case care must be taken to avoid excess dose variation at the junction of the lateral and anterior fields. The field size may be reduced during treatment to avoid overdosing critical normal tissues while giving a high dose to the site of maximum disease.

Treatments including surgery, radiotherapy or chemotherapy which reduce cell numbers can stimulate accelerated repopulation in tumours and normal tissues, and this can lead to a loss of tumour control. The overall duration of the total treatment is important particularly if it is longer than 4 weeks. A short delay in starting treatment appears to be less dangerous than unnecessary breaks once treatment has begun.

TYPE OF RADIATION

- Megavoltage X-rays are used for the majority of treatments.
- Electrons can be used to boost a small tumour volume or to cover nodes, especially those over the spinal cord.
- Superficial or deep X-rays are used for skin tumours.
- Brachytherapy can be used either as a continuous low dose rate treatment or as an intermittent high dose rate treatment. It can be particularly useful for small accessible tumours or in the salvage of radiation failures.

PREPARATION FOR RADIOTHERAPY

- Staging the tumour.
- Attention to general health, e.g. other medical conditions, weight loss, stopping smoking.
- Accommodation, transport, social support if needed.
- Dental assessment. Radiotherapy fields often cover the salivary glands, causing xerostomia which leads to accelerated dental caries. If the mandible is in the high dose region, dental infections or extractions after treatment can lead to osteonecrosis.
- Planning. In most cases a mask is made to immobilise the patient and to allow fields to be outlined without the need to draw or tattoo on the patient's face.
- A mouth block may be used to move structures out of the field and stabilise the patient. Shielding blocks are positioned to minimise the radiation dose to normal tissues.
- Wax is placed over scars and other areas if the full dose is needed on the skin.

SIDE EFFECTS OF RADIOTHERAPY

Acute

- Skin reactions
  — avoid hot water and soap, shave with electric razor

- — avoid sun and wind
- — use moisturising cream on dry areas

- Mucositis
  - — salt and bicarbonate mouthwash
  - — analgesics, e.g. soluble aspirin or paracetamol at first, narcotics if necessary
  - — local anaesthetics, e.g. diflam, xylocaine viscous
  - — antifungal treatment if necessary

- Loss of saliva and taste
  - — regular dental assessment during treatment
  - — referral to a dietician

Chronic

- Xerostomia.
- Skin changes: dryness, telangectasia, pigmentation.
- Sensitive mucosa.
- Osteonecrosis of mandible.
- Radiation myelitis. Spinal cord dose is usually kept to below 45 Gy but recent evidence suggests that this may be too conservative and that higher doses and even retreatment may be tolerated if necessary.
- Soft-tissue fibrosis.
- Eye: dry eye, cataract. The retina and optic chiasm may be damaged if dose is over 50 Gy.
- Chronic hearing loss due to conductive or sensory damage.

TREATMENT RESULTS OF INDIVIDUAL SITES

The reporting of results is difficult as these patients often have other serious illness and may die of these, rather than the tumour.

Mouth, oropharynx

- Early stages are usually treated by surgery, but radiotherapy can produce up to 80% local control.
- More advanced lesions can be controlled in 50% of cases with surgery and post- operative radiotherapy, and 20–30% with radiotherapy alone.

Larynx

- Early lesions radiotherapy alone 80–90% cure. Over 95% with salvage laryngectomy.
- In more advanced lesions, radiotherapy with or without chemotherapy produces 40–60% local control with preservation of the larynx.

Hypopharynx

- Early disease is uncommon. Radiotherapy produces up to 70% control.

- In more advanced disease there is 30–40% control with a combination of surgery, chemotherapy and radiotherapy.

Paranasal sinuses

- Early lesions are uncommon.
- In more advanced lesions, postoperative radiotherapy produces 40% control and radiotherapy alone 25%.

Parotid tumours

- Primary treatment is surgical. Postoperative radiotherapy is given if the margins are close or positive, the tumour is close to the facial nerve, in high grade tumours or recurrent disease.
- If inoperable, treatment is given with radiotherapy alone.
- Results vary according to tumour type, but local control is obtained in 70–80% of cases.

Skin

- Radiotherapy is used for larger tumours and those in which surgery would produce a poor cosmetic result or if the surgical margin is close or positive.
- Radiotherapy gives excellent control for BCCs but larger SCCs are more difficult to control.
- SCCs may also metastasise to the parotid region and other cervical nodes.

Unknown primary

- Enlarged cervical lymph nodes containing SCC can be found in the absence of a detectable primary site.
- Radiotherapy to the nodes and sometimes the likely primary sites can lead to 70% local control rate with a 50% survival rate at 3 years.

POSTOPERATIVE RADIOTHERAPY

There may be a need for radiotherapy if there is a high risk of recurrence at the primary site or in the neck after surgery. Radiotherapy is rarely successful if there is gross residual disease, but can be useful in the following circumstances:

- microscopic or close margins;
- large primary tumour;
- poorly differentiated tumour;
- perineural spread;
- several involved nodes; or
- extracapsular spread.

Large fields are usually required to cover the surgical bed and nodes, and a dose of 54–60 Gy is used.

RADIOTHERAPY IN COMBINATION WITH CHEMOTHERAPY

- Many small studies have suggested a significant improvement if chemotherapy is added to radiotherapy but results of larger randomised trials have been less definite.

- An overview suggests that any advantage is likely to be greatest with concurrent rather than sequential treatment.
- Side effects are also increased and an optimum regime has not yet been devised.
- The use of combined modality treatment in advanced laryngeal cancer can decrease the need for salvage laryngectomy.

ALTERED FRACTIONATION

If radiotherapy is given in smaller than 2 Gy fractions late normal tissue reactions can be reduced. To maintain effective tumour control, more than one fraction per day and usually a higher total dose are required. A gap of at least six hours between treatments is needed to allow repair of normal tissue damage. Randomised trials have shown better local control and survival, at the cost of greater acute toxicity. This approach has great promise for the future but the availability of machine time has limited its application to date.

CONFORMAL RADIOTHERAPY

Improvements in machine design and availability of more sophisticated computer planning systems allows the target volume to be more closely matched to the actual extent of the tumour. This allows sparing of critical normal tissues while giving a higher dose to the tumour. These techniques have great potential and will be developed for routine use in the near future.

PATIENT FOLLOW-UP

Regular follow-up by the surgeon and radiation oncologist is important to detect tumour recurrence and to manage the side effects of treatment. Most recurrences occur in the first two years, but second head and neck primaries and lung cancer can occur later. The need to stop smoking often needs frequent reinforcement.

REFERENCES

Dische, S., Saunders, M., Barrett, A., Harvey, A., Gibson, D. and Parmar, M. (1997) A randomised multicentre trial of CHART versus conventional radiotherapy in head and neck cancer. *Radiotherapy and Oncology*, 44(2), 123–136.

Horiot, J.C., Bontemps, P., van den Bogaert, W., Le Fur, R., van den Weijngaert, D., Bolla, M., Lusinchi, A., Stuschke, M., Lopez-Torrecilla, J., Begg, A.C., Pierart, M. and Collette, L. (1997) Accelerated fractionation (AF) compared to conventional fractionation (CF) improves loco-regional control in the radiotherapy of advanced head and neck cancers: results of the EORTC 22851 randomized trial. *Radiotherapy and Oncology*, 44(2), 111–122.

Munro, AJ (1995) An overview of randomised controlled trials of adjuvant chemotherapy in head and neck cancer. *Br J Cancer*, 71(1), 83–91

Stuschke, M & Thames, HD (1997) Hyperfractionated radiotherapy of human tumors: Overview of the randomised clinical trials. *Int J Radiation Oncology Biol Phys*, 37(2), 259–267.

Wang, C.C. (1997) *Radiation Therapy for Head and Neck Neoplasms*. New York: Wiley-Liss Inc.

CHAPTER 39

HEAD AND NECK CANCERS: SYSTEMIC THERAPY

Danny Rischin

INTRODUCTION

Head and neck cancers include squamous cell cancers of the upper aerodigestive tract arising in the oral cavity, oropharynx, hypopharynx and larynx. Smoking and alcohol are the major risk factors. Although distant metastases may occur, the initial presentation and subsequent clinical course is dominated by the primary site and nodal metastases.

The major curative modalities available for the treatment of head and neck cancers are surgery and radiotherapy. Chemotherapy has a limited role in the management of advanced head and neck cancer.

Nasopharyngeal carcinoma is a more chemosensitive tumour with different risk factors, and a greater propensity for distant metastases. As discussed in a separate chapter recent trials suggest a more definite role for chemotherapy in nasopharyngeal carcinoma.

RECURRENT OR METASTATIC DISEASE

Palliative chemotherapy has been used in patients with relapsed local disease that can not be salvaged with further surgery or radiotherapy, in patients with metastatic disease and in patients who present with locally advanced disease that is neither resectable nor suitable for radical radiotherapy.

Single agent methotrexate has been widely used with response rates reported of 10–30%. A recent large randomized trial that was restricted to patients in the above categories reported a response rate of only 10%[1]. It is usually started at a dose of 40 mg/m² weekly, and the dose may be escalated. It is generally well tolerated with possible side effects including mucositis, diarrhoea and myelosuppression.

Cisplatin and 5-fluorouracil (5-FU) is the most active regimen achieving objective responses in about one third of patients[1,2]. The dose of cisplatin is 100 mg/m² and 5-FU is given as a continuous intravenous infusion 1000 mg/m²/day for 4–5 days. In randomized trials this combination results in a higher response rate, but no improvement in survival when compared to single agent methotrexate, single agent cisplatin or single agent 5-FU. Possible side effects include nausea and vomiting, mucositis, diarrhoea, myelosuppression, nephrotoxicity, peripheral neuropathy and hearing impairment. It is of interest that patients with head and neck cancer who have a heavy alcohol intake tolerate cisplatin with less nausea and vomiting than is observed in other malignancies.

Carboplatin appears to be slightly less active than cisplatin in head and neck cancer but may be substituted for cisplatin in patients with renal impairment, peripheral neuropathy, or significant hearing impairment. The taxanes have activity in advanced head and neck cancer and are currently being investigated in clinical trials.

As chemotherapy has not been demonstrated to improve survival, it is primarily used for palliation of symptoms. Unfortunately, the impact of chemotherapy on symptom control and quality of life compared to best supportive care has not been adequately studied. As cisplatin and 5-FU may result in significant toxicity the decision to initiate or continue treatment is always a balance between symptomatic improvement and side effects that occur in the individual patient.

LOCALLY ADVANCED DISEASE

Standard surgical and radiotherapeutic techniques which yield good results for early stage head and neck cancer are much less effective for locally advanced disease. There has been considerable interest in determining whether the addition of chemotherapy may improve the outcome.

In patients with locally advanced disease that is resectable or suitable for radical radiotherapy, initial treatment using induction or neoadjuvant chemotherapy, with cisplatin and 5-FU results in response rates of 60–90%. However, numerous randomized trials have demonstrated no improvement in local control or survival with induction chemotherapy although distant metastases are decreased.

More encouraging results have been seen with the use of chemotherapy concurrent with radiotherapy. The results of a recent meta-analysis support further investigation of concurrent chemo-radiation rather than sequential treatment[3]. As the taxanes are potential radiosensitizers and have activity in head and neck cancer, concurrent taxane and radiation trials are in progress.

Another approach to combining chemotherapy and radiotherapy is to use drugs that target hypoxic tumour cells, as hypoxic cells are more resistant to radiotherapy. Hypoxia has been demonstrated in nodal metastases from head and neck cancer and appears to correlate with poor response to radiotherapy. Individual trials of hypoxic cell sensitizers have not demonstrated consistent benefit, though a recent meta-analysis has found a statistically significant improvement. A new approach under investigation is to use drugs such as tirapazamine, that are preferentially cytotoxic to hypoxic cells, in conjunction with radiotherapy.

At the present time the use of chemotherapy in patients receiving radical radiotherapy or undergoing surgery remains investigational and should not be part of routine practice.

LARYNX PRESERVATION

One indication where induction chemotherapy may have a role is in the area of larynx preservation. In patients with locally advanced glottic or supraglottic cancers initial chemotherapy with radiotherapy given to the responders has been demonstrated to be an alternative to total laryngectomy in two large randomized trials[4,5].

Patients who do not respond to two cycles of chemotherapy proceed to surgery, while responders receive a third cycle of chemotherapy. The criteria for proceeding with radiotherapy have varied with some trials requiring only a partial response to chemotherapy, while others mandating a complete response.

The percentage of survivors with a functional larynx at 3 years is approximately 65% in the patients randomized to initial chemotherapy, and survival is equivalent to patients who were randomized to initial surgery.

The contribution of chemotherapy to organ preservation remains unclear. As there is a correlation between chemosensitivity and radiosensitivity in head and neck cancer, chemotherapy may merely be predicting the patients who are destined to respond well to radiotherapy. Current randomized trials are addressing the question of whether similar rates of organ preservation may be achieved with initial radiotherapy without any preceding chemotherapy.

At the present time larynx preservation protocols with initial chemotherapy are an acceptable treatment option for many patients with locally advanced glottic and supraglottic cancer whose only surgical option is total laryngectomy.

CHEMOPREVENTION

Second Primary Cancers

Patients who have had a primary head and neck cancer are at significant risk of developing a second primary cancer of the upper aerodigestive tract, at a constant yearly rate of 2–5%. This is because the whole of the upper aerodigestive tract has been exposed to the same carcinogens.

The development of head and neck cancer, in this situation, is a multi-step process, with the pre-malignant lesions, leukoplakia and erythroplakia, having the potential to progress to invasive cancer at varying times. Cessation of smoking is an important component of any plan to reduce the risk of developing an upper aerodigestive tract malignancy.

Retinoids

Another approach currently being investigated is chemoprevention. This involves the use of natural or synthetic agents to prevent the development of an invasive cancer. Retinoids have been the most widely tested agents in head and neck chemoprevention trials, both in patients with oral premalignancy and in patients with a prior head and neck cancer.

Several randomised trials have demonstrated that retinoids can reverse oral leukoplakia, but there is a high risk of relapse following cessation of the drug[6]. Conflicting results have been reported in initial trials of retinoids for patients with a prior head and neck cancer. Current placebo controlled trials are evaluating further the role of retinoids in chemoprevention of second primary malignancies.

SALIVARY GLAND TUMOURS

Most salivary gland tumours are benign. Chemotherapy does not have any role in the management of localized malignant salivary gland tumours. Metastatic salivary gland tumours are uncommon but palliative chemotherapy may have a role. Response rates of 30–40% have been reported with platinum-based regimens. Some patients with pulmonary metastases may have a relatively indolent course, and hence chemotherapy is generally not given until significant symptoms develop.

KEY POINTS

- Surgery and radiotherapy are the major treatment modalities for head and neck cancer.
- Chemotherapy has a limited role in the palliation of patients with relapsed or metastatic head and neck cancer.
- Induction chemotherapy does not improve results in locally advanced disease, though it may have a role in permitting larynx preservation.
- Concurrent chemotherapy and radiotherapy is a more promising approach requiring further investigation.
- Retinoids can reverse oral premalignant lesions. The role of retinoids in chemoprevention of second primary tumours is being evaluated in ongoing clinical trials.

REFERENCES

1. Forastiere, A.A., Metch, B., Schuller, D.E., Ensley, J.F., Hutchins, L.F., Triozzi, P., Kish, J.A., McClure, S., VonFeldt, E., Williamson, S.K. and Von Hoff, D. D. (1992) Randomised comparison of cisplatin plus fluorouracil and carboplatin plus fluorouracil versus methotrexate in advanced squamous-cell carcinoma of the head and neck. *J Clin Oncol*, **10**, 1245–51.
2. Jacobs, C., Lyman, G., Velez-Garcia, E., Sridhar, K.S., Knight, W., Hochster, H., Goodnough, L.T., Mortimer, J.E., Einhorn, L.H. and Schacter, L. (1992)A Phase III randomised study comparing cisplatin and fluorouracil as single agents and in combination for advanced squamous cell carcinoma of the head and neck. *J Clin Oncol*, **10**, 257–63.
3. Munro, A.J. (1995) An overview of randomised controlled trials of adjuvant chemotherapy in head and neck cancer. *British Journal of Cancer*, **71**, 83–91.
4. The Department of Veterans Affairs Laryngeal Cancer Study Group (1991) Induction chemotherapy plus radiation compared with surgery plus radiation in patients with advanced laryngeal cancer. *New Engl J Med* , **324**, 1685–90.
5. Lefebvre, J.L., Chevealier, D., Luboinski, B., Kirkpatrick, A., Collette, L. and Sahmoud, T. (1996) Larynx preservation in pyriform sinus cancer: preliminary results of a European Organisation for Research and Treatment of Cancer phase III trial. *J Natl Cancer Inst*, **88**, 890–9.
6. Lippman, S.M., Batsakis, J.G., Toth, B.B., Weber, R.S., Lee, J.J., Martin, J.W., Hays, G.L., Goepfert, H. and Hong, W.K. (1993) Comparison of low-dose isotretinoin with beta carotene to prevent oral carcinogenesis. *N Engl J Med*, **328**, 15–20.

CHAPTER 40

NASOPHARYNGEAL CARCINOMA

John E.L. Wong

DIAGNOSIS

Early Clinical Presentation

When patients present early with nasopharyngeal carcinoma, they usually present with the following:

- epistaxis
- tinnitus
- cervical lymphadenopathy

Late Clinical Presentation

Late presenting signs and symptoms are those of more extensive infiltration:

- headache, often localised to the base of skull
- cranial nerve palsies
- metastatic disease, most often to bone, lung, and liver.

Investigations

The key to initial investigation of this disease is visualisation and biopsy:

- endoscopic examination of the nasopharynx with biopsy
- CT scan /MRI of the nasopharynx and neck

Once a diagnosis is made, more extensive work-up is indicated:

- Full blood count.
- Urea and electrolytes and liver function tests.
- Serologies for EBV IgA-VCA and IgA-EA are being evaluated in patients with undifferentiated nasopharyngeal carcinoma as a means for screening and as a marker for disease.

- Chest X-ray.
- CT abdomen.
- Bone scan.

STAGING

Two staging systems are commonly used: the International Union Against Cancer (UICC) TNM and the Ho staging system. Efforts are currently underway to attempt to integrate these two staging systems.

TREATMENT

T1-2, N0-1 Disease

For early stage, T1–2, N0–1 disease, radiation therapy is indicated. More than 80% will remain disease free in the long-term with this approach.

T3–4, N2–3 Disease

Radiotherapy with or without chemotherapy is usually indicated. An American Intergroup Trial, which has so far been published only in abstract form, showed that concurrent therapy with cisplatin combined with radiotherapy, followed by cisplatin plus 5-fluorouracil was superior to radiotherapy alone. In this study, the median progression-free survival was 52 months for chemo-radiation versus only 13 months for radiation alone. The median survival was not reached for the combined arm versus 30 months for radiation alone. The two-year survival rate was 80% for the combined arm versus 55% for radiation alone. The role of neo-adjuvant chemotherapy is still under evaluation.

Metaslatic or M1 Disease

Palliation with chemotherapy, such as cisplatin, 5-fluorouracil, methotrexate, anthracycline, bleomycin is usually indicated for metastatic nasopharyngeal cancer. Palliative radiotherapy is indicated for bone metastasis.

Locally Recurrent Disease

Consideration is given to further radiotherapy, surgery or chemotherapy as appropriate.

REFERENCES

Fandi, A., Altun, M., Azli, N., Armand, J.P. and Cvitkovic, E. (1994) Nasopharyngeal cancer: Epidemiology, staging, and treatment. *Semin. Oncol,* 21(3), 382.

Teo, P.M., Leung, S.F., Yu, P., Tsao, S.Y., Foo, .W. and Shiu, W. (1991) A comparison of Ho's, International Union Against Cancer, and American Joint Committee Stage Classification for nasopharyngeal carcinoma. *Cancer,* 67(2), 434.

Laramore, G.E. (ed.) (1989) *Radiation Therapy of Head and Neck Cancer.* Berlin: Springer-Verlag.

Al-Sarraf, M., LeBlanc, M., Giri, P.G.S., Fu, K., Cooper, J., Vuong, T., Forstiere, A., Adams, G., Sakr, W., Schuller, D. and Ensley, J. (1996) Superiority of chemo-radiotherapy versus radiotherapy in patients with locally advanced nasopharyngeal cancer: preliminary results of Intergroup (0099) randomized study. *Proc Amer Soc Clin Oncol.*, **15**, 882a.

International Nasopharynx Cancer Study Group (1996) Preliminary results of a randomized trial comparing neoadjuvant chemotherapy (cisplatin, epirubicin, bleomycin) plus radiotherapy versus radiotherapy alone in stage IV (>/= N2, M0) undifferentiated nasopharyngeal carcinoma: A positive effect on progression free survival. *Int J of Radiat Oncol Biol Phys,* **35**(3), 463.

Boussen, H., Cvitkovic, E., Wendling, J.L., Azli, N., Bachouchi, M., MahJouib, R., Kalifa, C., Wibault, P., Schwaab, G. and Armand, J.P. (1991) Chemotherapy of metastatic and/or recurrent undifferentiated nasopharyngeal carcinoma with cisplatin, bleomycin, and 5-fluorouracil. *J Clin Oncol* , **9**(9), 1675.

PART X

MELANOMA

FAST FACT SHEET 5

MELANOMA

H. L. Nguyen and Bruce K. Armstrong

WORLD IMPACT

In 1985, some 92,000 new cases of melanoma were diagnosed worldwide[1]. In the same year, melanoma caused an estimated 31,000 deaths[2].

The incidence of melanoma varies 100-fold among different countries. The highest incidence rates of melanoma in 1988–92 were recorded in Australia and New Zealand, North America and Europe, particularly the Scandinavian populations. Rates in Asian populations were very low[3].

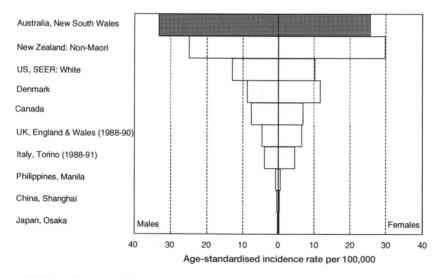

Figure FFS 5.1 Sex specific, age-standarised incidence rates of melanoma in selected countries, 1988–1992[3]

255

IMPACT IN AUSTRALIA

In 1990, 5,781 new cases of melanoma were registered in Australia, accounting for 10% of all registered cancers[4]. In 1994 in New South Wales[5], melanoma was the sixth most common cancer, after nonmelanocytic skin cancer and cancers of the prostate, colon and rectum, breast and lung. In 1995, 931 people died from melanoma in Australia, making it the ninth most frequent cancer causing death in males, and the thirteenth most frequent in females[6].

INCIDENCE BY SEX AND AGE

In 1992–95, incidence of melanoma in New South Wales, increased steadily and in parallel in males and females from 15–19 to 45–49 years of age[7]. Thereafter, rates rose much more rapidly with age in males than females, with rates in male patients aged in their 80s about double those in females. Over all ages, the incidence was 50% higher in males than in females.

INEQUALITIES IN INCIDENCE

Melanoma incidence increased steeply with increasing socioeconomic status in urban communities in New South Wales in 1983–95[7]. A weaker, opposite trend was observed in rural and remote communities. Incidence in Sydney was more than 50% higher in the highest quintile of socioeconomic status than in the lowest quintile in both sexes.

The death rate from melanoma in 1979–88 in people born in Australia was substantially higher than in Australian residents born in other countries[8]. The rate was almost twice that in migrants from the United Kingdom and Ireland and more than twice that in migrants from Southern and Eastern Europe.

Table FFS 5.1 Australian melanoma statistics

Statistics	Males	Females
Crude incidence 1990	36.7 per 100,000	31.0 per 100,000
Age adjusted incidence 1990	30.9 per 100,000	24.9 per 100,000
Cumulative incidence to 75 years of age 1990	3.3%	2.6%
Crude mortality 1995	6.7 per 100,000	3.6 per 100,000
Age adjusted mortality 1995	5.1 per 100,000	2.5 per 100,000
Person years of life lost to 75 years of age 1990	6 525 years	4 167 years
Trend in age adjusted incidence 1983 to 1995 in New South Wales	+3.6% p.a.	Stable
Trend in age adjusted mortality 1983 to 1995 in New South Wales	+0.9%p.a.	−1.4% p.a.
Five year relative survival 1977–94 in South Australia	85.8%	92.1%

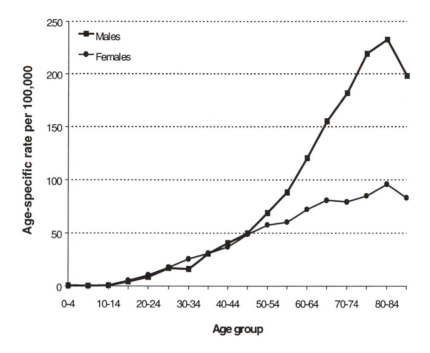

Figure FFS 5.2 Age-specific incidence rates of melanoma by sex and age in New South Wales, 1992–1995[7]

INCIDENCE AND MORTALITY TRENDS

Melanoma incidence in males in New South Wales increased irregularly from 1983 to 1995[7]. In females, incidence reached a peak in 1988, fell by 14%, and was then steady from 1989 to 1995. In Australia as a whole, mortality from melanoma increased steadily in males and females from 1931–34 to 1985–89, but at a higher rate in males than females. It increased further in 1991–94 in males but fell back a little in females[9].

SURVIVAL RATE

The five-year relative survival rate from melanoma in South Australia increased from 85.3% in those diagnosed in 1977–85 to 90.6% in those diagnosed in 1986–94[10]. Females diagnosed in 1977–94 had a higher five-year relative survival rate than males, the respective rates being 92% and 86%. In the same period, the relative survival rate was highest in those under 55 years of age (92.0%) and least in those 75 years of age and over (81.6%). People with thin melanomas (less than 0.76 mm in thickness) diagnosed in 1980–95 had a five-year relative survival rate of 99.0% compared with 65.0% in those with thick lesions (greater than 3.00 mm). Differences in survival rates among age groups could be explained by differences by age in the distribution of melanoma thickness.

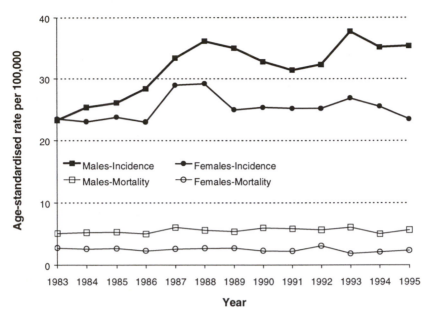

Figure FFS 5.3 Trends in annual age-standardised incidence and mortality rates of melanoma in New South Wales, 1983 to 1995[7]

RISK FACTORS

Exposure to ultraviolet radiation in sunlight is the main cause of melanoma. It has been estimated that 94% of all melanomas in Australia would not occur if there were no exposure to sunlight[11]. Risk of melanoma is thought to vary with both amount and pattern of sun exposure, with increasing intermittency of exposure being associated with increasing risk. Sun exposure in early life may be particularly important. In Australia, the risk of melanoma is highest in people who were born in Australia or who migrated to Australia in the first 15 years of life.

Genetic factors are also important. Risk is much higher in people of white, European origin than it is in black people and in people of Asian origin, and among people of white European origin, risk is highest in those with fair, sun sensitive skin. Mutation of the CDKN2 gene is associated with a greatly increased risk of melanoma.

The numbers of melanocytic naevi, particularly atypical naevi and freckles on the skin, are also independent, strong predictors of melanoma risk.

Other factors that may increase risk of melanoma are exposure to artificial sources of ultraviolet radiation, such as sun lamps, tanning booths and sun beds, occupational exposure to ionising radiation, immunosuppressive therapy such as following renal transplantation, and injury to the skin.

REFERENCES

1. Parkin, D.M., Pisani, P. and Ferlay, J. (1993) Estimates of the worldwide incidence of eighteen major cancers in 1985. *Int J Cancer,* 54, 594–606.

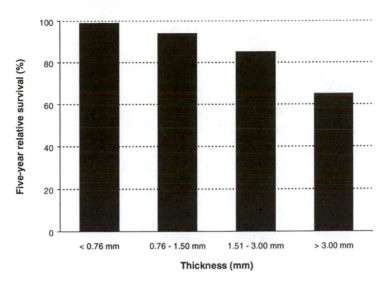

Figure FFS 5.4 Five-year relative survival by thickness of melanoma in South Australia, 1980–95[10]

2. Pisani, P., Parkin, D.M. and Ferlay, J. (1993) Estimates of the worldwide mortality from eighteen major cancers in 1985. Implications for prevention and projections of future burden. *Int J Cancer*, **55**, 891–903.

3. Parkin DM, Whelan SL, Ferlay J, Raymond L, Young J. (1997) *Cancer Incidence in Five Continents Volume VII*, Lyon, International Agency for Research on Cancer.

4. Jelfs, P., Coates, M., Giles, G., Shugg, D., Threlfall, T., Roder, D., Ring, I., Shadbolt, B. and Condon, J. (1996) *Cancer in Australia 1989–1990 (with projections to 1995)*. Canberra: Australian Institute of Health and Welfare.

5. Coates, M. and Armstrong, B. (1997) *Cancer in New South Wales Incidence and Mortality 1994*. Sydney: NSW Cancer Council.

6. Australian Bureau of Statistics (1996) *Causes of Death Australia 1995*. Canberra: Australian Government Publishing Service.

7. Nguyen, H.L., Armstrong, B. and Coates, M. (1997) *Cutaneous melanoma in NSW in 1983 to 1995*. Sydney: New South Wales Cancer Council.

8. Giles, G., Jelfs, P. and Kliewer, E. (1995) *Cancer mortality in migrants to Australia 1979–1988*. Canberra: Australian Institute of Health and Welfare.

9. Giles, G.G., Armstrong, B.K., Burton, R.C., Staples, M.P. and Thursfield, V.J. (1996) Has mortality from melanoma stopped rising in Australia? Analysis of trends between 1931 and 1994. *BMJ*, **312**, 1121–1125.

10. South Australian Cancer Registry (1996) *Epidemiology of Cancer in South Australia. Incidence, mortality and survival 1977 to 1995, incidence and mortality 1995 analysed by type and geographical location - nineteen years of data*. Adelaide: South Australian Health Commission.

11. Armstrong, B.K. and English, D.R. (1996) Cutaneous malignant melanoma. In *Cancer Epidemiology and Prevention*, edited by D. Schottenfeld and J.F. Fraumeni, pp. 1282–1312. New York: Oxford University Press.

CHAPTER 41

MELANOMA AND
OTHER SKIN CANCERS

William H. McCarthy

INTRODUCTION

Skin cancers are the most common cancers in the world but, fortunately, only melanoma has a high propensity to disseminate and cause death if not treated early and adequately. All skin cancers if treated early are curable.

MELANOMA

Classification

The morphological classification of melanoma includes superficial spreading melanoma, nodular melanoma, acral lentiginous melanoma and lentigo maligna melanoma (Hutchinson's melanotic freckle melanoma). However, the morphological classification has little practical value and has been superseded by the pTNM system based on Breslow tumour thickness.

Breslow thickness is the maximum vertical diameter of the melanoma measured from the granular cell layer of the epidermis to the deepest identifiable melanoma cell, ignoring tumour infiltration down hair follicles. The pTNM system classifies melanoma as:

- pTis: melanoma *in situ*
- pT1: melanoma ≤ 0.75 mm thick
- pT2: melanoma > 0.75–1.5 mm thick
- pT3a: melanoma >1.5–3.0 mm thick
- pT3b: melanoma > 3.0–4.0 mm thick
- pT4: melanoma > 4.0 mm thick

The AJCC/UICC staging system includes:

- Stage 1: pT1 or pT2 with no nodes or metastasis

- Stage 2: pT3 and pT4 with no nodes or metastasis
- Stage 3: Any patient with nodal metastasis and no systemic metastasis
- Stage 4: Any patient with any node metastasis but systemic metastasis detected

Clinical Diagnosis

The diagnosis of melanoma is made on the history of change in size or colour of a lesion, a change in surface characteristics or elevation of part of the lesion. Alternatively, a pigmented lesion may be noted to look different from other naevi even though there is no history of change.

Melanoma may arise from clear skin as well as from a pre-existing mole. While a change in pigmentation is usually apparent, it is wise to remember that some melanomas are amelanotic and present merely as a change in size or the appearance of a new non pigmented lesion.

The history of change is usually measured in months. Sometimes an intermittent itch is noted in association with melanoma development, but pain is not a feature of primary melanoma. Bleeding may occur but only in response to local trauma and in more locally advanced tumours.

The key to clinical diagnosis of a pigmented melanoma is irregularity of the lesion. Irregularity of colour is the most important, and the presence of a variety of colours in any one lesion is a key feature. While black or blue/black colour is the most usual feature, many other shades of brown, blue, red, grey or white are often seen. The irregularity of the outline is the second most common feature (see Colour Plates 3A to 3E, page 398).

The ABCDE system for the diagnosis of melanoma has gained general support and is defined as:

A: Indicates an asymmetrical lesion.

B: Indicates a border that is irregular, resembling a coastline with bays and promontories around the edge. Part of the border is usually well defined.

C: Defines colour variegation.

D: Indicates that melanomas are usually > 6.0 mm in diameter when first diagnosed but it is possible to diagnose smaller melanomas, particularly in nodular lesions.

E: Initially indicated elevation but the diagnosis of melanoma should be made when it is flat or with marginal elevation. E may be used to remind the clinician to examine a patient's other pigmented lesions to discern the difference in appearance of the suspicious lesion.

Biopsy of Suspicious Lesions

Where melanoma is suspected, referral for a second opinion or biopsy with a 2 mm margin is recommended. A clinically obvious melanoma may best be treated by referral to an appropriate specialist clinician.

Surgical Treatment of Primary Melanoma

Treatment of primary melanoma is based on the tumour thickness measurement. Generally accepted margins are:

- (pTis) melanoma *in situ*: margin 5 mm
- (pT1, pT2) melanoma 0–1.5 mm: margin 1 cm
- (pT3) melanoma > 1.5–4 mm: minimum margin 1 cm and maximum margin 2 cm

- (pT4) melanoma > 4.0 mm: minimum margin 2 cm and maximum margin 3 cm

There is no evidence that a margin >1 cm offers additional benefit for the patient in terms of survival but may decrease local recurrence. The depth of excision should equal the minimum excision margin where possible. It is not necessary to excise beyond the deep fascia.

Treatment of Lymph Nodes

Prophylactic lymph node dissection is not recommended for the majority of patients with melanoma. There are two randomised controlled trials which have suggested a marginal benefit for specific subsets of patients, but these subsets may better be treated with sentinel node biopsy and therapeutic lymphadenectomy where positive nodes are detected on sentinel node biopsy.

Sentinel Node Biopsy

Sentinel node biopsy is an unproven technique for the management of melanoma. However, preliminary studies have indicated a high degree of reliability for the technique and thus it may be recommended for specific groups of patients as an alternative to an observation policy or prophylactic node dissection for specific subsets of patients.

The sentinel node biopsy technique involves the identification of the 'sentinel node' by lymphoscintigraphy and biopsy of that specific node. Following histopathological examination of the sentinel node, radical lymph node dissection is recommended for those patients where melanoma is detected in the node.

Clinically Involved Node(s)

- Clinically involved nodes should be confirmed by needle biopsy rather than open excision biopsy to avoid the risk of tumour spillage at excisional biopsy.
- Radical lymph node dissection is recommended for confirmed lymph node involvement.
- A high risk of local recurrence in lymph nodes field exists without thorough formal dissection of all lymph nodes in the involved field.

Investigations

- Extensive investigation of patients with primary melanomas < pT4 is not necessary and it is rare to detect lymph node metastasis at the time of primary diagnosis.
- Chest X-rays, liver function tests and a full blood count, usually are adequate except for locally advanced tumours.
- Ultrasonography of the draining lymph node field for pT3 and pT4 tumours may be indicated.
- Bone scans, CT scans and magnetic resonance imaging (MRI) are only appropriate for clinically likely metastatic disease.

Outcome

Melanoma is curable if diagnosed early. T1 tumours carry a good prognosis with more than a 97% ten-year survival rate, but the survival rate drops to < 40% once tumour thickness exceeds 4 mm. The ten-year survival rate of patients with a single lymph node involved is 50% but drops to 10% when > 3 nodes are involved. Systemic metastases are almost invariably fatal with a < 5% five year survival rate regardless of therapy.

Desmoplastic Neurotropic Melanoma

Desmoplastic neurotropic melanoma has a higher risk of local recurrence, so an additional margin of excision of 1–2 cm is recommended for these primary melanomas. Radiotherapy is sometimes also used in an attempt to prevent local recurrence but as yet there is no evidence of the efficacy of this modality for this tumour.

Lentigo Malignant Melanoma

Lentigo malignant melanoma should be treated on the tumour thickness measurement (see Colour Plate 3C, page 398). However, these lesions are commonly on the face and narrow margins may be necessary to avoid damage to important structures such as the eyelids. Cosmetic considerations will determine the nature of the closure procedure for these facial melanomas.

Acral Lentiginous Melanoma

Acral lentiginous melanomas on the weight bearing areas of the foot require specialist reconstruction to enable comfortable walking following excision of the primary lesion (see Colour Plate 3D, page 398).

Melanoma in Childhood

Melanoma in childhood should be treated on the basis of tumour thickness, exactly as would be determined for the same lesion in the adult.

Non-Cutaneous Melanoma of the Mucous Surfaces of the Mouth, Nose, Anus, Vulva and Vagina

These lesions carry a poor prognosis but should be treated by surgical excision with appropriate local reconstruction determined by the site of the melanoma.

Follow-Up

All patients with invasive melanoma should be followed up for a period of at least 10 years. Patients with thicker melanomas, pT3, pT4, and Stage 3 melanoma require relatively close follow-up, while thin melanomas may be followed up less aggressively. A common regimen for thin tumours is a 6-monthly review for 2 years and then instructions to the patient to return if any untoward events, such as lumps under the skin or lumps in the lymph node field, become apparent. Patients with thicker melanomas may be followed on a 4-monthly basis for 2–3 years, 6-monthly basis for a further 2 years and yearly thereafter. Extensive investigation during the follow-up period is not required. All investigations should be done only on clinical suspicion of metastasis.

Radiotherapy for Melanoma

Radiotherapy is not recommended for the treatment of primary melanoma, but is used for local control of advanced primary lesions, the prevention of recurrence following a dissection of involved lymph nodes and for palliative treatment for metastases.

Locoregional Melanoma

Recurrence of melanoma in a limb, i.e. intransit metastasis, is best treated by isolation perfusion or infusion. In this procedure the limb is isolated by a tourniquet, catheters are placed in the artery and vein leading into the limb and high-dose chemotherapy is given. These treatments will achieve 60–70% complete remission but long-term control of only 25%.

NON-MELANOMA SKIN CANCER

Introduction

Squamous and basal cell carcinomas are the most common forms of skin cancer and are the most highly prevalent cancers in the world. In high sunlight countries such as Australia with a population with genetic susceptibility, such as Anglo-Saxon, Irish and Celtic populations, 2 in 3 such people will have at least 1 skin cancer during their lifetime. Fortunately both basal and squamous cell cancer are relatively simply treated and cured with an early diagnosis (see Colour Plates 1 and 2, page 397).

Basal Cell Carcinoma

Basal cell carcinoma (BCC) is the most common of the skin cancers with a high prevalence on sun-exposed areas of the body, particularly the face, shoulders and lower arms, and legs. Basal cell carcinoma presents as a small, pearly grey nodule in the skin, growing slowly over a period of 6–12 months, in some cases eventually becoming ulcerated, with the presence of minute blood vessels around the edge, or telangiectasia, and are known as nodular or cystic BCCs. These characteristics are more easily seen if the skin bearing the lesion is stretched (see Colour Plate 1A and 1B, page 397).

After a variable period of time, these nodular BCCs will ulcerate forming the well-known 'rodent' ulcer. The ulcerating BCC is characterised by an incomplete rim of pearly grey tissue with the ulcer base containing reddish granulation tissue. A third form of BCC, variously known as morphoeic, superficial spreading or sclerosing BCC presents as an ill-defined greyish patch in the skin, but the pearly appearance can usually be discerned and telangiectasia is often apparent around the edge. These lesions may have an inflammatory appearance with redness on the surface and develop scales on the surface.

Treatment

Early small BCCs are adequately treated by cryotherapy (cold therapy) or by diathermy curettage, but it is important to submit the curettings to histopathology to confirm the diagnosis. While cryotherapy may be done without a definitive diagnosis, should any evidence of local recurrence occur then a punch biopsy is necessary to confirm the diagnosis before further therapy (either by surgical excision or diathermy curettage) is undertaken. Larger BCCs are best treated by surgical excision with careful examination of the excised margins to determine the completeness of excision. The morphoeic BCC is prone to be more extensive than it appears on the surface so histological confirmation of the margins is important.

Moh's chemosurgery, which involves the serial excision with frozen section control of the BCC, has gained popularity for large BCCs and recurrent BCCs. The technique has the important advantage of careful examination of the edges to ensure completeness of removal. Repair of the residual defect is undertaken by primary closure if possible, but often a skin graft or rotation flap is necessary to close the defect. Moh's surgery requires experience and the availability of a histopathologist to assist with determination of the marginal clearance.

Squamous Cell Cancer

Squamous cell cancer (SCC) is approximately one-fifth as common as BCC and is strongly related to continuous chronic sun exposure. It is therefore more common on sun exposed skin and in white-skinned races.

Very early SCC is difficult to distinguish from BCC but it is more likely to have a scaly reddened surface or present as a hyperkeratosis, a sun cancer, which continues to develop over a period of 3–6 months (see Colour Plate 2A and 2B, page 397). Eventually the lesion will ulcerate forming a well-defined ulcer with raised, rolled and sometimes everted edges, and a base covered with a necrotic slough. A biopsy of the edge of the tumour is necessary to confirm the diagnosis before excision is contemplated. The treatment of SCC is essentially surgical with total removal, including an edge margin of at least 5 mm. Primary suture, local flap closure or skin graft are all appropriate for repair of the defect, the choice being based on size and cosmetic outcomes.

Rare Forms of Skin Cancer

Most of the rare forms of skin cancer are diagnosed only on histopathological examination of lesions suspected to be SCCs or BCCs. These rare forms of skin cancer are treated entirely by surgical excision.

REFERENCES

Australian Cancer Network (1997) *Guidelines for the Management of Cutaneous Melanoma*. Sydney: Stone Press.

Balch, C.M., Houghton, A.N., Milton, G.W., Sober, A.J. and Soong, S-J. (eds) (1992) *Cutaneous Melanoma*. Philadelphia: JB Lippincott Co.

Friedman, R.J., Rigel, D.S., Kopf, A.W., Harris, M.N. and Baker, D. (eds) (1991) *Cancer of the Skin*. Philadelphia: WB Saunders.

CHAPTER 42

MELANOMA: SYSTEMIC THERAPY

Richard F. Kefford

ADJUVANT THERAPY

A large variety of agents have been tested as adjuvant treatments following definitive surgical management of high-risk primary melanoma, including cytotoxic drugs, BCG vaccinations, levamisole, and vaccines prepared from cultured melanoma cells. The only form of adjuvant treatment to have shown a survival advantage in prospective randomised controlled clinical trials is recombinant interferon-α-2b (rIFN-α-2b).

In large doses (20 MU/m2/d intravenously (IV) for 1 month and 10 MU/m2 three times per week subcutaneously (SC) for 48 weeks), interferon-α produced a 12-month increment in median overall survival ($p < 0.02$). Although expensive, interferon treatment compares favourably with other cancer interventions in cost-effectiveness. Interferon therapy is toxic, with approximately one-half of the interferon-treated patients requiring major dose reductions. However, quality-of-life-adjusted time gained outweighed the reduced quality of life associated with treatment toxicity and relapse.

Further confirmation of this single study is recommended before standard adoption of this intensive and expensive adjuvant therapy. Meanwhile, wherever possible, eligible patients should be entered on randomised clinical trials of adjuvant therapy.

MANAGEMENT OF METASTATIC DISEASE

Philosophy of Treatment

There is no evidence that any form of systemic therapy prolongs overall survival for patients with disseminated metastatic melanoma. It is therefore advisable not to screen for asymptomatic visceral metastatic disease, and to reserve systemic therapy for patients who are either symptomatic, show early signs of weight loss, or who display rapid tumour progression. Regrettably, in a disease in which a principle objective is palliation, there are few studies of the effect of chemotherapy on quality of life. Such studies are now in progress.

Staging Procedures

Staging investigations should only be performed in relation to a defined management objective, or in accordance with the stratification requirements of prospective clinical trials. Magnetic resonance imaging (MRI) is the most sensitive test for cerebral metastases. When used with gadolinium the sensitivity for leptomeningeal disease is enhanced. Brain MRI is mandatory staging before planned surgical resection of metastatic disease. Positron emission tomography (PET) scanning is a highly sensitive tool for the detection of micrometastases, and is therefore useful in determining which patients might benefit from surgical excision of isolated metastatic deposits.

Chemotherapy

- Metastatic melanoma is relatively resistant to treatment with cytotoxic drugs. Partial responses to single agents occur in less than 25% of treated patients, and complete responses in less than 5%.
- The single agent with the highest reproducible response rate is dacarbazine (DTIC) with responses of 15–20%. These responses are usually short-lived (< 6 months). The usual schedule is 750 mg/m2 IV bolus every three weeks. The current first-line recommendation is single agent DTIC, outside clinical trials.
- Temozolamide is a new DTIC analogue which is administered orally and which may have equivalent efficacy. Other single agents with some activity against melanoma (15–20% response rate) are the nitrosoureas (BCNU, CCNU and fotemustine), the vinca alkaloids (vincristine, vinblastine and vindesine), cisplatin, and the taxanes (paclitaxel and docetaxel).
- Despite many initial reports of higher response rates in Phase II studies of a variety of combinations, there is currently no randomised controlled clinical trial evidence to support the superiority of any combination regime over single agent DTIC alone. Recent claims for high responses to a biochemotherapy regime utilising cisplatin, vinblastine and dacarbazine (CVD), followed by rIFN-α and rIL-2 (response rate of 60% and a CR rate of 20%), await the results of controlled trials comparing this regime to DTIC alone before this regime can be recommended as standard therapy.
- Such trials will require careful comparison of quality of life indices, as toxicity of biochemotherapy regimes is high and includes severe myelosuppression, infections, and IL-2 induced constitutional toxicity and hypotension, such that 15% of patients require intensive care support. Such toxicity is, of course, unacceptable when the principal objective of treatment is palliation and improvement in quality of life.

Predictors of Response to Chemotherapy

Predictors of response to chemotherapy in metastatic melanoma are shown in Table 42.1. Wherever possible, patients with metastatic melanoma should be referred for inclusion in clinical trials.

Table 42.1 Predictors of response to cytotoxic chemotherapy in metastatic melanoma

Response more likely	Response less likely
Subcutaneous metastases	Cerebral metastases
Cutaneous metastases	Liver metastases
Lymph node metastases	Bone metastases
Pulmonary metastases	Leptomeningeal metastases
Good performance status	Poor performance status

Experimental Immunotherapy

Spontaneous regression is common in primary melanomas. There are rare, well-documented observations of spontaneous regression of metastatic disease. There is *in vitro* and animal evidence for a cell-mediated immune response to melanoma cell surface antigens. These observations have acted to stimulate major international studies of immunotherapy strategies for both early and advanced disease. Many clinical trials of various immunotherapy strategies are currently being conducted in patients with advanced metastatic disease, but the fundamental principles of immunotherapy suggest that hints of activity in advanced disease may be most productively utilised in the adjuvant setting.

Immunotherapies which have shown some activity in metastatic disease in Phase II trials include the use of vaccination with melanoma cell-surface membranes or purified peptide components of common melanoma cell surface antigens, such as those of the MAGE family. Recent advances on these strategies include the addition of cytokines, such as GM-CSF, IL2 or interferon-α. Cytokines may be administered systemically by subcutaneous infusion, or locally in the site of vaccination utilising autologous melanoma cells, dendritic cells or tumour-infiltrating lymphocytes (TILs) transduced with a retroviral or adenoviral construct containing the cytokine gene. The latter approach constitutes the basis of a number of current gene therapy trials in metastatic melanoma. Whilst systemic IL2 has activity against metastatic melanoma, toxicity with the most effective high-dose regimens, including hypotension, pulmonary oedema and renal failure, has precluded its widespread use.

Other Experimental Approaches

Melanin synthesis utilises a relatively unique biochemical pathway in the melanocyte, and this has prompted biochemical and genetic attempts at targeted therapy. Melanoma cells *in vitro* accumulate toxic levels of hydroxyquinones when treated with L-DOPA. Clinical trials of high dose carbidopa failed to reach the required serum levels of DOPA before systemic toxicity was experienced.

The promoter regions of the genes for tyrosinase and tyrosinase-related protein (TRP) offer potential targets for gene therapy approaches, such as those utilising the thymidine kinase gene in virus-dependent enzyme prodrug therapy. The high frequency of defects in the p16-CDK4-pRb pathway in metastatic melanomas raises theoretical prospects for tumour suppressor gene therapy.

Surgery and Radiotherapy in Managing Systemic Disease

Surgical excision of metastatic melanoma has an established role in the palliation of specific problems, such as large painful haemorrhagic deposits, and in selected circumstances, long-term remissions are reported, particularly after excision of isolated pulmonary metastases. An experimental role exists for bulk reduction of more extensive metastatic disease in association with immunotherapy trials.

Radiotherapy is useful in palliating symptoms from local tumour effects, particularly in bone, subcutis, lymph nodes, mediastinum, and in spinal cord compression. Phase II studies have reported radiosensitising advantages of the use of concurrent procarbazine, cisplatin and fotemustine. Recommendations regarding the use of these and other radiosensitisers, such as tirapazamine, await evidence of efficacy in randomised studies. The management of specific metastatic problems in patients with disseminated melanoma is summarised in Table 42.2.

Table 42.2 Management of specific metastatic problems in disseminated melanoma

Problem	Treatment
Isolated cerebral metastases	Surgical excision and whole brain radiotherapy Stereotactic radiosurgery (selected cases)
Multiple cerebral metastases	Dexamethasone and whole brain radiotherapy Radiosensitising chemotherapy (experimental) Systemic fotemustine, procarbazine or CCNU (selected cases)
Extremity satellitosis (inoperable)	Cryotherapy Intralesional thio-TEPA Isolated limb perfusion/infusion (hyperthermic melphalan) Hindquarter amputation
Intestinal mucosal metastases with haemorrhage or obstruction	Surgical resection
Leptomeningeal metastases	Intrathecal thio-TEPA/methotrexate
Retro-orbital, retinal metastases	Radiotherapy
Bulky, unresectable symptomatic nodal or soft tissue disease	Radiotherapy Radiosensitising chemotherapy (experimental)

REFERENCES

Atkins, M.B. (1997) The treatment of metastatic melanoma with chemotherapy and biologics (see comments). *Curr Opin Oncol*, 9(2), 205–13.

Coates, A., Thomson, D., McLeod, G.R., et al. (1993) Prognostic value of quality of life scores in a trial of chemotherapy with or without interferon in patients with metastatic malignant melanoma (see comments). *Eur J Cancer*, 29a(12), 1731–4.

Cole, B.F., Gelber, R.D., Kirkwood, J.M., Goldhirsch, A., Barylak, E. and Borden, E. (1996) Quality-of-life-adjusted survival analysis of interferon alpha-2b adjuvant treatment of high-risk resected cutaneous melanoma: an Eastern Cooperative Oncology Group study (see comments). *J Clin Oncol*, 14(10), 2666–73.

Demierre, M.F. and Koh, H.K. (1997) Adjuvant therapy for cutaneous malignant melanoma. *J Am Acad Dermatol*, 36(5 Pt 1), 747–64.

Ewend, M.G., Carey, L.A. and Brem, H. (1996)Treatment of melanoma metastases in the brain. *Semin Surg Oncol,*12(6), 429–35.

Gurney, H., Coates, A. and Kefford, R. (1991) The use of l-dopa and carbidopa in metastatic malignant melanoma. *J Invest Dermatology,* 96, 85–87.

Hillner, B.E., Kirkwood, J.M., Atkins, M.B., Johnson, E.R. and Smith, TJ. (1997) Economic analysis of adjuvant interferon alfa-2b in high-risk melanoma based on projections from Eastern Cooperative Oncology Group 1684. *J Clin Oncol,* 15(6), 2351–8.

Houghton, A.N., Meyers, M.L. and Chapman, P.B. (1996) Medical treatment of metastatic melanoma. *Surg Clin North Am,* 76(6), 1343–54.

Kirkwood, J.M., Strawderman, M.H., Ernstoff, M.S., Smith, T.J., Borden, E.C. and Blum, R.H. (1996) Interferon alfa-2b adjuvant therapy of high-risk resected cutaneous melanoma: the Eastern Cooperative Oncology Group Trial EST 1684 [see comments]. *J Clin Oncol,* 14(1), 7–17.

Kirkwood, J.M., Wazer, D. and Rosenstein, M. (1997) Interferon adjuvant therapy of melanoma [letter; comment]. *Cancer,* 79(9), 1843–6.

Kirkwood, J.M., Resnick, G.D., and Cole, B.F. (1997) Efficacy, safety, and risk-benefit analysis of adjuvant interferon alfa- 2b in melanoma. *Semin Oncol,* 24(1 suppl. 4), S16–23.

Legha, S.S., Ring, S., Bedikian, A., et al. (1996) Treatment of metastatic melanoma with combined chemotherapy containing cisplatin, vinblastine and dacarbazine (CVD) and biotherapy using interleukin-2 and interferon-alpha. *Ann Oncol,* 7(8), 827–35.

Legha, S.S. (1997) Durable complete responses in metastatic melanoma treated with interleukin-2 in combination with interferon alpha and chemotherapy. *Semin Oncol,* 24(1 suppl. 4), S39–43.

Legha, S.S. (1997) The role of interferon alfa in the treatment of metastatic melanoma. *Semin Oncol,* 24(1 suppl. 4), S24–31.

Leong, S.P. (1996) Immunotherapy of malignant melanoma. *Surg Clin North Am,* 76(6), 1355–81.

Nathan, F.E., Berd, D., Mastrangelo, M.J. (1997) Chemotherapy of melanoma. In *The Chemotherapy Source Book* (2nd edn), edited by M.C. Perry, pp. 1043–1069. Baltimore: Williams and Wilkins.

Reintgen, D. and Kirkwood, J. (1997) The adjuvant treatment of malignant melanoma. J Fla Med Assoc, 84(3), 147–52.

Reintgen, D., Balch, C.M., Kirkwood, J., Ross, M. (1997) Recent advances in the care of the patient with malignant melanoma [see comments]. *Ann Surg,* 225(1), 1–14.

Rosenberg, S.A., Yang, J.C., Topalian, S.L., et al. (1994) Treatment of 283 consecutive patients with metastatic melanoma or renal cell cancer using high-dose bolus interleukin 2 [see comments]. *Jama,* 271(12), 907–13.

Rosenthal, M.A., Bull, C.A., Coates, A.S., et al. (1991) Synchronous cisplatin infusion during radiotherapy for the treatment of metastatic melanoma. *Eur J Cancer,* 27(12), 1564–6.

Thomson, D.B., Adena, M., McLeod, G.R., et al. (1993) Interferon-alpha 2a does not improve response or survival when combined with dacarbazine in metastatic malignant melanoma: results of a multi-institutional Australian randomized trial. *Melanoma Res,* 3(2),133–8.

PART XI

HAEMATOLOGICAL MALIGNANCIES

CHAPTER 43

MOLECULAR GENETICS OF HAEMATOLOGICAL DISEASES

Harry J. Iland

INTRODUCTION

Cancers result from acquired abnormalities of genes which code for proteins involved in the control of normal intracellular signal transduction, cell growth and differentiation. These abnormalities include point mutations, gene amplification, gene deletion, retroviral transactivation and gene rearrangements. Of these, gene rearrangements are fundamentally important in the pathogenesis of leukaemias and lymphomas, and generally result from reciprocal chromosomal translocations. Other structural cytogenetic lesions such as deletions and inversions occur less commonly. The techniques used to identify genetic abnormalities utilise whole chromosomes, genomic DNA or cellular RNA, and include:

- chromosome analysis (G-banding)
- fluorescence *in situ* hybridisation (FISH) — hybridisation of labelled DNA probes to metaphase or interphase chromosome preparations
- Southern (DNA) and northern (RNA) blotting — hybridisation of labelled gene-specific probes to genomic DNA or cellular RNA which has been transferred to membranes following size-separation by electrophoresis
- polymerase chain reaction (PCR) — amplification of genomic DNA using gene-specific primers
- reverse transcriptase-polymerase chain reaction (RT-PCR) — reverse transcriptase synthesis of a cDNA copy of RNA which can then be amplified by PCR

Since haematological malignancies are, with rare exceptions, monoclonal diseases, the genetic abnormalities which occurred at or before the onset of cell transformation will be present in the whole malignant cell population. Selected abnormalities can therefore be exploited as tumour markers which are disease-specific and, in some instances, patient-specific. The identification and characterisation of these genetic abnormalities has many applications:

273

- Improvement in the classification of leukaemias and lymphomas (with respect to treatment response and prognosis).
- Improvement in the detection of minimal residual disease (MRD) after conventional therapy.
- Facilitating the design of disease-specific therapy (e.g. antisense oligonucleotide technology).
- Selection of patients most likely to benefit from stem cell transplantation strategies.
- Evaluation of purging techniques and conditioning regimens used in transplantation.
- Evaluation of post-transplant strategies designed to enhance a graft-versus-tumour effect (e.g. donor lymphocyte infusions).

GENE REARRANGEMENTS

Translocations which cause gene rearrangements juxtapose sequences from two disparate genes. Over 60 different non-random chromosomal translocations have been recognised in haematological malignancies, and the number is steadily increasing. These translocations, their associated gene rearrangements, and the diseases in which they are found are tabulated in an exhaustive and excellent review by Drexler et al., 1995. The consequences of gene rearrangements are either:

- generation of a novel fusion gene derived from the two original genes, resulting in a novel chimaeric protein product, or
- altered expression of one of the rearranged genes resulting from the influence of regulatory regions belonging to the other rearranged gene.

Immunoglobulin genes and T-cell receptor genes also undergo rearrangement during the normal development of B-lymphocytes and T-lymphocytes respectively. These rearrangements cannot be recognised by chromosomal analysis and are not of pathogenetic importance. However, they are useful molecular markers of monoclonality in lymphoid malignancies and can be utilised in MRD assessment.

MYELOID MALIGNANCIES

Gene rearrangements in myeloid malignancies result in the formation of novel fusion genes.

Chronic Myeloid Leukaemia (CML)

In 95% of patients with chronic myeloid leukaemia (CML), cytogenetic analysis reveals a reciprocal translocation, t(9;22), resulting in rearrangement of the BCR and c-ABL genes on the long arms of chromosomes 22 and 9 respectively. The BCR-ABL fusion (Stam et al., 1985) on the derivative chromosome 22 (the Philadelphia chromosome) encodes a p210 protein with markedly enhanced tyrosine kinase activity. Cytogenetic analysis is useful in monitoring the response to alpha-interferon, since an interferon-induced reduction in the proportion of Philadelphia positive metaphases below 35% is associated with a significant prolongation of the chronic phase of the disease, and hence of overall survival. Several non-random cytogenetic abnormalities occur frequently in association with acute leukaemic transformation of the disease (e.g. second Philadelphia chromosome, trisomy 8, isochromosome 17, etc.). RT-PCR is used primarily to monitor MRD following allogeneic and autologous stem cell transplantation. The sensitivity of detection of the BCR-ABL fusion transcript by RT-PCR is around one leukaemic cell in 10^5–10^6 normal cells. Following transplantation, RT-PCR positivity may persist for up to 12 months. Patients who become and remain persistently

RT-PCR negative have a high probability of being cured, whereas persistence of, or reversion to, RT-PCR positivity generally heralds haematological and clinical relapse.

Acute Promyelocytic Leukaemia (APL)

Acute promyelocytic leukaemia (APL) is uniquely associated with a t(15;17) translocation. Two transcription factor genes, PML and RARα, are disrupted by the translocation which generates a PML-RARα leukaemia-specific fusion gene on the derivative chromosome 15. Accurate recognition of APL is essential, since optimal treatment (all-*trans* retinoic acid plus intensive anthracycline-based chemotherapy) is distinct from that used in other forms of acute myeloid leukaemia (AML). RT-PCR for the PML-RARα fusion transcript is the most reliable assay for establishing the diagnosis and for monitoring MRD. Published studies consistently demonstrate correlations between persistent or recurrent RT-PCR positivity and clinical relapse on the one hand, and between persistent RT-PCR negativity and continuing remission on the other (Miller et al., 1993).

Other Forms of AML

In addition to APL, two other subtypes of AML are associated with a relatively good prognosis. Both the t(8;21) translocation and the inv(16) (i.e. inversion of chromosome 16) produce abnormal chimaeric transcription factors which are derived from different DNA-binding subunits of a normal transcriptional regulator known as core binding factor (CBF). CBFα2 is encoded by the AML1 gene which is rearranged in t(8;21) leukaemias, and the gene encoding the CBFβ chain is rearranged in inv(16) leukaemias. Leukaemias carrying t(15;17), t(8;21) or inv(16) account for approximately 30–40% of all AML. In contrast with APL, virtually all patients with t(8;21), including those in long-term remission after allogeneic transplantation, remain positive for fusion transcripts by RT-PCR. The role of molecular monitoring for t(8;21) and inv(16) has not yet been adequately defined.

LYMPHOID MALIGNANCIES

Normal Immunoglobulin and T-cell Receptor Gene Rearrangements in Lymphoid Malignancies

The ability of the immune system to recognise a diverse range of antigens stems from a series of recombinase-mediated immunoglobulin and T-cell receptor (TCR) gene rearrangements which occur normally during B-cell and T-cell ontogeny. The immunoglobulin heavy chain (IgH) locus consists of approximately 100 variable (V_H) gene segments, approximately 30 diversity (D) segments, and six joining (J_H) segments. After rearrangement, a unique VDJ sequence is present and this codes for the variable region of the IgH polypeptide chain. The κ and λ immunoglobulin light chain (IgL) genes, as well as the α/δ, β and γ gene loci whose products constitute the TCR, undergo a comparable series of rearrangements. Further diversity arises from small deletions (exonucleolytic nibbling), non-templated additions mediated by terminal deoxynucleotidyl transferase, and somatic hypermutation. The final DNA sequence is unique to the lymphocyte in which these events occur, and also to all its progeny.

Although Southern blotting has traditionally been used to demonstrate monoclonal rearrangement of immunoglobulin and TCR genes, PCR strategies are becomingly increasingly popular. By sequencing the rearranged region, more sensitive clone-specific PCR systems can be developed (Jonsson et al., 1990) which are suitable for the study of MRD (~1 malignant cell in 100 000 normal cells). Several reports have shown that persisting PCR positivity in childhood acute lymphoblastic leukaemia (ALL) correlates with an increased likelihood of relapse, and quantitative studies have demonstrated that the extent of minimal residual disease in early remission is closely related to the probability of relapse.

Deregulated Gene Expression in Non-Hodgkin's Lymphomas and ALL

Errors in immunoglobulin and TCR recombination underlie many of the chromosomal translocations and associated gene rearrangements that are seen in lymphoproliferative disorders. In general, a gene involved in a critical cell function is rearranged into an IgH or IgL gene locus (in B-cell malignancies), or into a TCR locus (in T-cell diseases) (Korsmeyer, 1992). Its coding region remains intact, but its expression comes under the control of regulatory elements from the immunoglobulin or TCR gene. The resulting deregulation of gene expression may be quantitative or qualitative (i.e. expression in an inappropriate cell lineage).

The most common cytogenetic abnormality in B-cell non-Hodgkin's lymphomas is the t(14;18) translocation, found in 85% of follicular lymphomas and 20–30% of diffuse large cell lymphomas. The BCL-2 gene on chromosome 18 is translocated into the IgH gene locus on chromosome 14, resulting in high level deregulated expression of BCL-2, an inhibitor of programmed cell death (apoptosis). It therefore appears likely that this translocation prolongs survival of B-lymphocytes, predisposing them to additional mutations associated with lymphomagenesis. BCL-2 rearrangements are readily detectable by PCR amplification of genomic DNA. In mantle cell lymphoma, the Cyclin D1 gene (also known as BCL-1) is similarly rearranged into the IgH gene locus in association with a t(11;14) translocation.

The MYC oncoprotein, a member of the helix-loop-helix family of transcription factors, plays a central role in cell cycle progression. Recombination errors generate translocations which fuse all or part of the MYC gene on chromosome 8 with either the IgH or IgL genes, resulting in deregulated MYC expression. These rearrangements are found in B-cell ALL and high-grade B-cell non-Hodgkin's lymphomas, particularly the small, non-cleaved (Burkitt's and non-Burkitt's) varieties. Most rearrangements involve the IgH genes and are associated with t(8;14) translocations. Less commonly, MYC is rearranged with either the κ or λ IgL genes, characterised by t(2;8) and t(8;22) translocations respectively.

An analogous series of translocations involving components of the TCR gene complex occur in T-cell ALL, with deregulated expression of the relevant rearranged gene. The most common genetic abnormality in childhood T-cell ALL involves the stem cell leukaemia gene (SCL). An interstitial deletion of the short arm of chromosome 1, undetectable by cytogenetic analysis, results in juxtaposition of SCL with the regulatory region of the SIL (SCL interrupting locus) gene. Expression of SIL, but not SCL, normally occurs in T-cells, and aberrant SCL expression in T-cells resulting from this rearrangement is thought to be of major pathogenetic significance in the development of T-ALL.

Philadelphia Chromosome Positive ALL

Fusion genes also occur in lymphoid malignancies, and typically disrupt genes coding for transcription factors, tyrosine kinases or receptors (Drexler et al., 1995). The t(9;22) translocation seen in CML also occurs in approximately 25% of patients with adult ALL, and in a small proportion of childhood ALL. At a cytogenetic level the CML and ALL rearrangements are indistinguishable, and in about half of the ALL cases the molecular events are also indistinguishable from those seen in CML. In the remainder, the BCR gene is disrupted closer to its 5' end, resulting in a p190 BCR-ABL tyrosine kinase fusion protein. A large proportion of Philadelphia positive ALL patients remain RT-PCR positive after chemotherapy-induced complete remission, reflecting its poor prognosis. The results of RT-PCR assays in the post-transplant setting correlate closely with outcome.

ALL Associated with t(12;21)

The commonest abnormality in childhood pre-B cell ALL is the t(12;21) translocation, which generates a fusion transcription factor gene, ETV6-AML1. Preliminary reports suggest that this abnormality is associated with a good prognosis.

Abnormalities of Chromosome 11q23 in ALL and AML

A large number of translocations have been reported in which a specific region on the long arm of chromosome 11 (11q23) is consistently implicated. These leukaemias involve disruption of the MLL gene (also known as ALL-1 or HRX), with fusion to genes on chromosomes 4, 6, 9, and 19 being the most common. 11q23 abnormalities are most commonly seen in ALL and AML when it occurs during infancy, and a bilineage immunophenotype is frequently present. These leukaemias are associated with a bad prognosis. Secondary leukaemias (following topoisomerase II inhibitors such as etoposide and the anthracyclines) typically have abnormalities of 11q23 also.

POINT MUTATIONS

N-RAS Gene Mutations

The GTPase superfamily of RAS proteins act as membrane-bound signal transducers. Point mutations which generate amino acid substitutions in the guanine–nucleotide binding domains of RAS proteins are found in approximately 20% of all human cancers. N-RAS mutations are particularly common in AML and myelodysplasia (MDS). Most evidence suggests that RAS gene mutations are not early events in leukaemia, and their clinical significance remains uncertain. In MDS, the weight of evidence suggests that N-RAS mutations predict for shorter survival and increased risk of leukaemic transformation.

p53 Gene Mutations

Mutations of the p53 gene, which normally functions as a tumour suppressor gene, are the most frequent abnormality in cancer. p53 controls cell cycle progression and enables time for DNA repair processes to take place. This helps prevent accumulation of lethal replication errors, and hence p53 has been referred to as the guardian of the genome. Point mutations (and small deletions) in p53 occur in virtually all haematological malignancies and have universally been identified as an adverse prognostic factor. They are associated with lower remission rates and decreased responsiveness to chemotherapy in AML, MDS and chronic lymphocytic leukaemia, shorter survival in AML, ALL and MDS, and increased likelihood of progression to acute leukaemia in CML and MDS.

RETROVIRAL TRANSACTIVATION

HTLV-1 and Adult T-Cell Lymphoma/Leukaemia

The only well-documented example of retroviral-induced leukaemia or lymphoma in humans has a characteristic clinical presentation and follows HTLV-1 infection after a long latent period. While the mechanism of oncogenesis is complex, a key feature appears to be an autocrine loop resulting from increased expression of both cellular interleukin-2 (T-cell growth factor) and its receptor mediated by a viral transcriptional activating protein, Tax.

REFERENCES

Drexler, H.G., Borkhardt, A. and Janssen, J.W.G. (1995) Detection of chromosomal translocations in leukemia-lymphoma cells by polymerase chain reaction. *Leukemia & Lymphoma*, **19**, 359–380.

Jonsson, O.G., Kitchens, R.L., Scott, F.C. and Smith, R.G. (1990) Detection of minimal residual disease in acute lymphoblastic leukemia using immunoglobulin hypervariable region specific oligonucleotide probes. *Blood*, **76**, 2072–2079.

Korsmeyer, S.J. (1992) Chromosomal translocations in lymphoid malignancies reveal novel proto-oncogenes. *Annual Review of Immunology*, **10**, 785–807.

Miller Jr, W.H., Levine, K., DeBlasio, A., Frankel, S.R., Dmitrovsky, E. and Warrell Jr, R.P. (1993) Detection of minimal residual disease in acute promyelocytic leukemia by a reverse transcription polymerase chain reaction assay for the PML/RAR-alpha fusion mRNA. *Blood*, **82**, 1689–1694.

Stam, K., Heisterkamp, N., Grosveld, G., de Klein, A., Verma, R.S., Coleman, M., Dosik, H. and Groffen, L. (1985) Evidence of a new chimeric *bcr/c-abl* mRNA in patients with chronic myelocytic leukemia and the Philadelphia chromosome. New England *Journal of Medicine*, **313**, 1429–1433.

CHAPTER 44

HAEMATOPOIETIC GROWTH FACTORS IN ONCOLOGY

Guy C. Toner

INTRODUCTION

- All of the elements of the blood are derived from multipotent stem cells found primarily in the bone marrow. Large numbers of cells are constantly replenished. As the cells mature they become committed to a single lineage, creating a pool of progenitor cells that further mature to become the blood cells. This process is controlled by haematopoietic growth factors (HGFs), which are naturally occurring cytokines that regulate the proliferation, differentiation and activity of blood and bone marrow cells.

- There has been an explosion of information about haematopoiesis, HGFs and HGF receptors in the last 15 years (see Table 44.1). More than 20 HGFs have been identified, cloned and recombinant proteins produced. Many have been tested in clinical trials.

- HGFs which are in common clinical use include granulocyte colony-stimulating factor (G-CSF), granulocyte-macrophage CSF (GM-CSF) and erythropoietin (EPO). Only G-CSF and EPO are marketed in Australia at present. Thrombopoietin is being actively studied in clinical trials, and it and other HGFs may soon be more widely available (see Table 44.2).

- HGFs can have pleiotropic activities (e.g. interleukin-6 which has effects on multiple organ systems) or relatively lineage restricted activity (e.g. EPO mainly effects the red cell lineage).

- There remain many unanswered questions about the clinical uses of HGFs and the cost-effectiveness of these relatively expensive agents needs further study.

Granulocyte Colony-Stimulating Factor

- G-CSF is a relatively lineage specific cytokine controlling the proliferation, differentiation and function of the neutrophil lineage. G-CSF is the primary regulator of neutrophil production.

- The receptor for G-CSF is widely expressed but the function of non-haematopoietic receptors is unclear. Mutations in the cytoplasmic domain of the receptor have been demonstrated in a small number of patients with congenital neutropenia and acute myeloid leukaemia.

Table 44.1 Features of selected haematopoietic growth factors

HGF	Synonyms	Generic Name	Haematopoietic Effects	Endogenous Sources
Granulocyte colony-stimulating factor	G-CSF, CSF-β, CSF-3	Filgrastim Lenograstim	Neutrophil proliferation and function	Monocytes/macrophages, fibroblasts, endothelial cells, keratinocytes
Erythropoietin	EPO, hemopoietin	Erythropoietin Epoietin-α	Red cells	Renal cells, hepatocytes
Granulocyte-macrophage colony-stimulating factor	[a] GM-CSF, CSF-α, CSF-2	Sargramostim Molgramostim Regramostim	Neutrophils Eosinophils Monocytes	T lymphocytes, monocytes/macrophages, fibroblasts, endothelial and epithelial cells, osteoblasts
Thrombopoietin	TPO, MGDF[a] MPL ligand		Megakaryocytes, Platelets	Endothelial cells, fibroblasts, mRNA found widely including liver, kidney
Interleukin-11	IL-11		Megakaryocytes	Stromal fibroblasts, trophoblasts
Macrophage-CSF	M-CSF, CSF-1		Macrophage Osteoclast	Stromal cells, macrophages, fibroblasts, T and B lymphocytes, endothelium, keratinocytes
Stem cell factor	SCF, Steel factor, c-Kit ligand		Multilineage progenitors	Endothelial cells, fibroblasts, circulating mononuclear cells bone marrow stromal cells

[a] MGDF: Megakaryocyte growth and development factor

- Administration of G-CSF to humans results in a dose dependant increase in neutrophils accompanied by an expansion of the myeloid compartment of the bone marrow.

- G-CSF administered after chemotherapy reduces the severity and duration of neutropenia and has been associated with up to a 50% reduction in the frequency of admission for fever and neutropenia following intensive, standard-dose chemotherapy regimens.

- G-CSF has a less clinically significant benefit if administered after the onset of neutropenic sepsis but has been demonstrated to shorten the duration of neutropenia in this setting.

- G-CSF, either alone or with chemotherapy, mobilises bone marrow progenitor cells into the peripheral blood. These progenitors can be harvested and used to support high dose chemotherapy. Peripheral blood progenitor cells have been demonstrated to be superior to bone marrow harvested progenitors in the setting of autologous transplants.

- Two forms of G-CSF are marketed in Australia. Laboratory evidence suggests increased potency per unit weight for the glycosylated form. However, no clear differences in clinical activity have been demonstrated. The two forms are:

  1. Filgrastim produced in E. coli and non-glycosylated.
  2. Lenograstim produced in mammalian cells and glycosylated

- G-CSF is administered subcutaneously, usually daily, and has little toxicity. The most common side effect is bone pain for several hours after the injection, usually relieved by simple analgesia. The mechanism of bone pain is unknown but it is worse at the time of greatest myelosuppression and early recovery of blood counts.

Erythropoietin

- EPO is the primary regulator of the late stages of red cell development. Humans deficient in EPO production develop severe anaemia.

- EPO can reduce cancer-related anaemia and chemotherapy induced anaemia, particularly when associated with a low endogenous erythropoietin level. However, its use in this setting in Australia is relatively uncommon, at least partially due to cost and the availability and safety of transfusion services.

- The incidence of hypertension and thrombotic events observed with EPO treatment for chronic renal failure has not been observed in cancer patients. The side effects of EPO in cancer patients are generally minimal.

REFERENCES

Lieschke, G.J. and Burgess, A.W. (1992) Granulocyte colony-stimulating factor and granulocyte-macrophage colony-stimulating factor. Part 1: *New England Journal of Medicine,* **327**, 28. Part 2: *New England Journal of Medicine,* **327**, 99.

Lok, S. and Foster, D.C. (1994) The structure, biology and potential therapeutic applications of recombinant thrombopoietin. *Stem Cells,* **12**, 586.

Metcalf, D. (1989) The molecular control of cell division, differentiation commitment and maturation in haematopoietic cells. *Nature,* **339**, 27.

Petersdorf, S.H. and Dale, D.C. (1995) The biology and applications of erythropoietin and the colony-stimulating factors. *Advances in Internal Medicine,* **40**, 395.

Table 44.2 Selected Potential Clinical Applications of HGFs in Oncology

Potential Applications in Cancer	Relevant HGFs	Clinical Value	Comments
Reduction of chemotherapy induced neutropenia	G-CSF GM-CSF	+++ +	Mainly used to maintain dose intensity and reduce neutropenic complications where treatment is given with curative intent. Use limited partially by cost.
Mobilisation of peripheral blood progenitor marrow cells for harvesting to support high dose chemotherapy	G-CSF GM-CSF GM-CSF SCF, TPO	+++ ++ ?	Peripheral blood harvesting has largely replaced bone marrow as a source of progenitors. G-CSF and/or chemotherapy most commonly used.
Reduction of myelosuppression after high dose chemotherapy with progenitor cell support	G-CSF GM-CSF EPO, TPO	++ + ±, ?	G-CSF and GM-CSF hasten recovery from neutropenia. However, the main determinant of recovery is the quality and quantity of progenitor cells infused.
Reduction of anaemia associated with cancer and its treatment	EPO	+	Benefit demonstrated in some patients, particularly those with low endogenous erythropoietin. Further cost-effectiveness studies needed.
Treatment of established neutropenic sepsis (therapeutic not prophylactic)	G-CSF	+	Shortens duration of neutropenia
Reduction of chemotherapy induced thrombocytopenia	TPO IL-11	? ?	Clinical trials underway.
Amelioration of cytopenias associated with myelodysplastic syndromes and bone marrow failure states	G-CSF GM-CSF EPO	+ + +	Improved blood counts can be achieved in some patients while receiving HGF. Cost-benefit studies are required.
Increase the dose intensity of chemotherapy	GM-CSF TPO	++ ?	G-CSF has enabled increases in dose intensity up to 2-fold. The clinical value of this level of increase in most tumour types remains uncertain.
Stimulate leukaemic cells to proliferate prior to cell-cycle specific chemotherapy	G-CSF	±	Randomised trials have failed to demonstrate a clear benefit.
Treatment of non-neutropenic and fungal infections	G-CSF GM-CSF	?	Further trials required.
Direct anti-tumour effect or modulation of biologic response modifiers	IL-2, IL-4, IL-12	?	Further trials required.

CHAPTER 45

THE ACUTE LEUKAEMIAS

James F. Bishop

INTRODUCTION

Leukaemias are cloned, neoplastic proliferations of immature cells, or blasts, of the haematopoietic system. Leukaemic blasts rapidly populate the bone marrow and begin to circulate in the peripheral blood with associated bone marrow failure. If untreated, acute leukaemia is rapidly fatal with death within a few weeks. Acute leukaemia has had a large impact in oncology because it has been a prototype disease to develop the management of marrow failure and the principles of chemotherapy.

INCIDENCE

Leukaemias are uncommon diseases with an Australian incidence rate of 2.5 per 100 000 for acute myeloid leukaemia (AML) and 1.3 per 100 000 for acute lymphocytic leukaemia (ALL). AML is the usual acute leukaemia of adults and ALL in children. These diseases are a leading cause of cancer death for persons under 35 years of age.

AETIOLOGY

The cause of most leukaemia is not known. A small percentage of leukaemias are secondary leukaemias often associated with prior exposure to chemotherapy or radiotherapy. Such chemotherapy includes the use of long-term alkylating agents such as nitrogen mustard, procarbazine and chlorambucil to treat lymphomas such as Hodgkin's disease. Such leukaemias commonly have abnormalities of chromosome 5 and/or 7. Secondary leukaemia has also been associated with prior use of etoposide with an associated translocation of chromosome 11q23. Predispositions to increased risk of leukaemia include Down's Syndrome, Fanconi's anaemia, Bloom's Syndrome and ataxia telangiectasia.

DIAGNOSIS OF ACUTE LEUKAEMIAS

Symptoms

The symptoms of acute leukaemia may be non-specific with the diagnosis made on a full blood examination for an ill-defined illness or in an asymptomatic patient. Most symptoms are caused by anaemia, neutropenia and thrombocytopenia due to marrow failure. Thus symptoms commonly include fatigue, malaise, dyspnoea, easy bruising, weight loss, bone or abdominal pain and infections.

Signs

Anaemia causing pallor, neutropenia causing sepsis at any site with fever, thrombocytopenia causing epistaxis or other clinical bleeding, such as haematuria and a petichael rash, are the usual signs. Patients may present with a disseminated intravascular coagulation (DIC) syndrome which is usual in patients with acute promyelocytic leukaemia.

Diagnostic Work-Up

- Full blood examination and differential white cell count
- Coagulation profile including DIC screen and fibrinogen
- Blood electrolytes including creatinine, uric acid, potassium
- Septic work-up
- Bone marrow smear and biopsy
- Chest X-ray
- Leukaemia blast cell immunophenotyping and cytogenetics
- CSF examination in patients with ALL
- CT scan of the chest in patients with ALL
- HLA typing for younger, high risk patients considered for transplantation

CLASSIFICATION OF ACUTE LEUKAEMIAS

Acute leukaemia is, if possible, divided by lineage into AML or ALL. The common classification system used is the French American British (FAB) classification.

Acute Myeloid Leukaemia (AML)

For AML there are 8 categories: FAB M0 to M7. Classification is based on light microscopy, immunophenotyping, cytogenetics and, in some cases, molecular markers and electron microscopy. The latter is recommended when megakaryocytic leukaemia (FAB-M7) is suspected. On light microscopy AML frequently stains granules with myeloperoxidase, sudan black or AS-D chloroacetate, whereas monocytic cells stain with 2-naphthyl butyrate esterase.

Acute promyelocytic leukaemia (FAB M3) has large granules in the cytoplasm (not present in FAB-M3 variant), the cytogenetic translocation t(15:17)(q22:q11) and the molecular marker, PML-RAR a fusion transcript.

Acute Lymphocytic Leukaemia (ALL)

ALL is classified as FAB L1–3. Among the 3 types the classification FAB–L3 ALL (Burkitt type; mature B cell) is important since prognosis differs from the others. For light microscopy, these types of leukaemias are negative for the above myeloid stains; periodic acid-Schiff stain is too non-specific, but the acid phosphatase is most useful in T-cell ALL. Immunophenotyping with a panel of monoclonal antibodies will determine T- or B-cell lineage more precisely.

In a small subset of patients where lineage cannot be determined on morphology, immunophenotyping using monoclonal antibodies frequently determines myeloid lineage. These are designated FAB-M0 acute myeloid leukaemia.

CYTOGENETICS

In AML the translocations t (15:17), (t 8:21) and inversion of chromosome 16 have a favourable prognoses whereas t (9:11), + 8, deletion of 5q or 7, or deletion of 9q or multiple abnormalities have a poor prognosis. The presence of the translocation seen in CML, t (9:22), is found in 30% of adults with ALL and has a poor prognosis, as does t (8:14), diagnostic of mature B-cell ALL (FAB–L3).

PROGNOSIS

Clinical factors on presentation associated with a poor prognosis include older age, male sex, low haemoglobin, high peripheral leukaemic blasts, prior haematological disorder, the absence of Auer rods and the cytogenetic changes mentioned above. Patients with older age or FAB–M3 promyelocytic leukaemia are at high risk of dying in induction. More recently, it appears that leukaemic blast cells expressing the multi-drug resistant phenotype (MDR1) or bcl-2 may have a poorer prognosis.

GENERAL PRINCIPLES OF TREATMENT OF ACUTE LEUKAEMIA

The initial aim of management is to stabilise the patient with supportive measures required for bone marrow failure to control anaemia, neutropenia and thrombocytopenia.

One aim of the diagnostic work up is to identify a haemoglobin below 9.5 g/dl requiring a transfusion of packed red cells, a neutrophil $< 1 \times 10^6$/L commonly associated with infection, and platelets < 15–20×10^6/L requiring platelet transfusions. CMV-negative blood products should be given to CMV-seronegative patients who may require future transplantation.

For afebrile patients, platelet transfusion with counts of pooled non-HLA matched platelets may be required second daily when the platelet count is 15×10^6/L. For unwell patients, especially those with DIC or HLA antibodies, platelet counts of $< 20 \times 10^6$/L or below will require platelet transfusions. An important principle of platelet transfusion management is to check the platelet count preferably 1 hour after the transfusion to identify a clinically useful increase in platelet numbers to sustain the patient for the subsequent 24 hours. If unsuccessful, single donor, fresh HLA matched platelets should be considered.

INFECTION

Most patients with leukaemia who die in the first 3 weeks of diagnosis, die of infection or, less commonly, bleeding. Infection and fever occurs in the great majority of patients undergoing remission induction therapy for acute leukaemia. All patients with falling neutrophils below 0.5×10^6/L, and especially below 0.1×10^6/L, will get an infection. Signs may be minimal because of the lack of neutrophils.

The principles of management are to establish a large permanent indwelling (Hickman's) catheter, to know the frequent pathogenic organisms in the hospital or ward, to be vigilant to identify specific septic foci, to take appropriate swabs and blood cultures to identify the infecting organism, to initiate the standard institutional antibiotic policy for febrile neutropenia empirically without waiting for the microbiology. The specific antibiotics need to be reassessed each day. Antibiotics may need to be changed at 48 or 72 hours if infection persists.

The work-up should also establish the presence of DIC, high uric acid or renal failure. Following therapy, a tumourlysis syndrome may occasionally occur. More frequently the specific effects of chemotherapy must be managed. These include nausea and vomiting which may require a 5-HT$_3$ antagonist, anorexia, mucositis and enterocolitis. Cerebellar ataxia and conjunctivitis may accompany high-dose cytarabine therapy.

SPECIFIC TREATMENT FOR THE ACUTE LEUKAEMIAS

Acute Myeloid Leukaemia

- Large gains in survival in acute myeloid leukaemia came with the introduction of adequate supportive care above and combination chemotherapy. Drugs effective in combination include cytarabine (ara-c), anthracyclines (idarubicin), etoposide, mitoxantrone, amsacrine, 6-thioguanine and 5-azacytadine. In general, the first three are commonly used initially. Cytarabine dose has been escalated with some evidence of a dose effect relationship. Such programs have been successfully used in both induction and post-remission therapy.

- Intensive combination chemotherapy is applied for 1 or 2 courses until a complete remission (CR) occurs with < 5% leukaemia blasts in marrow. Following CR some controversy exists as to the most effective therapy. High-dose ara-c programs as post-remission therapy appear to improve outlook if such therapy has not been given initially.

- The treatment of FAB–M3 or acute promyelocytic leukaemia has differed in recent years with the introduction of all-trans-retinoic acid (ATRA) for its treatment. ATRA will cause good leukaemia control but may increase white cell count, causing a pulmonary distress syndrome. ATRA appears insufficient without associated chemotherapy.

- Younger patients with an HLA-identical sibling should be considered for allogeneic transplantation if they have poor or standard risk of relapse and obtain a CR initially. For good prognosis, patients allogeneic transplantation is often reserved for first relapse or second remission following further chemotherapy. The use of autologous transplantation in first CR is controversial and requires further evidence.

- For older patients, over 60 years, standard dose therapy or slightly attenuated dose therapy is used for remission induction. Results are inferior possibly due to poor tolerance of intensive chemotherapy, more induction deaths and a higher expression of multi-drug resistant phenotype in older patients.

Outcome for AML

With optimal combination chemotherapy, about 70% of patients with AML obtain a CR with an overall median survival of about 18 months. However, only 20% of patients are long-term survivors with standard dose chemotherapy alone. High dose cytarabine in induction or post-induction is associated with a 40% leukaemia-free survival at 5 years in patients less than 60 years. Allogeneic transplantation in first CR is associated with 50% long-term survival in patients under 45 years.

Acute Lymphocytic Leukaemia

The regimens used to treat adult ALL borrow heavily from successful regimens developed for the better prognosis childhood ALL. The mainstay of therapy has been the use of vincristine, prednisone, L-asparaginase, anthracycline and cyclophosphamide. These drugs have been combined into a number of intensive, successful programs. The drug most commonly used in post-remission is cytarabine often combined with etoposide and anti-metabolites such as methotrexate.

In contrast to AML, adults with ALL require protracted maintenance therapy and the use of prophylactic treatment to the CNS. The incidence of CNS disease in ALL at presentation is about 10% with a higher percentage with relapse in the meninges. Thus, adult ALL patients receive prophylactic intrathecal methotrexate with prophylactic whole brain radiation given less frequently in recent times.

Outcome for ALL

The 2-year survival rate for adults with ALL is nearly 50%. However, only 24% of adult patients are alive at 6 years. The use of early transplantation in ALL is controversial. Most recommend transplantation in first CR for patients with quite adverse prognostic signs but otherwise reserve allogeneic transplantation for younger patients following first relapse.

REFERENCES

Bishop, J.F. (1997) The treatment of adult acute myeloid leukemia. *Semin Oncol*, **24**(1), 57–69.

Bloomfield, C.D., Herzig, G.P. and Caligiuri, M.A. (1997) Actue leukemia: recent advances. *Semin Oncol*, **24**(1), 1–147.

Clift, R.A., Buckner, C.D., Thomas, E.D. (1987) The treatment of acute non-lymphoblastic leukemia by allogeneic marrow transplantation. *Bone Marrow Transplantation*, **2**, 243–258.

Hoelzer, D., Ludwig, W.D., Thiel, D., Gassmann, W., Loffler, H., Fonatsch, C., Rieder, H., Heil, G., Heinze, B., Arnold, R., Hossfed, D., Buchner, T., Koch, P., Freund, M., Hiddemann, W., Maschmeyer, G., Heyll, A., Aul, C., Faak, T., Kuse, R., Ittel, T.H., Gramatzki, M., Diedrich, H., Kolbe, K. and Uberla, K. (1996).Improved outcome in adult B-cell acute lymphoblastic leukemia. *Blood*, **87**, 495–508.

Mrosek, K., Heinonen, K., de la Chapelle, A. and Bloomfield (1997) Clinical significance of cytogenetics in acute myeloid leukemia, *Semin Oncol*, **24**(1), 17–31.

Van Leeuwen, F.E., Chorus, A.M.J., Van den Belt-Dnoebout, A.W., Hagenbeek, A., Hoyon, R., van Kerkhoff, E.H., Pinedo, H.M. and Somers, R. (1994) Leukemia risk following Hodgkin's Disease: relation to cummulative dose of alkylating agents, treatment with teniposide combinations, number of episodes of chemotherapy and bone marrow damage. *J Clin Oncol*, **12**, 1063.

CHAPTER 46

CHRONIC LEUKAEMIAS AND MYELODYSPLASTIC DISEASE

Peter Mollee and Kerry Taylor

CHRONIC MYELOID LEUKAEMIA

Biology

Chronic myeloid leukaemia (CML) is a clonal haemopoietic stem cell disorder with a cytogenetic hallmark — the Philadelphia (Ph) chromosome. The Ph chromosome, a reciprocal translocation between chromosomes 9 and 22, transposes the c-abl proto-oncogene from chromosome 9 next to the breakpoint cluster region (bcr) on chromosome 22 to form a new hybrid BCR-ABL oncogene. This BCR-ABL transcript is present in over 95% of CML cases, and encodes for a novel protein with tyrosine kinase activity which is involved in the genesis of CML. Perturbation of apoptosis, the normal mechanism of myeloid cell death, may be important in the pathogenesis of CML.

Diagnosis

Clinical Features

- Median age approximately 50 years.
- Fatigue, anaemia, progressive splenomegaly and leukocytosis usually develop gradually.
- Symptoms of hypermetabolism (e.g. night sweats, weight loss), gout, hyperleukocytosis (e.g. priapism, tinnitus) and splenic infarction are less common.

Investigations

- Increased total white cell count with morphologically normal granulocyte precursors present in the blood.
- Basophilia.
- Thrombocytosis in 50%.
- Low or absent neutrophil alkaline phosphatase.
- Increased vitamin B_{12}, urate and lactate dehydrogenase.

- Bone marrow is hypercellular with increased myeloid to erythroid ratio and predominance of the myelocyte.
- Ph positivity demonstrated by cytogenetics or identification of BCR-ABL transcript

Disease Course

CML has a characteristic triphasic course. It usually presents in an indolent or chronic phase, which is easily controlled with therapy. Typically after about three years the disease progresses, sometimes through an accelerated phase, to acute leukaemia or blast crisis, and death ensues within months.

Prognostic factors include age, percentage of blasts in the blood, degree of splenomegaly, thrombocytosis, total basophils and development of additional cytogenetic abnormalities.

Treatment

Recent improved outcomes for CML have occurred, with median survival time now greater than five years. Treatment options include the following.

Standard Chemotherapy

Oral agents such as hydroxyurea and busulphan provide good chronic phase control, but do not appear to alter disease course, survival time, or induce Ph suppression. Hydroxyurea is favoured because of lesser short- and long-term toxicity and possible improved survival rate.

Allogeneic Bone Marrow Transplantation

About 40–60% of patients can be cured with this modality which is most efficacious earlier in the disease course and in younger patients. With refinement unrelated donor transplants may increase the fraction (15–20%) of CML patients able to have this curative therapy.

α-Interferon

Interferon is administered at the maximal tolerated dose (up to 10,000,000 u/day) subcutaneously. α-interferon affords haematological control in the majority of patients and induces substantial Ph suppression (decrease in Ph+ metaphases to < 35% and frequently 0%) in 20–40%, especially in the early chronic phase of CML. Randomised studies have confirmed survival benefit, and while therapy related toxicity is not insubstantial, α-interferon is now first line therapy for all new CML cases without a related matched allograft donor. The addition of parenteral cytarabine may further improve cytogenetic response rates and overall survival rates.

Other Modalities

Homoharringtonine, intensive chemotherapy ± autologous stem cell transplantation may suppress the Ph+ clone, allowing temporary restoration of normal haemopoiesis. These options increasingly play a role in those intolerant or unresponsive to α-interferon who do not have an allogeneic transplant option or whose disease is progressing.

CHRONIC LYMPHOCYTIC LEUKAEMIA

Biology

Chronic lymphocytic leukaemia (CLL) is a clonal expansion of malignant lymphocytes. These cells have enhanced survival and accumulate in the blood, bone marrow and lymphatic tissues. It is not associated with ionising radiation, drugs, chemicals or a viral aetiology, but there is an increased familial incidence. Clonal chromosomal abnormalities, most commonly involving chromosomes 12,13 and 14, have been noted in over 50% of patients, but their role in the pathogenesis of CLL is undetermined. BCL-2(proto-oncogene) and p53(tumour suppressor gene) expression is sometimes found in CLL and may correlate with more advanced disease and chemotherapy resistance.

Diagnosis

Clinical Features

- Median age approximately 60 years.
- Asymptomatic in over 25%.
- Fatigue and malaise early symptoms.
- Weight loss, recurrent infections, bleeding, anaemia, lymphadenopathy (80%), splenomegaly (50%) and extra nodal infiltration with advancing disease.

Investigations

- Sustained lymphocytosis > 5 $\leftrightarrow$ 10^9/L with morphologically mature appearing cells.
- Bone marrow usually > 30% replacement by small lymphocytes.
- Immunophenotyping showing: (1) coexpression of B-cell markers CD19, CD20, CD23 together with the T-cell marker CD5; (2) low density surface immunoglobulin expression; and (3) monoclonality with kappa or lambda light chain restriction.
- Anaemia common and usually normochromic, normocytic, but may be autoimmune in approximately 8%.
- Thrombocytopenia due to hypersplenism and/or marrow replacement, but may be autoimmune.
- Hypogammaglobulinaemia common, but approximately 5% have a monoclonal paraprotein.

Staging

Two major staging systems have been developed in CLL to assist in determining prognosis and survival: the Rai Clinical Staging System (Table 46.1) and the Binet Clinical Staging System (Table 46.2).

Other indicators of a poorer prognosis include diffuse pattern of marrow involvement, lymphocyte count doubling time of < 12 months, an abnormal karyotype, high serum beta 2 microglobulin and increasing age.

Treatment

Due to the relatively indolent course of early stage CLL, the elderly nature of the population and the inability to cure the disease with current treatment, therapy is usually instituted for symptomatic disease only. Indications for therapy include: anaemia or thrombocytopenia; bulky disease (symptomatic lymphadenopathy or splenomegaly, high or rising lymphocyte count); constitutional symptoms; and disease transformation.

Chemotherapy is the principal treatment modality although maintenance therapy has not been shown to improve survival. Radiotherapy is useful to palliate bulky lymphoid masses or massive splenomegaly in selected cases. Splenectomy in the setting of severe thrombocytopenia with resistant or advanced disease is sometimes indicated, and prednisone may be used by itself for immune phenomena.

- *Chlorambucil*: used alone or with prednisone; may be given in a continuous or intermittent schedule.
- *Nucleoside analogues*: Fludarabine and cladribine are newer drugs with pronounced anti-CLL activity. Fludarabine, the most efficacious agent in CLL, has a high complete response rate and a proven role in salvage therapy. It may be an appropriate initial drug of choice although this is not yet proven.
- *Combination chemotherapy*: used in progressive or advanced stage CLL, but has not shown consistent benefit over single agent therapy
- *Transplantation*: Bone marrow transplantation has been shown to induce a long-term disease-free survival rate of approximately 40% at five years, especially in younger patients. Monoclonal antibody purged autologous transplants also show promising results.

Special Considerations

- *Infection*: Major cause of morbidity and mortality due to hypo-gammaglobulinaemia and impaired antibody mediated response. Streptococcal, staphyloccal, E. coli and herpes zoster virus are the main pathogens. Monthly intravenous gammaglobulin decreases the frequency of bacterial infections.
- *Autoimmune phenomena*: Prednisone is used to control immune thrombocytopenia and autoimmune haemolysis. Treatment of the underlying disease will not necessarily resolve the autoimmune features.

Table 46.1 Rai Clinical Staging System

Stage	Clinical features at diagnosis	Median survival
0	Blood and marrow lymphocytosis	>150 mo
I	Lymphocytosis and lymphadenopathy	101 mo
II	Lymphocytosis and enlarged spleen and/or liver	>71 mo
III	Lymphocytosis and Hb< 11g/dL	19 mo
IV	Lymphocytosis and platelets < 100 x 10^9/L	19 mo

Table 46.2 Binet Clinical Staging System

Stage	Clinical features at diagnosis	Median survival
A	Blood and marrow lymphocytosis < 3 areas of lymphadenopathy	> 7 yrs
B	Blood and marrow lymphocytosis < 3 areas of lymphadenopathy	< 5 yrs
C	As per B with anaemia or thrombocytopenia	< 2 yrs

- *Richter's transformation*: Development of a high-grade B-cell lymphoma occurs in 3–15% of patients at any time from diagnosis. Prognosis is generally poor with a median survival time of five months.

HAIRY CELL LEUKAEMIA

Hairy cell leukaemia (HCL) is a lymphoproliferative disorder of late lineage B cells with distinctive morphology. There is a male predominance, with an average age of onset of 55 years.

Clinical presentation is of splenomegaly and cytopenias, with the bone marrow and peripheral blood showing characteristic 'hairy' cells with sky blue, agranular cytoplasm and numerous cytoplasmic projections. The cytoplasm stains positively for tartrate-resistant acid phosphatase (TRAP). Immunophenotyping is positive for pan B-cell markers and surface immunoglobulin.

In the last decade, the prognosis of HCL has improved dramatically due to the interferons and nucleoside analogues; 2CdA is now the first line therapy with prolonged disease-free survival times recorded.

PROLYMPHOCYTIC LEUKAEMIA

Prolymphocytic leukaemia (PLL) is a B- or T-cell disorder with the cells appearing more immature than in CLL. Clinical presentation is primarily of splenomegaly, with hepatomegaly, marrow involvement and minimal or absent lymphadenopathy. The disease course is typically aggressive and is poorly chemo-responsive.

MYELODYSPLASTIC DISEASES

Myelodysplastic syndrome (MDS) is an acquired, progressive, clonal disorder of marrow proliferation characterised by dysplasia of the peripheral blood and marrow, cytopenias, and a high risk of transformation to acute leukaemia. The FAB (French, American, British) classification separates *de novo* MDS into five morphologic subtypes, predominantly on marrow blast percentage (Table 46.3):

Table 46.3 FAB Classification

Subtype	Frequency	Peripheral Blood (monocytes)	Bone Marrow	Median Survival (months)
RA	35%	$< 1 \times 10^9$/L	blasts $< 5\%$ ringed sideroblasts $< 15\%$	30–60
RARS	20%	$< 1 \times 10^9$/L	blasts $< 5\%$ ringed sideroblasts $> 15\%$	30–70
RAEB	20%	$< 1 \times 10^9$/L	blasts 5–20%	9–20
CMML	15%	$> 1 \times 10^9$/L	blasts $< 20\%$	12–30
RAEB-t	15%		blasts 20–30%	5–10

1. refractory anaemia (RA)
2. refractory anaemia with ringed sideroblasts (RARS)
3. refractory anaemia with excess blasts (RAEB)
4. chronic myelomonocytic leukaemia (CMML)
5. refractory anaemia with excess blasts in transformation (RAEB-t)

Diagnosis

Clinical features:

- Median age 60–65 years.
- Initial symptoms are those of anaemia and, less commonly, bleeding or infection.
- Splenomegaly is present in 10–20% (more common in CMML).

Investigations:

- Anaemia is the most common finding, often associated with thrombocytopenia and neutropenia. Isolated neutropenia or thrombocytopenia are uncommon.
- Morphology of the peripheral blood and marrow shows characteristic dysplastic features.
- Cytogenetic abnormalities are frequent, and in addition to marrow blast percentage, have prognostic significance.

Treatment

Therapy needs to be individualised, and in the elderly supportive care is preferred. In younger patients (< 65 years) with increased blast percentage, AML induction chemotherapy may achieve complete remission and improve survival. Transformation to frank leukaemia is treated with standard AML induction therapy if indicated, although it carries a poor prognosis.

- Supportive care:
  — aggressive treatment of infections
  — platelet transfusions in event of bleeding or preoperatively
  — blood transfusions to prevent symptomatic anaemia (consideration of iron chelation therapy in chronically transfused with predominant anaemia)
- *Growth factors*: No cytokine (erythropoietin, G-CSF, GM-CSF, IL-3) has yet been proven to improve survival or reduce morbidity, but colony stimulating factors may have a role in management of severe infections due to their ability to improve the neutrophil count.
- *Allogeneic bone marrow transplantation*: may be curative in young patients.

Special considerations

- *CMML*: a subset of MDS patients with myeloproliferative features (increased circulating monocytoid cells and hepatosplenomegaly). It is considered as part of the spectrum of MDS because of the presence of trilineage dysplasia, cytopenias, and its rate and pattern of leukaemic transformation.
- *5q- syndrome*: While the 5q- karyotype is not specific for MDS, when seen it defines patients with a syndrome characterised by macrocytic anaemia, leucopenia, and normal or raised platelet count with uncommon progression to leukaemia.

- *Therapy-related MDS (t-MDS)*: best considered a separate entity, most commonly complicating alkylating agent therapy and carrying a poorer prognosis.

REFERENCES

Chronic Myeloid Leukaemia

Sokal, J.E., Cox, E.B., Baccarani, M., Tura, S., Gomez, G.A., Robertson, J.E., Tso, C.Y., Braun, T.J., Clarkson, B.D., Cervantes, F., Rozman, C. and The Italian Cooperative CML Study Group (1984) Prognostic discrimination in 'good-risk' chronic granulocytic leukemia. *Blood*, **63**, 789–99.

The Italian Cooperative Study Group on Chronic Myeloid Leukaemia (1994) Interferon alfa-2a as compared with conventional chemotherapy for the treatment of chronic myeloid leukaemia. *N Engl J Med*, **330**, 820–825.

Chronic Lymphocytic Leukaemia

Cheson, B.D., Bennett, J.M., Grever, M., Kay, N., Keating, M.J., O'Brien, S. and Rai, K.R. (1996) National Cancer Institute-sponsored Working Group Guidelines for chronic lymphocytic leukemia: revised guidelines for diagnosis and treatment. *Blood*, **87**, 4990–7.

O'Brien, S., Kantarjian, H., Beron, M., Smith, T., Koller, C., Estey, E., Robertson, L.E., Lerner, S. and Keating, M. (1993) Results of fludarabine and prednisone therapy in 264 patients with chronic lymphocytic leukemia with multivariate-analysis derived prognostic model for response to treatment. *Blood*, **82**, 1695–1700.

Myelodysplastic Diseases

Bennett, J.M., Catovsky, D., Daniel, M.T., Flandrin, G., Galton, D.A.G., Gralnick, H.R., Sultan, C. and the French-American-British (FAB) Co-operative Group (1982) Proposals for the classification of the myelodysplastic syndromes. *Br J Haematol*, **51**, 189–99.

CHAPTER 47

LYMPHOMA

Graham A.R. Young

INTRODUCTION

Lymphomas are cancers of the lymphatic system. Traditionally, they have been divided into two main types: Hodgkin's disease (HD) and non-Hodgkin's lymphoma (NHL).

HODGKIN'S DISEASE

Hodgkin's disease was named after Dr Thomas Hodgkin from St Bartholomew's Hospital, London whose article entitled 'On some morbid appearances of the absorbent glands and spleen' was published in 1832.

Epidemiology

- Hodgkin's disease is an uncommon malignancy with an age-adjusted rate of 3/100,000 in the US. The incidence appears to have decreased by 10% in the last 20 years.
- The male to female ratio is 2:1.
- It has an interesting age distribution and ethnic variation, for example, in California the white population shows a bimodal incidence with peaks at ages 15–40, and in those aged over 55. The young adult peak is much lower for Blacks and hardly seen for patients of Hispanic or Asian origin.

Risk factors

- In general, the risk factors are not clearly defined but interesting associations exist.
- Incidence higher in upper social classes (infective aetiology?).
- Incidence lower in women (hormonal influence?).
- Risk increases with HIV infection.
- Genetic susceptibility.

- Epstein-Barr virus (EBV) may be associated with some cases.

Diagnosis

- Diagnosis must be made by tissue biopsy, and is usually made on morphological and immunohistochemical grounds.
- Hallmark of the disease is the large, often mutlinucleated cell; this is the classical Hodgkin (H) or Reed-Sternberg (RS) cell.
- Important to have 'background' reactive lymphoid cells and histocytes.
- Currently five histological types are recognised (incidence in brackets):
    1. lymphocyte predominant (5%)
    2. nodular sclerosis (60%)
    3. mixed cellularity (30%)
    4. lymphocyte depleted (< 5%)
    5. lymphocyte rich classical HD (< 5%)

Clinical Features

- Patients typically present with painless cervical lymphadenopathy (80% of cases); often with non-specific malaise.
- 'B symptoms' — fever (> 38°C), weight loss (> 10% in preceding 6 months) and night sweats — influence prognosis
- Pruritus, although sometimes present, is not a 'B' symptom.

Approach to Management

An approach to the managment of lymphoma is illustrated in Figure 47.1.

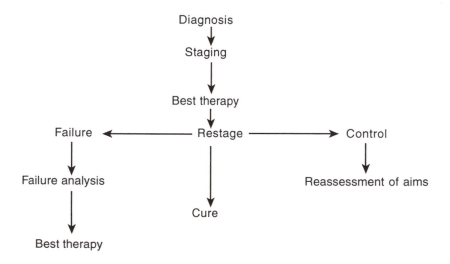

Figure 47.1 An approach to the management of lymphoma

Staging

The Ann Arbor system

- Stage I: Single nodal area or structure
- Stage II: Two or more nodal areas on the same side of diaphragm
- Stage III: Nodal areas on both sides of diaphragm
- Stage IV: Visceral involvement
- B = symptoms as noted previously
- A = absence of such symptoms
- E = extranodal involvement by contiguity

Staging Procedures

- Patient and family history and clinical examination is performed.
- FBC, ESR, LDH, liver function tests.
- CXR, CT scan of neck, chest, abdomen and pelvis.
- Gallium scan.
- Bone marrow biopsy if FBC abnormal.
- A laparotomy is probably no longer recommended.

Treatment

Treatment is controversial and evolving. Traditionally treatment was based on stage of disease but now there is recognition of other biological factors such as age, sex, FBC, lymphocyte count, and LDH. There is a tendency to try to reduce long term sequelae as the majority of patients are long-term survivors.

Risk Factors in Treatment

Factors recognised as conferring a poor prognosis include stage ($\pm$ B symptoms), bulk disease, especially mediastinal mass and spleen, age, ESR, anaemia and LDH as a probable surrogate of bulk of disease.

Treatment Guidelines (based on German studies)

- Stage I/II with no risk factors or early stage disease: Extended field radiotherapy.
- Stage I/II with 1 risk factor or intermediate stage disease: Combined chemotherapy/RT, e.g. 2 $\leftrightarrow$ (COPP+ABVD) + 20Gy EF.
- Stage IIB/IIIA with risk factor, all IIIB/IV or advanced stage disease: Anthracycline based, e.g. ABVD/RT or Stanford V.

NON-HODGKIN'S LYMPHOMA

Epidemiology

- Non-Hodgkin's lymphoma is more common than Hodgkin's disease. In the US the age-adjusted incidence rate is 25/100,000. The incidence has increased by 75% in the last 20 years.
- The male to female ratio is 2:1.
- In general, incidence increases with age.

- There is a geographical variation with a higher incidence of T-cell disease in Asia.

Risk factors

- Congenital immunodeficiency states.
- Acquired immunodeficiency states such as post-organ transplantation, HIV infection, HTLV1 infection.
- AIDS: Approximately 30% of AIDS patients will develop NHL.
- Pesticides and herbicides.

Diagnosis

- Diagnosis must be made by tissue biopsy and is usually made on morphological and immunohistochemical grounds.
- At least 15 types of non-Hodgkin's lymphoma can be identified on morphological grounds.
- Several classification systems exist, e.g. Working Formulation, Keil classification and REAL (Revised European American Lymphoma) classification (see Table 47.1).
- In general lymphomas are classified by:
  — cell phenotype (B, T or null cell type)
  — cell size (small or large cell)
  — presence or absence of follicles
  — genetic abnormalities
  — clinical behaviour

Table 47.1 REAL (Revised European American Lymphoma) classification

B-cell neoplasms	T-cell neoplasms
Precursor B-cell neoplasms	Precursor T-cell neoplasms
Precursor B lymphoblastic leukaemia/lymphoma	Precursor T lymphoblastic leukaemia/lymphoma
Peripheral B-cell neoplasms	Peripheral T cell and NK cell neoplasms
B-cell chronic lymphocytic leukaemia/ prolymphocytic leukaemia/small lymphocytic	T-cell chronic lymphocytic leukaemia/ prolymphocytic lymphoma leukaemia
Immunocytoma/lymphoplasmacytic	Large granular lymphocyte lymphoma leukaemia (LGL)
Mantle cell lymphoma	Mycosis fungoides/Sezary syndrome
Follicle centre cell lymphoma, follicular	Peripheral T-cell lymphomas unspecified
Marginal zone B-cell lymphoma	Angioimmunoblastic T-cell lymphoma (AILD)
Hairy cell leukaemia	Angiocentric lymphoma (nasal NK/T cell lymphoma)
Plasmacytoma/plasma cell myeloma	Intestinal T cell lymphoma
Diffuse large B-cell lymphoma	Adult T cell lymphoma/leukaemia (ATL/L)
Burkitt's lymphoma	Anaplastic large cell lymphoma (ALCL)

Clinical Features

NHL is a heterogenous group of diseases and the clinical presentations reflect this. Although lymphadenopathy is common, patients often present with disease in extranodal sites, e.g. the gastrointestinal tract, skin, bone, etc. Non-specific malaise, fever, weight loss and night sweats also commonly occur.

Approach to Management and Staging

In principle the approach to the management and staging of NHL is as with Hodgkin's disease.

Treatment

- Treatment is controversial and evolving.
- Traditionally based on histology and stage of disease, but now includes recognition of the importance of biological factors.

Risk Factors in Treatment

Age, stage of disease, performance status, LDH and number of extranodal sites are recognised as influencing outcome from therapy.

Treatment Guidelines

Treatment for NHL remains controversial and complex (see references). In general treatment is as follows.

Low-grade Lymphoma

- Early stage: observe /RT.
- Advanced stage: alkylating agent.
- Possible options: purine analogues or high-dose chemotherapy with rescue.

Gastric MALT lymphoma

- Often associated with *Helicobacter pylori* infection.
- Eradication of *H. pylori* with omeprazole, amoxycillin and metronidazole can cause regression of lymphoma.

Mantle Cell lymphoma

- Aggressive lymphoma.
- Median survival 3–4 years.
- Management difficult with transplantation being studied.

Intermediate Grade Lymphoma

- CHOP probably remains gold standard.
- Results of dose escalation studies awaited with anticipation.

Table 47.2 Survival rates for Hodgkin's disease and non-Hodgkin's lymphoma (NHL)

	Hodgkin's disease	NHL
1 year	90%	70%
5 years	80%	50%
10 years	65%	45%
15 years	60%	35%

High-grade Lymphoma (lymphoblastic lymphoma and Burkitt's lymphoma)

- Treated with multiagent chemotherapy as in lymphoblastic leukaemia
- CNS prophylaxis required

Survival Rates

Survival rates for Hodgkin's disease and NHL are listed in Table 47.2.

REFERENCES

Hodgkin's Disease

Diehl, V. (1996) Hodgkin's Disease. Bailliere's Clinical Haematology. International Practice and Research. 9:3. London: Bailliere's Tindall.

Yuen, A.R. and Horning, S.J. (1996) Recent advances in Hodgkin's disease. *Current Opinion in Haematology*, **3**, 273–278.

Non-Hodgkin's Lymphoma

Bierman, P.J. and Armitage, J.O. (1996) Non-Hodgkin's lymphoma. *Current Opinion in Haematology*, 3, 266–272.

Harris NL, Jaffe ES, Stein, H., Banks, P.M., Chan, J.K., Cleary, M.L., Delsol, G., DeWolf Peters, C., Fallini, B. and Gutter, K.C. (1994) A revised European-American classification of lymphoid neoplasms: a proposal from the International Lymphoma Study Group. *Blood*, **84**, 1361–1392.

Press, O.W., Horning, S. and Vose, J. (1995) Evaluation and Management of the 'New' Lymphoma Entities: Mantle Cell Lymphoma, MALT Lymphoma, Monocytoid B Cell Lymphoma, and Anaplastic Large Cell Lymphoma Education Program. The American Society of Haematology.

The International Non-Hodgkin's Lymphoma Prognostic Factors Project (1993) A Predictive model for aggressive non-Hodgkin's Lymphoma. *N Engl J Med*, **329**, 987–994.

CHAPTER 48

MULTIPLE MYELOMA

Douglas E. Joshua

INTRODUCTION

Multiple myeloma is the most common plasma cell dyscrasia and a paradigm of a B-cell tumour. Clinical manifestations of the disease are a direct reflection of disease pathophysiology including the following:

- Disease due to growth of the malignant plasma cell and associated bony destruction.
- The effects of the secreted paraprotein either in the serum or the urine.
- Marrow infiltration leading to bone marrow failure.
- Immunosuppression caused by hypogammaglobulinaemia and an associated primary immune deficit.
- Renal disease, which has a multifactorial aetiology.

The incidence of myeloma in Caucasians is approximately 4 per 100 000. There does appear to be a racial variation in the incidence in Afro-Americans of 10–12 per 100,000 and an incidence in Asians of 1–2 per 100 000. The disease is sporadic with only occasional reports of family associations or geographical clusters. Both radiation and benzene exposure have been implicated in its aetiology, and a number of occupational associations, including agricultural work, rubber, wood, leather and textile manufacturing industries, have also been reported.[1]

DIAGNOSIS

- Myeloma usually involves the axial skeletons and the proximal ends of the long bones. Lytic bone lesions detected radiologically are often associated with general osteoporosis. Thus, the most common presenting symptom is usually bone pain, often back pain, associated with crush fractures of vertebrae.
- Other presenting symptoms include the symptom complex associated with hypercalcaemia, renal failure, or unexplained severe infections in previously well patients.

- The unequivocal diagnosis requires the combination of lytic bone lesions in association with a monoclonal infiltrate of plasma cells in the marrow and a paraprotein or M component in either the serum or the urine. Many patients, however, do not show all these characteristics and marrow infiltration in a normal skeletal survey is not an uncommon clinical finding.

- An important clinical distinction is to differentiate between active myeloma and MGUS or smouldering myeloma. In the latter conditions treatment is not usually considered immediately necessary. The distinction relies upon the amount of the serum monoclonal protein, the percentage of infiltrated plasma cells in the bone marrow and, importantly, the absence of anaemia, renal failure, hypercalcaemia, and a low beta 2 microglobulin and plasma cell labelling index.

- Electrophoresis is used to detect the presence of monoclonal proteins in the serum or urine. Immunofixation is used to identify these proteins.

- The most commonly found paraprotein is IgG, which occurs in approximately 40–50% of cases. IgA- and Bence Jones-only myeloma are each approximately 20% of cases and IgE, IgD, IgM, myelomas are rare.

PROGNOSIS

Prognostic Factors

Prognostic factors are of importance in the evaluation of patients with myeloma. The important prognostic factors relate to the intrinsic proliferative capacity of the myeloma clone, tumour bulk, renal function, and host-tumour interaction.

Plasma Cell Labelling Index and Serum Thymidine Kinase

Intrinsic properties of the malignant clone include the plasma cell labelling index and the serum thymidine kinase level. The plasma cell labelling index is one of the most significant prognostic tools so far identified and can be used to differentiate MGUS, smouldering myeloma, and active myeloma. It is highly correlated with the serum thymidine kinase level and neither the serum thymidine kinase level, nor the labelling index correlate with beta 2 microglobulin, another important measure of prognosis.

Beta 2 Microglobulin

The two important and widespread methods for assessing myeloma tumour mass are the beta 2 microglobulin level and clinical staging systems. However, the clinical staging system is used less commonly these days as the combination of beta 2 microglobulin and the plasma cell labelling index provides the best prognostic information.

Clinical Staging System

The Durie-Salmon three-stage system, was developed by analysis of presenting the clinical features, the response to treatment and the survival of a cohort of patients with multiple myeloma in whom indirect measurements of total body myeloma has been made. The three stages, I, II, and III, are sub-classified into A and B, depending on the presence of renal failure. The Durie-Salmon staging system clearly identifies Stage 1A, which is a group of good prognostic patients with smouldering myeloma. There is, however, considerable overlap in the prognosis of Stage II and Stage III disease.

Renal Failure

The importance of renal failure in myeloma has been widely reviewed. It is present in approximately 30% of patients at diagnosis, and it is important to appreciate that correction of hypercalcaemia, dehydration, hyperviscosity and acidosis can lead to significant correction of renal function in a large percentage of these patients, without the need for immediate chemotherapy.

THERAPY

General Considerations

The therapy of myeloma is complex and requires many patient-specific decisions. Factors such as the patient's general state of health and the presence of disease complications and co-morbidity are often more important than the chemosensitivity of the tumour.

A particular problem has been the management of bony disease, and measures to prevent progression of bony destruction by using agents such as the bisphosphonates has recently been introduced into management protocols. Such drugs appear to be able to reduce the subsequent incidence of skeletal events in patients with myeloma. Management of hypercalcaemia has also been vastly improved recently by the introduction of bisphosphonates.[2]

Hyperviscosity

Hyperviscosity is another acute management problem which can occur in patients with myeloma and especially in patients with IgA or IgM paraproteins. Hyperviscosity causes central nervous system symptoms and can lead to an exacerbation of renal failure.

Plasma exchange is the management of choice for patients with symptomatic hyperviscosity, and it can be a lifesaving procedure. A 4–5 litre exchange with normal plasma or albumin replacement is required and needs to be repeated as frequently as indicated by clinical features.

Chemotherapy

Melphalan, with or without prednisone, is the traditional therapy for myeloma and has been used for over 30 years. A number of combinations of drugs (used at non-ablative doses) have been compared to melphalan in a large number of trials without clear evidence of superiority.

Commonly used doses of melphalan are 8 mg/m^2 for 5 days every 6 weeks together with prednisone 50 mg/m^2 for days. Combinations of drugs such as VMCP/VBAP (vincristine, melphalan, cyclophosphamide, BCNU, doxorubicin and prednisone) or ABCM (doxorubicin, BCNU, cyclophosphamide and melphalan) have also been extensively used.

Transplantation

Allogeneic Transplantation

Allogeneic transplantation is likely only to play a small role in patients with myeloma because the requirements for allogeneic transplantation are rarely met. These requirements, which include age and fitness of the recipient, a suitable sibling donor, minimal disease at transplantation, and sensitivity of the tumour to dose escalation, are such that only 2–3% of patients are eligible.[3]

Autologous Transplantation

A large number of studies involving autologous transplantation have been carried out, including randomised studies which have shown the benefit of autologous transplantation over conventional therapies. The major challenge when managing patients involves the selection and timing of appropriate therapy.[4]

Given the age distribution the majority of patients will receive conventional chemotherapy, and for elderly patients Melphalan is still the treatment of choice. More intensive combination therapies are attractive for younger patients who should be considered for both autologous and, if appropriate, allogeneic transplantation.

Interferon

The role of interferon remains unclear despite many years of evaluation, but its most beneficial role is in the maintenance of plateau phase rather than as an induction or co-induction agent where the addition of interferon to induction therapy seems to have little role.[5]

New Therapies

The difficulty of obtaining a cure in myeloma has led to a number of new avenues being explored. These include mechanisms which explain the pathogenesis of the escape from plateau phase and the possibility of any idiotypic vaccination using either DNA or protein vaccines. It has been demonstrated recently that the presence of the expanded T-cell clones in myeloma is of prognostic significance, and such avenues as augmenting T-cell responses are being actively studied.[6]

OUTCOMES

Myeloma, however, remains an incurable disease. It is incurable with conventional chemotherapy, incurable with autografting, including double transplant programmes, and the vast majority of patients who receive allogeneic transplants also fail to be cured of their disease. The median survival remains at 3–4 years despite the advent of transplantation protocols.

REFERENCES

1. Joshua, D.E. and Gibson, J. (1996) Diagnosis and treatment of multiple myeloma. In *Neoplastic Diseases of the Blood* (3rd edn), edited by P. Wiernik, G. Canellos, J. Dutcher and R. Kyle, pp. 561–584. New York: Churchill Livingstone Inc.
2. Berenson, Jr, Lichtenstein, A., Porter, L., Dimopoulos, M.A., Bordoni, R., George, S., Lipton, A., Keller, A., Ballester, O., Kovacs, M.J., Blacklock, H.A., Bell, R., Simeone, J., Reitsma, D.J., Heffernan, M., Seaman, J. and Knight, R.D. (1996) Efficacy of pamidronate in reducing skeletal events in patients with advanced multiple myeloma: Myeloma Aredia Study Group. *N Eng J Med.*, 334(8), 488–493.
3. Gahrton, G. (1996) Allogeneic bone marrow transplantation in multiple myeloma. *Brit J Haematol*, 92(2), 251–4.
4. Attal, M., Harousseau JL, Stoppa, A.M., Sotto, J.J., Fuzibet, J.G., Rossi, J.F., Casassus, P., Maisonneuve, H., Facon, T., Ifrah, N., Payen, C., Bataille, R. for the Intergroupe Francais du Myelome (1996) A prospective randomized trial of autologous bone marrow transplantation and chemotherapy in multiple myeloma. *N Eng J Med*, 335, 91–97.

5. Joshua, D.E., Penny, R., Matthews, J.P., Laidlaw, C.R., Gibson, J., Bradstock, K., Wolf, M., Goldstein, D. for the Australian Leukaemia Study Group (1997) Australian Leukaemia Study Group Myeloma II: a randomized trial of intensive combination chemotherapy with or without interferon in patients with myeloma. *Br J Haematol,* **97**, 38–45.

6. Brown, R., Yuen, Y., Nelson, M., Gibson, J. and Joshua, D. (1997) The prognostic significance of T cell receptor b gene rearrangements with idiotype-reactive T cells in multiple myeloma. *Leukemia,* **11**, 1312–1317.

CHAPTER 49

BONE MARROW AND STEM CELL TRANSPLANTATION

Ken F. Bradstock

INTRODUCTION

Bone marrow transplantation (BMT) has evolved from attempts to treat radiation accident victims 40 years ago. Effective development was delayed until the discovery of human histocompatibility antigens in the 1960s. Early transplants, carried out for aplastic anaemia and end-stage leukaemia, demonstrated the feasibility of the technique, but highlighted a number of major problems, particularly the syndrome of acute graft-versus-host disease.[1] Improved results were obtained in the following decade with better patient selection. A major advance in the late 1970s was the use of *autologous* (self) marrow as a substitute for *allogeneic* (from other donors) cells.

In the mid 1980s, it was realized that marrow stem cells could be collected from blood by apheresis following myelosuppressive chemotherapy and/or administration of growth factors, and that these blood stem cells gave rise to faster engraftment than marrow.[2] This has led to a rapid increase in the number of auto-transplants being carried out worldwide, and to the use of BMT in a wider range of diseases, including solid tumours sensitive to cytotoxic drugs.[3] In this chapter, the term BMT is used generically to describe blood or marrow transplantation.

RATIONALE

Use of Blood or Marrow Transplantation

Transplantation of blood or marrow cells may be used for one or more of the following reasons:

- To allow delivery of supralethal doses of chemotherapy and radiotherapy to patients with malignant disease. Infusion of marrow cells after completion of high dose anti-cancer therapy allows reconstitution of bone marrow function, and normalisation of blood counts.
- To generate an allogeneic immune response against tumour cells to eradicate minimal residual disease. Cytotoxic T lymphocytes and other immune effector cells generated from infused bone marrow can recognize and kill malignant cells surviving high-dose chemotherapy.[4]

- To replace defective marrow stem cells in inherited and aquired non-malignant disorders. Infusion of histocompatible marrow cells from a normal donor can correct a number of conditions due to marrow stem cell defects, including aplastic anaemia, immunodeficiency states, and myelodysplasias.
- To deliver intensive immune suppression in auto-immune disorders. A proportion of cases of aplastic anaemia have an underlying immunological basis and can be cured by BMT. Other auto-immune disorders may also be amenable to the same approach.

WHO SHOULD RECEIVE BMT?

Selection of Patients for Blood or Marrow Transplantation

Age

Age is a major predictive factor for successful outcome, particularly in allogeneic BMT. Patients aged less than 20–30 years have been found to have a better transplant outcome than older patients, particularly those over 40 years. Many BMT centres impose upper age limits at 50 to 55 years for allogeneic BMT. Age appears to be less important in autologous BMT, where successful transplants for patients over 60 years of age are not unusual.

Medical and Psychological Fitness

The physical and mental fitness to withstand the effects of high dose anticancer treatment, and the absence of major co-morbid medical conditions, is an important factor predicting transplant outcome.

Disease Type and Status

BMT is used strictly as curative, rather than palliative, therapy. Therefore the patient's tumour must be amenable to near or complete eradication by high dose therapy, with a steep dose-response to cytotoxic agents. This excludes some, but not all, of the common epithelial cancers, as well as initially sensitive tumours that have aquired drug resistance during the course of previous treatment.

Stem Cell Availability

Allogeneic BMT

For patients to receive allogeneic BMT, a compatible donor must be identified. Traditionally, this has been a fully histocompatible sibling (matched for all 6 histocompatibility antigens). In typical Western families, the chances of identifying a fully matched sibling donor are only 30%. This can be improved by about 5–10% by accepting siblings with a 1 antigen mismatch, or by searching the family (first-degree relatives) for a fully matched or 1 antigen mismatched relative.

An alternative option is to search for an *unrelated* volunteer fortuitously matched with the patient.[5] Over 3 million tissue-typed donors are accessible on international volunteer registries. The chances of finding such a donor are directly related to the patient's ethnic background (registries are currently biased towards Caucasoid donors) and the commoness or rarity of their histocompatibility antigens. As a general rule of thumb, matched unrelated donors can be found for about one-third of patients on international searching.

Autologous BMT

Marrow stem cells, derived from bone marrow harvests or from blood apheresis, must be available in sufficient numbers, with excellent viability, and relatively free of contaminating malignant cells, before autologous BMT can be considered.

THE PROCESS OF BMT

Preassessment

The BMT procedure is a complex process that varies according to the disease being treated and the type of marrow cells (autologous versus allogeneic) being used. Patient selection is the initial crucial step, which, in addition to the issues outlined above, involves extensive counselling and education of the patient, their family, and (where appropriate) the donor. The risks of the procedure, chance of cure, and alternative options must be fully discussed. The patient must be carefully assessed to document the disease status pre-BMT, and measure baseline vital organ function (cardiac, renal, liver, pulmonary function). Central venous access must be available.

Autologous transplantation

Over 75% of autologous transplants are now carried out using marrow stem cells collected from apheresis of blood. These stem cells are usually collected on recovery from a course of myelosuppressive chemotherapy, followed by daily injection of a growth factor such as granulocyte colony-stimulating factor (G-CSF).

Typically, leucocyte recovery is seen 10 to 14 days after treatment, and marrow stem cells can be collected by leucapheresis on 1–3 successive days, when small numbers of stem cells expressing the CD34 marker appear in the blood. The apheresis collections are frozen, stored in liquid nitrogen, and samples tested for viability and stem cell content by CD34 and colony assays.

Allogeneic transplantation

The identification of a suitable histocompatible donor is a critical step in proceeding with allogeneic BMT. In addition to tissue typing, donors must be carefully assessed for medical fitness to undergo the donation procedure.

In the past, donation has been carried out by bone marrow harvest under general anaesthesia, with collection of 0.5 to 1.5 litre of marrow from the pelvis. Increasingly now, however, marrow stem cells are being collected from the blood of allogeneic donors by 1–2 leucaphereses after 4 daily injections of G-CSF, thus eliminating the risks of general anaesthesia.

Pre-BMT treatment

Typically, pre-BMT treatment is given in the week prior to infusion of marrow cells, and is commonly called conditioning therapy. This consists either of combinations of cytotoxic agents in extremely high doses, or chemotherapy in conjunction with total body irradiation. The purpose of conditioning therapy is to:

• create space in the marrow for engraftment of the infused marrow cells;
• kill all or the majority of malignant cells;
• immunosuppress the recipient sufficiently to accept the marrow graft (for allogeneic BMT).

An outline of commonly used protocols is given in Table 49.1. Following the completion of conditioning therapy, marrow cells are infused intravenously, either freshly collected from an allogeneic donor, or cryopreserved autologous cells thawed at the bedside and infused immediately.

POST-BMT MANAGEMENT

Complications

- Infection: Severe neutropenia occurs predictably in all patients and carries a significant risk of bacterial and fungal infection. Preventative strategies consist of scrupulous oral, skin, and perianal hygeine, the use of colony stimulating factors to hasten neutrophil recovery, and prophylactic oral antibacterial (e.g. quinolones) and antifungal agents. Fever during neutropenia is treated promptly with broad spectrum intravenous antibiotics.
- Mucositis: Oropharyngeal mucositis is very frequent, and often requires parenteral nutrition and opiate, analgesics.
- Bleeding: Thrombocytopenia < 20 x 10^9/L is usual and requires prophylactic platelet concentrate transfusions.
- Renal failure: Renal impairment, due to the use of nephrotoxic antibiotics, such as aminoglycosides, amphotericin B and cyclosporin, is commonly seen after BMT.
- Hepatic venoocclusive disease (VOD): This syndrome of jaundice, hyperbilirubinaemia, weight gain, ascites, and tender hepatomegaly has been reported in 5% to 30% of BMT patients, and can lead to liver failure and death. Centrilobular hepatocyte damage and associated central sinusoidal thrombosis is thought to be due to conditioning regimen toxicity. Prophylactic strategies include low-dose heparin during and after conditioning therapy, and prostaglandin infusion. Established VOD sometimes responds to fibrinolytic therapy with tissue plasminogen activator.
- Haemorrhagic cystitis: Uroepithelial damage from alkylating agent metabolites in the urine leads to this syndrome in about 10% of BMT recipients. Preventative measures consist of hyperhydration with intravenous fluids and Mesna during conditioning therapy.
- Graft-versus-host-disease (GVHD): This is a complex multi-system inflammatory disease occurring in approximately one-third of recipients of matched sibling transplants, and over 80% of unrelated allogeneic transplants, due to the infusion of alloreactive T lymphocytes and their precursors in marrow grafts.
- Acute GVHD occurs in the first 100 days post-transplant, and is graded according to the severity of involvement of skin (exfoliative dermatitis), liver (hepatitis), and gastrointestinal tract (diarrhoea and bleeding). Prophylaxis against GVHD consists of intravenous Cyclosporin, given

Table 49.1 Commonly used BMT conditioning regimens

Allogeneic	Autologous
1. Busulphan/Cyclophosphamide (Bu/Cy)	BCNU, Etoposide, Cytarabine, Melphalan (BEAM)
2. Cyclophosphamide/total body irradiation (Cy/TBI)	Cyclophosphamide, BCNU, Etoposide (CBV)

from the day before marrow infusion for 3 to 6 months post-BMT, combined with either low-dose IV Methotrexate (days 1, 3, 6, 11) or IV methylprednisolone from day +7.[6] Removal of the majority of T cells from the graft is also an effective preventative measure. Treatment of established GVHD includes the continued use of Cyclosporin, high doses of corticosteroids, and antibodies to human T cells (antilymphocyte globulin, monoclonal antibodies).

- Chronic GVHD occurs after 100 days post BMT, and has features of a number of autoimmune diseases, including scleroderma, oral lichen planus, Sjogren's syndrome, and biliary cirrhosis. Thrombocytopenia and severe immunosuppression are common problems. Chronic GVHD occurs in up to 50% of allogeneic BMT recipients, and frequently requires treatment with oral corticosteroids, Cyclosporin, and prophylactic antibiotics.

- Relapse: Relapse of the underlying malignancy is a major cause of late treatment failure after BMT. Factors increasing the risk of relapse include more advanced disease stage at BMT, absence of acute or chronic GVHD, and T cell depletion of allogeneic grafts. Relapse is more common after autografts.

- Late complications of BMT: A variety of problems have been described in long-term survivors of BMT, including cataracts, growth retardation in children, endocrine insufficiency, particularly hypothyroidism, second cancers, and infertility.

INDICATIONS FOR BMT AND OUTCOME

Acute Myeloid Leukaemia (AML)

Allogeneic BMT in first complete remission using a matched sibling donor has proved superior to chemotherapy in all reported studies, and should be offered to all patients under 40–45 years (with the possible exception of cases with favourable cytogenetic abnormalities). International Bone Marrow Transplant Registry (IBMTR) data indicate a leukaemia-free survival (LFS) rate of 60% in first CR. Allogeneic BMT is also indicated in relapsed AML patients with matched donors, although LFS is inferior (35% relapse 1, CR2, CR3; 15–20% resistant relapse)

The role of autologous BMT in AML in CR1 is controversial. LFS rates of 45–50% have been reported, and appear marginally superior to the use of conventional consolidation therapy. Autologous BMT or unrelated allogeneic BMT may be used to salvage patients with relapsed AML, who do not have a matched related donor.

Acute Lymphoblastic Leukaemia (ALL)

The use of related allogeneic BMT and autologous BMT for ALL patients in CR1 is reserved for cases with adverse progostic factors (adverse cytogenetics, particularly Philadelphia chromosome; hyperleucocytosis in pre-B disease; slowness to remit). Results are comparable to AML in CR1. Matched related or unrelated allogeneic BMT, or autologous BMT, produce LFS in 25–35% of patients with recurrent ALL.

Chronic Myeloid Leukaemia (CML)

Allogeneic BMT remains the only proven curative therapy for CML, and is usually offered to younger patients with matched family donors during first chronic phase, with LFS of 55–70% in large registry studies. Unrelated allogeneic BMT is also being used increasingly in patients under 30 years of age in early phase CML. Allogeneic BMT can also be used in patients with transformed CML, but with inferior results (LFS 35% for accelerated phase, 15% blast crisis). Auto BMT is an experimental procedure for CML.

Non-Hodgkin's Lymphoma (NHL)

Autologous stem cell transplantation is the treatment of choice for chemosensitive relapsed intermediate grade NHL, with a disease-free survival rate of 45–50% commonly reported. Allogeneic BMT also results in comparable disease-free survival rate, but with higher toxicity. Increasing numbers of transplants are being performed for low-grade lymphoma, although the long-term curative effect is still uncertain.

Hodgkin's Disease

Autologous stem cell transplantation is a recognised form of salvage therapy for patients with relapsed Hodgkin's disease, although the precise timing of its application remains contraversial. Disease-free survival rates of approximately 40–60% are reported in patients transplanted after failing radiotherapy and chemotherapy, or two chemotherapy modalities.

Multiple Myeloma

Although younger patients with myeloma can be cured by allogeneic BMT, registry data indicate disappointingly low disease-free survival rates of only 30–35%. More interest has been focussed on the use of single or multiple autologous stem cell transplants during first plateau phase, with superior results to conventional chemotherapy.

Solid Tumours

Autologous stem cell transplantation is now widely used for treatment of a variety of common solid tumours, including breast, small cell lung, ovarian, and soft tissue sarcomas. With the exception of paediatric tumours, results are generally disappointing.

Breast cancer is currently the major reason for autologous stem cell transplantation in the USA at present, although the scientific evidence to support this trend is weak.[3] A small proportion of patients with advanced metastatic disease can achieve a complete response and prolonged survival after auto BMT, but long-term cure remains unproven. Current interest is focussed on the adjuvant role of high dose chemotherapy and auto BMT in patients with high-risk Stage 2 disease at diagnosis.

REFERENCES

1. Thomas, E.D., Storb, R., Clift, R.A., A. Fefer, Johnson, F.L., Neiman, P.E., Lerner, K.G., Glucksberg, H. and Buckner, C.D. (1975) Bone Marrow Transplantation. *New Engl J Med*, **292**, 832–43.
2. Juttner, C.A., To, L.B., Haylock, D.N., Dyson, P.G., Throp, D., Dart, G.W., Ho, J.Q.K., Horvath, N. and Bardy, P. (1989) Autologous blood stem cell transplantation. *Transplant Proc*, **21**, 2929–31.
3. Antman, K.H., Rowlings, P.A., Vaughan, W.P., Pelz, C.J., Fay, J.W., Fields, K.K., Freytes, C.O., Gale, R.P., Hillner, B.E., Holland, H.K., Kennedy, M.J., Klein, J.P., Lazarus, H.M., McCarthy Jr, P.L., Saez, R., Spitzer, G., Stadtmauer, E.A., Williams, S.F., Wolff, S., Sobocinski, K.A., Armitage, J.O. and Horowitz, M.M. (1997) High dose chemotherapy with autologous hematopoietic stem cell support for breast cancer in North America. *J Clin Oncol*, **15**, 1870–9.

4. Weiden, P.L., Sullivan, K.M., Flournoy, N., Storb, R. and Thomas, E.D. (1981) Antileukemic effect of chronic graft-versus-host disease. *New Engl J Med*, **304**, 1529–33.

5. Ash, R., Casper, J.T., Chitambar, C.R., Hansen, R., Bunin, N., Truitt, R.L., Lawton, C., Murray, K., Hunter, J., Baxter-Lowe, L.A., Gottschall, J.L., Oldham, K., Anderson, T., Camitta, B. and Menitove, J. (1990) Successful allogeneic transplantation of T cell depleted bone marrow from closely HLA-matched unrelated donors. *New Engl J Med*, **332**, 485–94.

6. Storb, R., Deeg, M.J., Pepe, M., Appelbaum, F., Anasetti, C., Beatty, P., Bensigner, W., Berenson, R., Buckner, C.D., Clift, R., Doney, K., Longton, G., Hansen, J., Hill, R., Loughran Jr, T., Martin, P. Singer, J., Sanders, J., Stewart, P., Sullivan, K., Witherspoon, R. and Thomas, E.D. (1989) Methotrexate and cyclosporine versus cyclosporine alone for prophylaxis of graft-versus-host disease in patients given HLA-identical marrow grafts for leukemia:long-term follow-up of a controlled trial. *Blood*, **73**, 1729–34.

PART XII

MISCELLANEOUS CANCERS

CHAPTER 50

SARCOMAS:
DIAGNOSIS AND SURGERY

Paul D. Stalley

INTRODUCTION

Sarcomas are primary malignancies of bone and soft tissues (voluntary muscles, fat, fibrous tissue and accompanying vessels and also by convention the peripheral nervous system). These tumours are rare, with primary bone sarcoma accounting for 0.3% of new cancer notifications per year and soft tissue sarcomas 0.8% of new cases.

Sarcomas are usually classified according to the presumed primary cell of origin. Osteosarcomas must by definition produce osteoid and are bone forming tumours. Chondrosarcomas originate in primitive cartilage cells and liposarcomas originate in lipoblastic cells. The more common sarcomas include:

- Bone sarcomas
  - Osteosarcomas
  - Chondrosarcomas
  - Malignant fibrous histiocytoma
  - Ewing's sarcoma
  - Chordoma

- Soft tissue sarcomas
  - Fibrosarcoma
  - Malignant fibrous histiocytoma
  - Liposarcoma
  - Leiomyosarcoma
  - Rhabdomyosarcoma

Sarcomas are of variable aggression, but most bone sarcomas are of high-grade malignancy with often late presentation being an important feature. They form a relatively higher percentage of malignancy in childhood than cancer in the population at large.

Metastases predominently involve the lung with other bones the next most common site for metastatic disease. Spread by lymphatics is a late phenomenon.

PRESENTING SIGNS AND SYMPTOMS

A mass or swelling is the most common presentation of sarcoma. Pain or diffuse ache, particularly in a weight bearing bone, is the next most common presenting feature, with a predilection for pain to be worse at night. Some tumours present with a systemic illness, mimicking infection, and Ewing's sarcoma is the most common tumour to do this. Children particularly present with an apparent febrile illness of unknown aetiology. Pathological fracture of long bones or symptomatic pulmonary metastases are less common presentations.

DIAGNOSTIC WORK-UP

- Local imaging: Plain X-ray and/or CT scan are required of the affected area for bone anatomy, whereas MRI scans will show soft tissue extent and any soft tissue masses and the relationship to adjacent neurovascular structures.
- Systemic assessment: To determine if metastases are present, chest X-ray and CT scan of the lungs for pulmonary secondaries and a bone scan for bone secondaries.
- Haematological and biochemical analyses play only a minor role. The ESR will be elevated in many sarcomas and in bone forming tumours an elevation in the alkaline phosphatase is demonstrable.

STAGING

Once the extent of tumour has been determined by the diagnostic investigations, a biopsy is performed to confirm the histological nature of the tumour. This is performed by a true cut needle biopsy or a formal open biopsy to obtain adequate material for a definitive histological diagnosis. The histology and the radiology allow the tumour to be accurately staged.

GRADING

The grade is based on the behaviour of specific histological sub-types.

- Grade I (low grade) examples are parosteal osteosarcoma, chordoma and low-grade chondrosarcoma but high-grade tumours.
- Grade II (high grade) osteosarcoma, Ewing's sarcoma, malignant fibrous histiocytoma.
- Grade III are metastatic tumours.

All Grade I and II tumours are also characterised by their location, being: A intracompartmental or B extracompartmental. For a bone tumour this means that Stage A would be intra-osseous with no soft tissue mass, but Stage B would be where the tumour extends beyond the normal confines of the bone.

Soft Tissue Sarcomas

Soft tissue sarcomas have a multitude of staging systems, but basically they are similar to the Enneking system for primary bone malignancies with more subdivisions according to histological grade, size of tumour at the time of diagnosis, the presence of nodal secondaries and the presence of distant metastases.

MANAGEMENT

- The principle of management is to obtain remissions or cure of the tumour, and requires both local and systemic treatment.
- Where no distant metastases can be identified, treatment usually involves chemotherapy or radio-therapy, followed by resection of the affected area with limb salvage and reconstruction, where possible. This form of treatment is the basic format for the management of osteosarcoma, Ewing's sarcoma, malignant fibrous histiocytoma of bone and most soft tissue sarcomas.
- Chondrosarcoma responds very poorly to either chemotherapy or radiotherapy, and the primary modality of treatment for chondrosarcoma is surgical resection.

Surgical Management

The improvement of the surgical management of bone sarcoma in the last thirty years has occurred with the development of new regimes of chemotherapy and/or radiotherapy to achieve better tumour control. Amputation for most sarcomas was the treatment of choice before it became possible to achieve local surgical resection and limb salvage without increasing the likelihood of local recurrence. To perform a limb salvage procedure and resect only the bone tumour and have higher mortality rates from local recurrence, is not acceptable and amputation is preferable.

Studies of amputation versus limb salvage with appropriate chemotherapy and radiotherapy, however, have shown that patients can retain their limbs without increasing the likelihood of local recurrence. The indication for amputation is where limb salvage would leave a defunctioned limb because of sacrifice of neurovascular structures, or where the amount of tissue to be resected would not leave enough soft tissue cover to performe a limb reconstruction. Amputation rates for primary bone tumours are now only 15%. The remaining tumours can be managed with limb salvage.

The tumour bed should be removed because chemotherapy and/or radiotherapy cannot guaran-tee to have obliterated all viable tumour cells. In addition, trials have shown that disease-free survival is enhanced by resecting the tumour bed even where there has been an excellent response to chemo-therapy.

Resection of large tumours may be indicated for palliation even in the presence of multiple pulmonary secondaries and a limited prognosis. Sarcomas may reach such a size that they produce local effects or ulcerate or block vascular structures, resulting in distal ulceration. The quality of life of the patient is of paramount importance in the presence of metastatic disease and, although mutilating amputation surgery is not an attractive proposition, it may well be better than the mass effects of a huge local sarcoma in some cases.

In other tumours, chemotherapy and radiotherapy alone are indicated. Extensive involvement of the spine, base of skull, or pelvis are examples where resection is not possible.

Types of Surgery

Most sarcomas, both of bone and soft tissue, have around them a marginal zone which may contain small satellite tumour lesions. For this reason, any excision of a tumour bed requires an adequate cuff of normal tissue to ensure tumour eradication. A 2 cm margin appears to be the arbitrary accepted margin for most soft tissue sarcomas and also for bone sarcomas. The marginal zone around the main tumour is usually assessed by the MRI study and then a 2 cm margin distal to this is resected.

This may mean sacrifice of segments of bone, segments of artery and sacrifice of peripheral nerves. In the latter case, where a nerve is a major structure such as the sciatic nerve and the patient will, therefore, be left with an insensate distal limb, prone to ulceration and injury, amputation may be preferable. In most other situations, reconstruction can be performed to save a limb which, while not normal, is preferable to a prosthesis.

For bone reconstruction massive tumour prostheses replacing not only hip or knee joints but segments of long bone are available. Allograft banked bone is widely used for reconstructions, particularly of the pelvis, and for long bone replacement vascularised fibula grafts from the patient's own leg are increasingly being utilised.

Each operation must be tailormade to suit the particular patient and the anatomy of their tumour. No two patients will be identical and variations in technique of reconstruction must be a feature of the dexterity of the surgeon.

In some patients with isolated pulmonary metastases there can be a role for pulmonary segment resection or lobectomy, or partial lobectomy depending on the number of metastatic deposits.

Palliative internal fixation for pathological fractures prior to radiotherapy or for the treatment of bony secondaries is an integral part in the management of the whole patient with malignant disease.

Outcomes

Surgery for sarcoma is relatively uncommon and this has hampered an adequate collection of outcome information. However, in the last two decades there has been a worldwide effort to develop bone and soft tissue sarcoma tumour registers which has allowed compilation of large numbers of these rare tumours from multiple centres. These results have shown that cure rates for specific tumours significantly improved with advances in surgery, and also in chemotherapy and radiotherapy. Combination chemotherapy in Ewing's sarcoma has improved the survival rate from less than 10% to in excess of 70%. Overall, sarcomas now have a 5-year survival rate of 40–60%.

New Developments

Advances in the management of sarcomas have occurred with the development of more successful regimes and, in the future, new cytotoxic agents should further improve results. The development of more accurately targeted radiotherapy using sophisticated radiotherapy planning is likely to produce further improvements in overall results.

Surgery is developing limb salvage reconstructions that will last the rest of the patient's life. Many patients are children and if they obtain a cure they are then left with the problems of the salvaged limb. Growth in children must be mimicked in the limb salvage and may, on current techniques, require multiple procedures.

Implantable devices which can be stimulated to extend in length without surgery are being developed, and a move away from mega-prostheses is being sought as all tumour prostheses, like any hip or knee replacement, can, and probably will, become loose in a patient's lifetime. The use of vascularised fibular grafts overcomes this in many situations, as the reconstruction is living viable bone which should last forever. In many situations, as in children in pelvic surgery, there is not an adequate vascular replacement available, and the use of extra-corporeal irradiation and intra-operative irradiation are being explored.

CHAPTER 51

SARCOMA: SYSTEMIC TREATMENT

Martin H. N. Tattersall

INTRODUCTION

Sarcomas (fleshy tumours) were distinguished from carcinomas in antiquity. The primitive mesoderm is the common embryonic origin of sarcomas. Sarcomas are relatively more common in children than adults, with 15% of cancers in children and only 1% in adults.

The histological classification of sarcomas has evolved in recent years with an increasing proportion of malignant fibrous histiocytomas, rather than fibrosarcoma, leiomyosarcoma, liposarcoma, etc. Traditionally, the classification has subdivided sarcomas into bone and soft tissue tumours, but the distinction is increasingly blurred, and the 'biology' of the cancer is the main discriminate, i.e. what is the length of history? the age of the patient? the predominant tissue involved? the cell type?

A relatively new variant of sarcoma is Kaposi's sarcoma. The classic or Mediterranean form was initially described in 1872 by a dermatologist as an indolent skin lesion particularly in elderly men of Jewish or Mediterranean descent. An African variant was described some years later, occurring in young males with nodular or exophytic tumours sometimes with bone involvement. Kaposi's sarcoma was reported in renal transplant recipients and more recently in association with HIV only in the past 30 years, and the lesions associated with AIDS can be very widespread affecting skin, gastrointestinal and pulmonary systems.

BIOLOGY OF SARCOMAS

One common feature of the biology of sarcomas is their tendency to spread via the blood stream and, relatively less commonly than carcinoma, via the regional lymphatics.

The context is which the sarcoma is diagnosed is important.

- Is the patient immune compromised (e.g. HIV positive)?
- Are there possible aetiological factors, e.g. a family history of unusual cancers, possible aetiological agent exposure, e.g. radiation, herbicides, etc.?

- How long is the antecedent history?
- Are there 'embryonic' or well-differentiated histopathological features?

The relevance of these factors relates to the probably efficacy of systemic therapy in patients with metastatic or locally advanced sarcoma and also the possible benefit of adjuvant chemotherapy in patients who have had the primary site treated by surgical excision or radiation.

CHEMOSENSITIVE SARCOMAS

- Empiricism has been the main basis for gauging/predicting the chemosensitivity of sarcomas.
- Sarcomas with embryonal histology, those with a rapid growth rate and those occurring in young children or adolescents are very responsive to a range of chemotherapy drugs, including doxorubicin, actinomycin D, cyclophosphamide/ifosfamide, etoposide, and cisplatin.
- Tumours occurring in patients with HIV, particularly Kaposi's sarcoma, are also commonly responsive to chemotherapy and the most effective drugs are doxorubicin, vinca alkaloids, and alkylating agents.
- In slowly growing soft tissue sarcomas in adults, tumour regression following chemotherapy is reported in only 30%, with doxorubicin being the most effective agent, but cyclophosphamide/ifosfamide, DTIC and platinum analogues also have some activity.
- In primary bone sarcomas, there is a range of chemosensitivity, with Ewing's sarcoma being very responsive to several drugs notably doxorubicin, cyclophosphamide/ifosfamide, vinca alkaloids, and etoposide.
- Osteogenic sarcoma is responsive to drugs, notably doxorubicin, high-dose methotrexate, cyclophosphamide and to a lesser extent platinum analogues, perhaps particularly when given regionally.
- Chondrosarcomas are particularly chemoresistant.

HORMONE SENSITIVE SARCOMAS

In soft tissue sarcomas of the uterus, tamoxifen and progestin therapy sometimes cause tumour regression. Indeed these tumours commonly contain oestrogen and/or progesterone receptors, though their presence does not predict tumour responsiveness.

PRIMARY CHEMOTHERAPY IN SARCOMAS

- For locally advanced or metastatic chemosensitive sarcomas, initial chemotherapy is used because tumour response may reduce the extent of subsequent surgery or radiotherapy.
- If the tumour is chemosensitive, the patient can be treated with curative intent with adjuvant systemic treatment after local treatment has been completed. This strategy is widely used in children or young adults with Ewing's sarcoma and extra-cranial neuroectodermal tumours, in embryonal rhabdosarcoma and other sarcomas of childhood.
- In children and adults with osteogenic sarcomas, and in adult-type soft tissue sarcomas in the extremities who are candidates for limb conserving surgery, primary chemotherapy may be used.
- Such chemotherapy, most commonly doxorubicin, cisplatin ± other drugs may reduce the need for mutilating surgery or amputation.

- The limited randomised trials performed do not suggest that intra-arterial chemotherapy is more effective, or has less side effects than intravenous treatment using the same drugs. Nevertheless, intra-arterial chemotherapy is widely used.
- In osteogenic sarcoma, the degree of necrosis in the primary tumour after chemotherapy is of prognostic importance and implies that primary chemotherapy influences outcomes in this disease.

ADJUVANT CHEMOTHERAPY IN SARCOMAS

- In patients with chemosensitive sarcoma, chemotherapy is usually given as primary treatment and subsequent to surgery. It is also usual for adjuvant chemotherapy to be given for several months following local therapy.
- The total duration of treatment is characteristically longer in children than adults. However, there is no good clinical evidence on the optimal duration of systemic adjuvant treatments in either adults or children.
- In adults with soft tissue sarcomas, adjuvant chemotherapy with doxorubicin containing regimens may be beneficial although the evidence is not well established.
- In children and adults with osteogenic sarcoma, there is evidence that adjuvant chemotherapy is effective, prolong survival. The most active drugs in osteogenic sarcoma are doxorubicin, methotrexate, cyclophosphamide/ifosfamide, but the optimal duration and schedule of systemic treatment is not certain.

REFERENCES

1. Antman, K.H. (1992) Chemotherapy of advanced sarcoma of bone and soft tissue. *Semin Oncol* **19** (6 Suppl 12), 13–20.
2. Bramwell, V., Rouesse, J., Steward, W., Santoro, A., Schrattorat-Koops, H., Buesa, J., Raka, W., Priavio, J., Wagener, T., Burgers, N., Unnik, J.V., Contesso, G., Thomas, D., um Glabbelle, N., Markham, D. and Pinedo, H. (1994) Adjuvant CYVADIC chemotherapy for adult soft tissue sarcoma—reduced local recurrence but no improvement in survival: a study of the EORTC Soft Tissue and Bone Sarcomas Group. *J Clin Oncol,* **12**, 1137–49.
3. Daugaard, S., von Glabbeke, M., Schiodt, T. and Mouridsen, H.T. (1993) Histological grade and response to chemotherapy in advanced soft tissue sarcoma. *Eur. J Cancer*, **29A(6)**, 811–813.
4. Mazanet, R. and Antman, K.H. (1991) Sarcomas of soft tissue and bone. *Cancer*, **68(3)**, 463–473.
5. Verweij, J., van Oosterom, A.T., Somers, R., Santoro, A., Rouesse, J., Keizer, J., Tursz, T., Woll, P., Steward, W. and Buesa, J. (1992) Chemotherapy in the multidisciplinary approach to soft tissue sarcoma: EORTC Soft Tissue and Bone Sarcoma Group studies in perspective. *Ann. Oncol.*, **3** (suppl 2), S75–80.

CHAPTER 52

TUMOURS OF THE CENTRAL NERVOUS SYSTEM

Jane Beith

INTRODUCTION

There are a wide variety of primary brain tumours whose incidence varies with age.

- CNS tumours are the most prevalent solid neoplasm of childhood, the second leading cancer-related cause of death in children younger than 15 years of age, and the third leading cause of death from cancer in persons 15 to 34 years of age.
- Most intracranial tumours occur in people older than 45 years. The incidence of high-grade astrocytomas, glioblastoma multiforme, increases with age.
- Medulloblastomas are predominantly a tumour observed in children and account for 20% of tumours in this age group, whereas in the adult these are extremely rare.

CLASSIFICATION

Polednak and Flannery have reported the incidence of brain tumours as summarized in Table 52.1.

AETIOLOGY

There is little evidence pointing to causes of brain tumours. Exposure to certain pesticides, herbicides, fertilizers and petrochemicals have been purported to increase the incidence of brain tumours but there is little evidence to support this. Simultaneously there has been concern about electromagnetic fields causing glial tumours but most studies do not support this hypothesis.

CLINICAL PRESENTATION

- Headache is the most common symptom which has classically been described as occuring in the early morning hours or on waking.
- Gastrointestinal symptoms including anorexia, nausea and vomiting are common.

- Sometimes the only presenting symptoms are changes in personality, mood, mental capacity and concentration.
- Seizures are a presenting symptom in approximately 20% of patients with supratentorial tumours.
- Less commonly, patients present with focal neurological symptoms.

DIAGNOSIS

MRI and CT scanning are the major techniques used to demonstrate cerebral lesions. MRI is more sensitive, especially for low-grade and posterior fossa tumours.

ASTROCYTOMAS

Prognosis

Low-grade astrocytomas have 10-year survival rates of 6% to 35% dependent on extent of resection. The median survival for high-grade astrocytomas is 2 to 3 years for anaplastic astrocytomas and 8 to 9 months for glioblastomas. Apart from histology, there are several other major prognostic factors which predict for outcome in malignant astrocytoma, such as age, performance status, extent of surgery and a long history of fits.

Treatment

Surgery

Surgery is part of the initial management of gliomas to establish the diagnosis and quickly relieve mass effect. Extensive resection allows improvement in focal as well as global symptoms and also increases survival in both low- and high-grade astrocytomas.

A median survival of 14 to 22 weeks with surgery alone reflects the unique infiltrative growth characteristics of malignant gliomas. This makes true 'total resection' impossible without causing unacceptable neurological damage to the patient.

Table 52.1 Frequency of primary central nervous system tumours

Type	Frequency (%)
Glioblastoma multiforme	40.6
Infiltrative astrocytoma	42.4
Pilocytic astrocytoma	1.5
Oligodendroglioma	3.5
Mixed oligoastrocytoma	1.7
Ependymoma	3.0
Medulloblastoma	3.6
Others	3.9

Source: Data from Polednak, A.P. and Flannery J.T. (1995) Brain, other central nervous system and eye cancer. *Cancer*, **75**, 330.

Radiotherapy

Radiation therapy has a central role in the management of malignant gliomas. For malignant gliomas, the usual treatment regimen of 50 to 60 Gy delivered over a period of 5 to 6 weeks at the time of initial diagnosis unequivocally prolongs survival. A randomised prospective study by the Brain Tumour Cooperative reported a median survival time of 14 weeks with surgery alone and 36 weeks with surgery and radiotherapy.

However, despite aggressive radiotherapy, 80% to 90% of patients die from local disease. Primary brain tumours rarely metastasize. To date, the use of radiation sensitisers, hyperbaric oxygen or hyperfractionated schedules as modifiers of the radiation therapy have not resulted in significant improvement in survival. The role of radiotherapy in low-grade gliomas is less well defined and usually used for incompletely resected tumours.

Chemotherapy

Chemotherapy in patients with high-grade gliomas has had little impact on survival. The most active drugs include chloroethylnitrosoureas, procarbazine and vincristine. The chloroethylnitrosoureas which are highly lipid-soluable, generally non-ionised compounds that readily cross the blood-brain barrier, have received the most attention.

Individual studies assessing the use of chemotherapy in high-grade gliomas have found no significant increase in survival. A meta-analysis of large prospective randomised chemotherapeutic trials of malignant gliomas found a consistent beneficial effect for chemotherapy. The mean 12-month survival rate among 884 patients with radiation therapy alone was 41.2%, as compared with 53.5% among 1,538 patients who received radiation therapy and chemotherapy. At 24 months there was a persisting absolute increase in the survival rate of 8.6%, with the mean 24-month survival rate being 15.9% with radiation alone and 23.4% with radiation and chemotherapy. These results show a significant benefit of chemotherapy. Despite these results chemotherapy is not often used routinely as adjuvant treatment.

Treatment of Recurrent Malignant Astrocytomas

At the time of recurrence, surgery is often limited by tumour involvement of the functional brain or diffuse brain infiltration. Radiation may be contraindicated because of constraints such as the normal tissue tolerance from prior radiation exposure. Thus, chemotherapy is often the only standard treatment option available. However, its effectiveness is limited by excessive tumour burden, problems of drug delivery, and acquired drug resistance. The management of recurrent gliomas remains palliative with complete responses infrequent.

New drugs continue to enter clinical trials for treatment of high-grade astrocytomas. Initial studies with temozolomide have shown partial response rates of 40% to 50% in patients with newly diagnosed and recurrent high-grade gliomas. High-dose chemotherapy with autologous bone marrow rescue or intra-arterial therapy have not been very effective and have had significant toxicity. Potentially promising approaches include interstitial chemotherapy using surgically implanted polymers, continuous infusion of chemotherapeutic agents and modulation of drug resistance in these tumours.

Other therapeutic modalites such as radioactive seed implants, stereotactic radiosurgery, conjugation of radio-isotopes to antibodies against the epidermal-growth factor receptor, and gene therapy are also being evaluated.

OLIGODENDROGLIOMAS

- Treatment of oligodendrogliomas is similar to malignant gliomas which involves initial debulking surgery followed by radiotherapy for high-grade oligodendrogliomas.
- For low-grade tumours the role for radiotherapy is controversial and tends to be administered to those patients with incompletely resected tumours.
- Chemotherapy is usually reserved for recurrence and these tumours have shown better response rates than astrocytomas.
- Similar chemotherapeutic agents are utilised. Median survival in these tumours has been reported 4–5 years.

MEDULLOBLASTOMAS

- Surgery is initial treatment followed by craniospinal radiotherapy, as medulloblastomas commonly infiltrate the subarachnoid space and spread through the the CSF.
- The five-year survival rate ranges from 50% to 65%.
- These tumours are responsive to chemotherapy and the benefit of its use in combination with radiotherapy at initial diagnosis is controversial.
- For children aged under two years there is increasing tendency to use combination chemotherapy as primary therapy instead of radiotherapy.

EPENDYMOMAS

- Ependymomas tend to arise in the cerebral ventricles and occasionally in the spinal canal. Maximal surgical debulking is initial treatment followed by radiotherapy.
- Local radiotherapy is given and consideration for craniospinal irradiation is done because of the tendency for these tumours to seed the subarachnoid area.

MENINGIOMAS

- Meningiomas are the most common benign brain tumour.
- After complete surgical excision there is a recurrence rate of 8–11% at 10 years and for incomplete resection 29–44%.
- The role of radiotherapy for incompletely resected tumours is controversial.
- These tumours may have oestrogen and progesterone receptors.
- They are twice as frequent in females, may enlarge during pregnancy and are more common in patients with breast carcinoma.

REFERENCES

Black, P.M. (1991) Brain Tumours. *New England Journal of Medicine*, **324**, 1471–1476.
Black, P.M. (1991) Brain Tumours. *New England Journal of Medicine*, **324**, 1555–1564.
Fine, H.A., Dear, K.B., and Loeffler, J.S. (1993) Meta-analysis of radiation therapy with and without adjuvant chemotherapy for malignant gliomas in adults. *Cancer*, **71**, 2585–2597.

Levin, V.A., Leibel, S.A. and Gutin, P.H. (1997) Neoplasms of the Central Nervous System in Cancer. In *Principles and Practice of Oncology* (5th edn), edited by DeVita, pp. 2022–2082. Philadelphia: Lippincott-Raven.

Walker, M.D., Alexander, E., Hunt, W.E., MacCarty, C.S., Mahaley, M.S. Jr, Norrell, H.A., Owens, G., Ransohoff, J., Wilson, C.B., Gehan, E.A. and Strike, T.A. (1978) Evaluation of BCNU and/or radiotherapy in the treatment of anaplastic gliomas, a cooperative trial. *J Neurosurg*, **49**, 333–343.

FAST FACT SHEET 6

TUMOURS OF THE ENDOCRINE SYSTEM

Elizabeth Chua and John R. Turtle

THYROID CARCINOMA

Table FFS 6.1 Classification of thyroid carcinoma

Type	Distribution	Mortality Rate
Papillary	70–80%	10% at 10 years
Follicular	10–20%	20–40% at 10 years
Medullary	5–10%	30–40% at 10 years
Anaplastic	1–3%	100% at 3 years

Risk Factors for Thyroid Cancer

- history of neck irradiation
- family history of thyroid cancer
- rapid tumour growth

PARATHYROID TUMOURS CAUSING PRIMARY HYPERPARATHYROIDISM

- parathyroid adenoma (80%)
- parathyroid hyperplasia (20%)
- parathyroid carcinoma (< 1%)

FUNCTIONING PITUITARY TUMOURS

- prolactin (30–40%)
- growth hormone (2–17%)

- adrenocorticotrophic hormone (2–10%)
- follicle stimulating hormone and luteinizing hormone (10%)
- thyroid stimulating hormone (1%)

TUMOURS PRODUCING GLUCOCORTICOID EXCESS

- ACTH-secreting pituitary adenoma (70–80%)
- ectopic ACTH from non-pituitary tumours (10%)
- adrenal adenoma (10–20%)
- adrenal carcinoma (10%)

PANCREATIC ENDOCRINE TUMOURS

- insulinoma
- glucagonoma
- gastrinoma

CHAPTER 53

TUMOURS OF THE ENDOCRINE SYSTEM

Elizabeth Chua and John R. Turtle

THYROID TUMOURS

Introduction

Thyroid nodules are extremely common. Evaluation and management remain a challenging task despite the numerous diagnostic resources available to the clinician. An accurate assessment of the risk of malignancy is crucial for the treatment plan. The classification of thyroid carcinoma is listed in Table FFS 6.1.

Diagnosis

- When assessing a thyroid nodule, factors such as history of neck irradiation, positive family history, rapid nodule growth, and presence of lymph nodes increase the risk for malignancy.
- Thyroid function test is usually normal.
- Ultrasound and radionuclide scans offer little discriminatory value in distinguishing benign from malignant lesions.
- Although fine needle biopsy is used extensively to guide the diagnosis, aspirates may be insufficient or diagnosis inconclusive even in experienced hands.

Management

- Patients with malignant results on biopsy should have total thyroidectomy, while patients with benign results should have a repeat biopsy if any risk factors arise. Those with suspicious findings however, should proceed to surgery, the extent of which may be determined by a frozen section analysis.

Papillary Carcinoma

The diagnosis of papillary carcinoma can be made by fine needle biopsy or at surgery. Surgical excision is the primary treatment followed by radioactive iodine (I^{131}) therapy 4–12 weeks post-operatively to ablate surgical remnants. Subsequently, patients are permanently maintained on thyroxine to suppress thyroid stimulating hormone (TSH), as this hormone can stimulate growth of thyroid tumours and/or metastases. Patients are monitored with radionuclide scans and thyroglobulin levels (marker for recurrent or residual disease), and treated with I^{131} until there is no scan evidence of malignancy and thyroglobulin levels are undetectable. Thereafter, most patients are monitored on a yearly basis with clinical examination and thyroglobulin levels.

Due to the associated risk of hypoparathyroidism and recurrent laryngeal nerve injury with total thyroidectomy, some centres advocate minimal thyroid surgery for papillary carcinoma that are < 1 cm, unifocal and intrathyroidal in young patients. The drawback with this approach is the possibility of missing multifocal or microcarcinoma in the other lobe and the difficulty of subsequently utilizing adjuvant radionuclide scanning/treatment and thyroglobulin level monitoring.

Metastasis is by local lymph node invasion, but may spread to the lungs. It is usually slow growing and is not associated with death or significant morbidity.

Follicular Carcinoma

Follicular carcinoma is frequently indistinguishable from follicular adenoma based on fine needle cytology or frozen section analysis. Vascular and capsular invasion, which are used as markers of malignancy, may be missed on the two procedures.

A hemithyroidectomy is performed initially, followed by a more extensive surgery if indicated. Patients are treated with I^{131} after surgery to ablate remnants and metastases, and are maintained on thyroxine suppression.

Metastases, which occur through haematogenous routes, involve bones or lungs. Tumour recurrences in distant sites occur in aggressive cases.

Medullary Carcinoma

Medullary carcinoma, which arises from the calcitonin-secreting cells of the thyroid gland, may occur in the following settings:

- sporadic medullary thyroid carcinoma
- multiple endocrine neoplasia type II (MEN II) syndromes
- familial non-MEN medullary carcinoma

Patients may present with a thyroid nodule or as part of the familial syndrome. Elevated calcitonin levels, either basal or after pentagastrin stimulation, are highly suggestive of the diagnosis of medullary carcinomas. Considering the possibility of MEN II in a patient, the presence of phaeochromocytoma should be checked prior to surgery.

Early detection and adequate therapy results in a good prognosis. Total thyroidectomy with or without neck dissection is the primary treatment. Cervical node metastases occur early and may be present at time of diagnosis. Calcitonin levels and other imaging modalities such as CT scan or MRI are used for monitoring after surgery. As medullary carcinoma is not responsive to I^{131} treatment, external beam radiation may be given for metastatic disease.

Anaplastic Carcinoma

Anaplastic carcinoma usually occurs in elderly patients with longstanding history of goitre or it may arise from differentiated carcinoma. Treatment consists of surgery and radiation therapy. The prognosis is very poor with death occurring in 6–36 months.

PARATHYROID TUMOURS

Primary hyperparathyroidism may result from a single parathyroid adenoma or from hyperplasia of all four glands. Those associated with MEN syndrome almost always involve multiple glands.

Patients with parathyroid tumours may present with asymptomatic hypercalcaemia, bone disease, nephrolithiasis, or as part of the MEN syndrome. Serum calcium and intact parathyroid hormone (PTH) levels are both elevated.

Successful parathyroidectomy is achieved, without preoperative imaging, in > 90% of cases in the hands of an experienced parathyroid surgeon. In patients whose initial neck exploration is unsuccessful or in those with recurrent disease, further imaging using ultrasound, CT scan, MRI or technetium-99m sestamibi scan may be necessary to aid the surgeon in localizing the tumour.

Although surgery is curative in > 90% of cases, controversy still exists for managing patients with mild asymptomatic hypercalcaemia. Guidelines for surgery established by the Consensus Development Conference on the management of asymptomatic primary hyperparathyroidism include:

- serum calcium > 2.99 mmol/L (12 mg/dl)
- marked hypercalciuria (> 9.98 mmol/day)
- overt manifestation of hyperparathyroidism (nephrolithiasis, bone disease)
- markedly reduced cortical bone density (radius z score < –2)
- reduced creatinine clearance in the absence of other cause
- age < 50 years

Patients with parathyroid carcinoma may have symptoms and signs secondary to the hypercalcaemic state and not necessarily from enlargement of the tumour. Debulking of the tumour helps in the control of hypercalcaemia.

PITUITARY TUMOURS

Pituitary tumours are almost always benign. They can be classified either as:

1. functioning (oversecretion of a specific hormone) or nonfunctioning
2. microadenoma (< 1 cm) or macroadenoma.

Diagnosis

Clinical presentation varies depending on the hormone that is hypersecreted. On the other hand, patients with non-functioning tumours may present with hypopituitarism due to progressive loss of function from pressure on adjacent areas of the gland or pressure on the stalk resulting in impaired flow of releasing factors. Large tumours may cause visual impairment ranging from bitemporal hemianopia to complete visual loss. Radiologic evaluation includes CT scan of the pituitary region or MRI.

Treatment

- Treatment of pituitary adenomas includes surgery, radiotherapy and drugs to suppress hormone hypersecretion.

- Surgery is the primary treatment in most cases, with transphenoidal approach as the procedure of choice.
- Patients presenting with visual impairment should have surgery as early as possible in an attempt to reverse any visual loss.
- Surgical complications including cerebrospinal fluid leak, meningitis, visual impairment, and diabetes insipidus (transient or permanent) occur mostly in patients with large tumours.
- Patients with large tumours which are not completely resected are given radiotherapy.
- Bromocriptine, a dopamine agonist, has been used extensively in patients with hyperprolactinaemia, both as the initial and primary treatment, or as a supplementary treatment after surgery.
- Octreotide, a long-acting somatostatin analogue, is used in patients in whom surgery or radiotherapy fail to reduce growth hormone levels to normal.
- After surgery, patients' hormonal reserve should be assessed with stimulation tests and deficient hormones should be replaced.

ADRENAL TUMOURS

Glucocorticoid-secreting Tumours

Glucocorticoid-secreting adrenal tumours (adenoma or carcinoma) result in Cushing's syndrome, commonly presenting with truncal obesity, moon facies, buffalo hump, and purplish striae.

Documentation of endogenous hypercortisolism is done by an overnight 1 mg dexamethasone suppression test or a 24-hour urine free cortisol determination. Simultaneous determination of plasma corticotrophin (ACTH) levels and serum cortisol levels helps localize the source of hypercortisolism. In glucocorticoid secreting adrenal tumours, the plasma ACTH levels will be suppressed. Patients with adrenal carcinomas usually have high levels of DHEA in addition to cortisol excess. CT scan of the abdomen will show a unilateral adrenal tumour, usually 2 cm or larger, and the uninvolved contralateral gland will be normal or atrophic.

Patients with adrenal adenomas are treated with unilateral adrenalectomy resulting in an excellent outcome. Because of suppression of the other gland, patients should be covered with steroids both during and after surgery until the other gland recovers which may take up to 6 months or longer. In patients with adrenal carcinoma, surgery reduces the tumour mass and medical treatment (mitotane) is given in an attempt to block corticosteroid hormone production.

Aldosterone-producing Adenomas

Aldosterone-producing adenomas are usually small and unilateral. Patients present with low serum potassium, low plasma renin activity and borderline or high aldosterone levels. A unilateral adenoma can be picked up by CT scan 80% of the time. The most reliable means of establishing hyperaldosteronism and distinguishing unilateral from bilateral overproduction is bilateral catheterization of adrenal veins. The preferred treatment for patients with aldosterone producing adenoma is unilateral adrenalectomy.

Phaeochromocytoma

Phaeochromocytoma presents classically with headaches, sweating and palpitations with a background of hypertension. It may be associated with MEN II syndromes. Diagnosis depends on demonstration of high levels of plasma and urine catecholamines, followed by localization of the tumour by CT scan or MRI, with or without metaiodobenzylguanidine (MIBG) scan.

Preoperative adequate alpha followed by beta blockade should be achieved to prevent perioperative morbidity and mortality. Plasma and urine catecholamines should be repeated 1–3 months post-operatively and patients followed-up long term because of the possibility of metastases occurring several years later.

Incidental Adrenal Tumours

Unsuspected adrenal masses have been identified by abdominal CT scans. Full clinical assessment and hormonal screening should be done initially, followed by serial CT scan monitoring for non-functioning tumours < 3 cm.

PANCREATIC TUMOURS

Insulinomas

Insulinomas are the most common type of islet cell tumour; 90% are single and benign, 10% are multiple and may occur in association with MEN I. Patients often present with neurological symptoms associated with hypoglycemia, such as confusion, lightheadedness, loss of consciousness or aberrant behaviour.

The hallmark of an insulin-secreting tumour is failure of endogenous insulin to be suppressed in the presence of hypoglycaemia. This can be done either by a supervised prolonged fast (72 hours) or by an insulin infusion keeping the blood glucose levels < 2.5 mmol/L. Since most tumours are small (< 2 cm in 80%), a negative CT or MRI imaging is not conclusive. Arteriography and transhepatic portal vein sampling may aid the localization of the tumour.

The treatment of choice is surgical resection done by surgeons with extensive experience with islet cell tumours. Palpation and intra-operative ultrasound localization of tumours have 85–90% success rate. Diazoxide is the treatment of choice for inoperable patients, or for patients whose tumours are not found intra-operatively.

MULTI-SYSTEM TUMOURS

MEN I

MEN I is characterised by tumours of the pituitary, parathyroids and pancreas. The pituitary lesion is usually a benign adenoma, the parathyroid involvement is multiglandular and the most common pancreatic tumour involved is gastrinoma.

MEN II

MEN IIA is associated with medullary thyroid carcinoma, phaeochromocytoma and hyperparathyroidism. On the other hand, MEN IIB consist of medullary thyroid carcinoma, phaeochromocytoma, multiple mucosal ganglioneuromas and marfanoid habitus. Surgery is the treatment of choice for the neoplasias.

Since MEN syndromes are dominantly transmitted, evaluation of family members should be instituted. Now that the MEN I gene has been cloned, its role in identifying individuals at risk are being studied.

REFERENCES

Dulgeroff, A.J. and Hershman, J.M. (1994) Medical therapy for differentiated thyroid carcinoma. *Endocrine Reviews*, **15**, 500–515.

Gifford, R.W., Manger, W.M. and Bravo, E.L. (1994) Phaechromocytoma. *Endocrinology and Metabolism Clinics of North America*, **23**, 387–40.

Hammond, P.J., Jackson, J.A. and Bloom, S.R. (1994) Localization of pancreatic endocrine tumours. *Clinical Endocrinology*, **40**, 3–11.

Hennessey, J.V. and Jackson, I.M.D. (1995) Clinical features and differential diagnosis of pituitary tumours with emphasis on acromegaly. *Bailliere's Clinical Endocrinology and Metabolism*, **9**, 271–314.

Samuels, M.H. and Loriaux, D.L. (1994) Cushing's syndrome and the nodular adrenal gland. *Endocrinology and Metabolism Clinics of North America*, **23**, 555–569.

Silverberg, S.J. and Bilezikian, J.P. (1996) Evaluation and management of primary hyperparathyroidism. *Journal of Clinical Endocrinology and Metabolism*, **81**, 2036–2040.

CHAPTER 54

PAEDIATRIC CANCER

Keith Waters

INTRODUCTION

Cancer is a rare disease in childhood but is the second most common cause of death after accidents in children aged 1–14 years. The annual incidence rate is 130 per million children. Leukaemia and lymphoid malignancy account for 40–50% and primary central nervous neoplasms for 20% (Table 54.1). Overall the expected survival rate is 80% and it is projected that 1 in 1000 young adults will be cancer survivors by early next century.

AETIOLOGY

The aetiology of most childhood cancer is unknown. There is a slight male preponderance. Certain rare genetic disorders are associated with an increased risk of malignancy, e.g. Down syndrome, Fanconi's aplastic anaemia, ataxia telangiectasia, WAGR syndrome: Wilms' tumour, aniridia, genital abnormalities and mental retardation. Bilateral retinoblastoma has an autosomal dominant pattern of inheritance requiring loss of both copies of the rb1 gene for tumour development. Germline mutations of p53 have been found in association with the Li-Fraumeni syndrome and some cases of soft tissue sarcoma and osteosarcoma. An increased incidence of Wilms' tumour, hepatoblastoma and adrenal cortical carcinoma occurs in children with Beckwith-Wiedemann syndrome, as does optic glioma and malignant schwannoma in those with neurofibromatosis type I.

OUTCOMES IN PAEDIATRIC CANCER

Paediatric cancer differs from adult cancer in that the expectation is of cure and hopefully cure without cost. In some tumours, e.g. medulloblastoma, the tumour may have produced symptoms such as ataxia and cranial nerve palsies which do not recover completely after surgery, and long-term complications of therapy necessary for cure include growth failure and poor school performance secondary to irradiation therapy.

Table 54.1 Frequency of malignant disease in childhood

Malignant disease	Frequency (%)
Leukaemia	30
Primary CNS tumours	20
Lymphoma	10
Wilms' tumour	6–8
Neuroblastoma	6–8
Soft tissue sarcoma	5
Bone sarcoma	4
Histiocytosis	5
Teratoma	2
Retinoblastoma	1
Others	5

Potential long-term complications of chemotherapy include cardiomyopathy due to anthracyclines, infertility due to alkylating agents and renal dysfunction due to cis-platinum or ifosfamide. Some of these problems may not become evident for many years after treatment has ceased indicating the importance of long-term follow-up of children cured of cancer.

LEUKAEMIA

Acute lymphoblastic leukaemia (ALL) accounts for approximately 80%, acute myeloid (AML) for 20% and chronic myeloid for 1–2% of childhood leukaemia.

Acute Lymphoblastic Leukaemia (ALL)

Presentation

ALL has a peak incidence at 4 years of age. Presenting symptoms include pallor (commonest), easy bruising, fever and limp and reluctance to walk due to bone pain. Signs include painless lymphadenopathy and hepatosplenomegaly of variable extent. CNS, testicular and other extramedullary involvement is rare at presentation. Differential diagnoses includes infectious mononucleosis, juvenile rheumatoid arthritis, aplastic anaemia, lymphoma and neuroblastoma. Anaemia and thrombocytopenia are usually present, 50% having an elevated white cell count.

Bone marrow aspirate confirms the diagnosis, allows cytogenetic analysis and immunophenotyping — 80% of cases are of precursor B-cell origin and 20% of T-cell origin.

Prognostic Factors

Clinical features predicting a poor prognosis are age < 1 year or > 10 years and WCC > 50 $\leftrightarrow$ 10^9/L but have become less important with improved therapy. Genotypic abnormalities are of most prognostic significance and now are used to determine risk groups and thus the intensity of therapy (Table 54.2).

Table 54.2 Risk group classification for acute lymphoblastic leukaemia (ALL)

Risk Group	Clinical Features	Cytogenetic/Molecular Features

Low risk	1. Age 1–10 years
	   WCC < 50 x 10⁹/L
	2. Not T-cell phenotype
	3. No CNS or testicular
	   leukaemia
	4. Rapid response to
	   initial therapy
		1. DNA index ⊕ 1.16
		2. Absence of — t(9;22) BCR/ABL
		                    — t(4;11) MLL/AF4
		                    — t(1;19)
		                    — MLL rearrangement
		
		3. t(12;21) TEL/AML1
		4. t(8;14), t(2;8) or t(8;22)
		   (with short-term intensive therapy)

High risk	Those not in low or very high risk groups	
Very high risk	1. Induction failure 2. Age <12 months	1. t(9;22), t(4;11) 2. MLL rearrangements

Treatment

- Remission induction — Vincristine, prednisolone, L-asparaginase ± daunomycin and intrathecal methotrexate (IT MTX) gives a 98% remission induction rate.
- CNS preventative therapy — IT MTX ± high-dose IV MTX together with consolidation therapy with cyclophosphamide, Ara-C, 6-Mercaptopurine (6-MP), vincristine. Cranial irradiation reserved for cases at very high risk of CNS relapse. Not given below 4–5 years due to risk of intellectual impairment. CNS relapse rate now <10%.
- Interim maintenance therapy is usually oral 6-mercaptopurine (6-MP) and methotrexate (MTX). Reinduction-reconsolidation — similar to initial therapy. Maintenance chemotherapy with monthly vincristine and prednisolone pulses and daily 6-MP, weekly MTX, both orally. Treatment for 2 years provided remission maintained. Ten to fifteen percent risk of relapse once therapy is stopped extending over 2 years. Relapse during therapy portends a poor outlook (10–20% cure) and stem cell transplantation recommended to improve chance of cure (40–50% cure).

Acute Myeloid Leukaemia (AML)

- AML requires intensive myelosuppressive induction and consolidation therapy utilising a combination of Ara-C, daunomycin or idarubicin, 6-thioguanine, etoposide (VP-16), amsacrine and intrathecal (MTX).
- Remission induction rate is 85–90%. Cure rate is 50–60%.
- Role of growth factor support remains uncertain.
- Probable equivalent cure rate for autologous or allogeneic transplantation.
- Use of retinoic acid as differentiating agent in acute promyelocytic leukaemia.
- Total length of therapy six months.

NON-HODGKIN'S LYMPHOMA

- Staging is clinical with organ imaging, bone marrow and CSF examination.
- Treatment of Stage I and II with Vincristine, cyclophosphamide, prednisolone, intermediate dose methotrexate and occasionally anthracyclines. Cure rate is 80–90%.
- Stage III and IV:
  — Thoracic primary (mediastinal) of T-cell origin, treated as ALL.
  — Abdominal primary of B-cell origin require a highly intensive, short, six-month course utilising vincristine, prednisolone, cyclophosphamide, high dose MTX and Ara-C, doxorubicin and intrathecal MTX.
- Cure rate is 70–80%. There is no role for XRT.

HODGKIN'S DISEASE

- Hodgkin's disease is treated with chemotherapy alone.
- Irradiation therapy avoided because of effects on growth and development.
- Cure rate is 90% irrespective of Stage.
- Universal infertility occurs in males, less so in females, secondary to MOPP.
- ABVD is equally effective, less toxic.

NEUROBLASTOMA

Presentation

Primary sites are adrenal, abdominal non-adrenal, thoracic, pelvic, cervical, in decreasing frequency. Neuroblastoma metastasises to bone, bone marrow, lymph nodes, liver, skin. It presents with abdominal mass, proptosis and/or eyelid bruising, node enlargement, fever, bone pain, signs of spinal cord compression (thoracic). Staging is performed clinically and with organ imaging, multiple bone marrow aspirates and MIBG scan.

Treatment

Surgery alone is used for Stage I and II where the cure rate is 90–100%. Intensive chemotherapy ± autologous stem transplant is used for Stage III and IV where the cure rate is 10–20%. Increased N-myc copy number and 1p chromosome deletions predict for a poor prognosis, irrespective of Stage. Stage IVS defines an infant with metastases to skin and/or liver and/or bone marrow but not bone. Spontaneous regression has been reported. Screening has not decreased incidence of Stage III or IV but detects tumours likely to undergo spontaneous remission with normal or low N-myc copy numbers.

WILMS' TUMOUR (NEPHROBLASTOMA)

Presentation

Wilms' tumours present as an abdominal mass but rarely haematuria. Staging is performed clinically on abdominal ultrasound or CT specifically to exclude renal vein or IVC extension. Chest X-ray and CT of the lung is also performed.

Treatment

The treatment for Wilms' tumour is surgical with a nephrectomy, adjuvant chemotherapy with vincristine, actinomycin-D for Stages I and II plus doxorubicin added for Stages III and IV. Abdominal irradiation is given for Stage III. Radiation is not given to the lungs in Stage IV if complete clearing of pulmonary metastases has occurred on CT with initial chemotherapy. Chemotherapy prior to nephrectomy is the European approach compared to immediate nephrectomy which is the North American approach. Cure rate for Stages I and II is 90–100% and for III and IV is 80%.

RHABDOMYOSARCOMA

- Primary sites are genitourinary, extremity, parameningeal, orbit, other.
- Accurate staging is important.
- Alveolar histology has a worse outlook than embryonal.
- Avoid mutilating surgery in the management, e.g. pelvic exenteration.
- Chemotherapy remains the mainstay of treatment.
- The European approach avoids irradiation wherever possible, although it is widely used in North America.
- Cure rate for group I and II is 80–90%, group III is 50% and for IV, 20%.

OSTEOSARCOMA

- Primary treatment is with Cis-platinum, doxorubicin, high-dose methotrexate then limb preserving surgery if possible.
- Histologic response of primary predicts prognosis.
- Resection of pulmonary metastases where possible.
- Overall cure rate is 70%.

EWING'S SARCOMA

- Ewing's sarcoma can occur in any bone. Pelvic primaries are very large.
- Metastases to lung, bone and marrow are commonly seen.
- Chromosome translocations, t(11;22), are diagnostic.
- Tumour volume and histologic response predict prognosis.
- Chemotherapy is given to resolve the soft-tissue component.
- Resection of involved bone is indicated whenever possible.
- Irradiation for non-resectable or with residual soft-tissue tumour.
- High-dose chemotherapy and stem cell support is considered in poor prognosis cases.
- Cure rate is 60–70%.

HEPATOBLASTOMA

Hepatoblastoma presents with an enlarged liver and raised alphafetoprotein. Initial chemotherapy is given to shrink the tumour, then delayed surgery. Cure rate with this approach is 60–80% even in patients with pulmonary metastases.

LANGERHAN'S CELL HISTIOCYTOSIS

Langerhan's cell histiocytosis is possibly a defect of immune regulation. It involves bone, skin, liver, marrow and the GI tract. Clinical presentation is with pain, bony swelling, chronic otitis, diabetes insipidus and diarrhoea. Treatment of choice is vinblastine, prednisolone, MTX, 6-MP or etoposide. While there is high cure rate, it often recurs.

PRIMARY CENTRAL NERVOUS SYSTEM TUMOURS

Surgery alone is used for low-grade astrocytoma. Irradiation is added to diseases like high-grade astrocytoma. Role of chemotherapy is less certain. Chemotherapy is used to delay or avoid irradiation in children < 4 years with medulloblastoma. Intensive chemotherapy is indicated prior to XRT in medulloblastoma with residual tumour post-surgery or spinal metastases and in primitive neuroectodermal tumour. Poor prognosis is associated with brain stem glioma. Endocrine problems occur, such as growth hormone or thyroid, gonadal insufficiency, if pituitary or hypothalamus in the irradiation field.

RETINOBLASTOMA

Classically the disease retinoblastoma presents as the cat's eye reflex (leukokoria) or squint. Family history must be obtained. Enucleation of the eye is indicated in unilateral cases or the most affected eye in bilateral cases. Cryotherapy and photocoagulation may be used. Irradiation is indicated in larger tumours. There is a possible role for chemotherapy which is yet to be determined. There is a risk of osteosarcoma at any site later in life.

REFERENCES

Pappo AS, Shapiro DN, Crist WM, Maurer HM. (1996). Biology and therapy of paediatric rhabdomyosarcoma. *Journal of Clinical Oncology*, **13**(8), 2123–2129.

Piu, C-H. (1995) Childhood leukaemias. *New England Journal of Medicine*, **332**(24), 1618–1630.

Piu, C-H. (1996). Acute leukaemia in children. *Current Opinion in Haematology*, **3**, 249–258.

Pizzo, P.A. and Poplack, D.G. (1997) *Principles and Practice of Paediatric Oncology*. Philadelphia: Lippincott-Raven.

Sandlund, J.T., Downing, J.R. and Crist, W.M. (1996) Non-Hodgkin's Lymphoma of Childhood. *New England Journal of Medicine*, **334**(19), 1238–1248.

Woods, W.G., Tuckman, M., Robison, L.L., Bernstein, M., Leclerc, J.M., Brisson, J.C., Bossard, J., Hill, G., Shuster, J., Luepker, R., Byrne, T., Weitzman, S., Bunin, G. and Lemieux, B. (1996) A population-based study of the usefulness of screening for neuroblastoma. *The Lancet*, **348**(9043), 1682–1687.

CHAPTER 55

CANCERS IN AIDS PATIENTS

Sam Milliken and Ronald Penny

INTRODUCTION

Cancer is an important association of chronic immunodeficiency states. In human immunodeficiency virus (HIV) infection, the virus causes a slow relentless deterioration in T-cell immune function with an average of 10 years from primary infection until acquired immunodeficiency syndrome (AIDS), develops. As helper T cells (CD4) decline the immune system fails leading to the well-recognised complications of AIDS occurring, such as opportunistic infections and cancer.

Cancer associated with HIV infection and AIDS is a major problem. In the USA, HIV/AIDS is the major cause of cancer death in men less than 45 years. It is estimated by the World Health Organisation that currently there are approximately 20 million people infected with HIV and 8 million people with AIDS worldwide. In Australia, which has successfully contained the epidemic, there are still approximately 11,000 people with HIV infection, with over 500 new HIV and over 600 new AIDS cases each year.

Initially, Kaposi's Sarcoma (KS) and primary central nervous system (CNS) lymphoma were recognised as AIDS-defining conditions. Subsequently, systemic non-Hodgkins lymphoma (NHL) and carcinoma of the uterine cervix became AIDS defining.

More recently, Hodgkin's disease, squamous cell carcinoma (SCC) of the conjunctiva, soft tissue sarcoma in children, testicular carcinoma and SCC of the oral cavity and anus in adults have been associated with HIV infection, but are not AIDS defining diagnoses. Many case reports have appeared in the literature for many other cancer types, but these appear to be coincidental. However when these cancers do occur, they run a more aggressive course, particularly in patients who are severely immunosuppressed.

HIV infection may be a major complicating factor in determining appropriate treatments. With progression of HIV disease, pancytopenias become more common (due to the effects of HIV infection on the bone marrow) making therapy for cancer more difficult.

Generally the risk of cancer increases with worsening immune function, being greatest in AIDS patients. Such patients have the greatest risk of impaired bone marrow function, opportunistic infections, generalised debility and wasting. Recent advances in antiretroviral therapy (ART) may result in prolonged periods of reduced immunosuppression but could be associated with an increased cancer risk.

AETIOLOGY

An increased risk of cancer in people with rare inherited forms of immunodeficiency and with prolonged iatrogenic immunodeficiency following organ transplantation has long been recognised. Generally these cancers are of unusual type, e.g. KS and high-grade NHL, rather than the common types seen in society such as lung, colon and breast cancer.

Co-infection with oncogenic viruses may explain these differences. Latent or chronic infection with Epstein-Barr virus (EBV) has been strongly linked to NHL, both systemic and CNS lymphomas. Human Papilloma virus, especially the highly oncogenic subtypes, numbers 16, 18, 31, 33, 35 and 51, are strongly linked to cervical (CIN) and anal intraepithelial neoplasia (AIN), precursor lesions to SCC of these organs.

Recently KS associated Herpes virus (KSHV), also termed human herpes virus type 8 (HHV8), has been strongly implicated as a causative infection for KS in both HIV-seropositive and -seronegative patients and a subgroup of HIV-seropositive patients with high-grade NHL presenting as effusions in body cavities (pleural, pericardial and peritoneal spaces).

KAPOSI'S SARCOMA

Kaposi first described KS in its classic form in 1872 as violaceous, pigmented and raised sarcomatous tumours of the skin, usually on the lower limbs of elderly middle-European, Jewish men. These usually have an indolent course and respond well to local therapies such as radiotherapy.

Subsequently three other more aggressive clinical types of KS have been described:

1. Iatrogenic KS is seen after immunosuppressive therapy usually following organ transplantation. It has a less indolent course and may spontaneously resolve on withdrawal of immunosuppression.
2. An endemic form occurs in young males in equatorial Africa.
3. Epidemic disease commonly occurs in HIV/AIDS and has an aggressive course. Over one-third of AIDS patients, predominantly homosexual men and equatorial Africans, will develop KS.

Presentation

- The disease most commonly presents with typical skin lesions, often occurring in widespread clusters involving any part of the body.
- Biopsy is important to establish the diagnosis, especially in patients without a prior AIDS-defining event, and to exclude other diseases such as Bacillary Angiomatosis or cutaneous NHL, the main differential diagnoses.
- Cutaneous, oral and gastrointestinal tract lesions are most common in that order although often asymptomatic.

- Systemic lesions occur in the lungs, liver and spleen. Approximately 10% of cases involve the lungs, usually with reticulonodular parenchymal lesions and pleural effusion is common. Pulmonary KS is usually rapidly progressive and fatal if unresponsive to therapy.
- Limb and face oedema due to lymphatic obstruction and generalised lymphadenopathy are not uncommon and may occur without obvious cutaneous KS.
- Unusual presentations such as lesions in the heart have been reported. CNS involvement has not been reported.
- Skin lesions may be macules, nodules or plaques and with time may coalesce into large lesions covering the skin surface. Fortunately this type of disease is becoming rarer with recent chemotherapeutic advances.
- Systemic symptoms, fevers, sweats and weight loss may occur with advanced disease.

Kaposi's Sarcoma as the First AIDS Diagnosis

KS occurs more commonly as immune function fails but can occur in patients with normal CD4 cell counts. Although decreasing as a first AIDS diagnosis (< 15%) it may occur in as many as a third of homosexual men with AIDS overall. It has a large psychological impact because it is a prominent, persistent and visible hallmark of HIV/AIDS.

Treatment

Treatment approaches depend on many factors including the psychological impact of the disease on the patient, the extent of disease, the severity of immunodeficiency, and the presence of complicating factors such as systemic symptoms, severe tumour associated oedema and other HIV/AIDS complications. The disease may take a variable course and this also influences treatment decisions.

Observation

Patients with preserved immune function and only a few asymptomatic skin lesions may not require therapy, opting for careful observation with treatment only when more widespread or symptomatic disease arises. Recent advances in combination ART significantly improve immune function with sporadic reports of spontaneous remissions or slowing of KS progression. With dramatic improvements in ART, this may become the treatment of choice.

Local Treatment

- For patients with more widespread cutaneous disease or cosmetically unacceptable lesions, local or topical therapies may be beneficial together with ART.
- Local radiotherapy is very successful but durations of response may be short and facilities for treatment are usually limited to tertiary referral centres.
- Cryotherapy may be successful for smaller lesions (< 2 cm).
- Early studies with topical retinoid creams show some promise with good responses in about one-third of patients.
- Other therapies such as laser, intralesional chemotherapy, alpha interferon or sclerosants have been used with success but are more uncomfortable.

Systemic Treatment

For patients with more widespread disease, particularly causing oedema, systemic symptoms or involving internal organs, more aggressive therapy is warranted.

- For such patients with preserved immune function (CD4 > 300 cells/uL) systemic alpha interferon has a high response rate with durable responses. However high doses are required (> 18 million units s.c. daily), which are expensive and may be toxic. Response rates are slow (1 to 2 months) making this therapy inappropriate for rapidly progressing disease. Smaller doses of alpha interferon may be effective if given in combination with ART.

- For patients with lower CD4 counts the mainstay of treatment is chemotherapy. Protocols utilising agents such as the vinca alkaloids, vincristine and vinblastine, bleomycin and adriamycin are effective but durations of response are short. The newer liposomal preparations of the anthracyclines, adriamycin, and daunorubicin, and the relatively new agent taxol have demonstrated high response rates and durable responses with little toxicity. These drugs have become the treatments of choice for rapidly progressive and life-threatening KS.

NON-HODGKIN'S LYMPHOMA

Presentation

Non-Hodgkin's lymphoma occurs in all HIV groups and presents as systemic disease or primary cerebral lymphoma.

Primary Cerebral Lymphoma

Primary cerebral lymphoma presents with signs and symptoms of raised intra-cranial pressure or with focal neurological signs in patients with severe immunosuppression (CD4 counts < 100 and usually < 50 cells/uL). The main differential diagnosis is with cerebral toxoplasmosis which is more common in this population. Consequently, most clinicians advocate an empiric trial of antibiotics and consider CNS biopsy for patients who do not respond.

Systemic Lymphoma

Systemic lymphoma has more protean presentations, and while it occurs more commonly in patients with low CD4 cell counts, may occur at any level of suppression and rarely with normal counts (CD4 > 500 cells/uL). Lymphadenopathy is a common presentation but unlike HIV seronegative lymphoma patients extra-lymphatic presentations are also very common. These occur in the GIT, lungs, skin and serosal surfaces. The majority have advanced disease with 90% Stage III or IV on presentation. CNS involvement is common but as leptomeningeal involvement rather than a solid lesion. Pyrexia of unknown origin may be the first manifestation of systemic NHL.

There may be a number of differential diagnoses, mostly infections and other tumours. Lymphadenopathy, hepatosplenomegaly and night sweats occur in AIDS patients due to CMV or atypical mycobacteria. Biopsy of a mass lesion and tissue culture for infection are important to establish the diagnosis. Systemic NHL may be the first AIDS diagnosis, whereas most with primary CNS lymphoma already have a prior AIDS diagnosis.

Management of Primary Cerebral Lymphoma

Management of primary cerebral lymphoma is difficult. These are aggressive, rapidly growing high-grade tumours causing major morbidity such as coma or hemiparesis and rapidly progress to death in a matter of a few weeks or months. The main therapies are measures to reduce intra-cranial pressure, such as corticosteroids or osmotic agents (mannitol) and radiotherapy. Treatment is palliative and may be futile in patients who deteriorate rapidly.

Patients commonly are already debilitated by pre-existing AIDS diagnoses. Careful assessment of the goals of therapy and expectations of outcome are essential and need to be discussed with the patient or their significant others before considering therapy. Many patients will already have formulated concepts for their preferred care in the event of such a diagnosis.

Most radiotherapists advocate careful treatment to a total dose of 30 Gray in 10 fractions over 2 weeks. Treatment usually improves neurological impairment and reduces the need for corticosteroids. In approximately 20% of patients, signs progress and treatment is discontinued.

Toxicity of treatment is usually modest despite the poor performance status of many patients. Complete alopecia is usual as is scalp erythema but it is rarely severe. Most experience transient worsening of tiredness and lethargy.

Management of Systemic NHL

Systemic NHL is also an aggressive disease, but not to the same degree as primary CNS lymphoma. With systemic NHL there is usually time to assess and stage the disease. Patients prognosis will vary according to many factors not all directly related to the lymphoma, such as the degree of immunodeficiency.

For the majority of patients, chemotherapy is necessary for effective palliation. At present the most effective treatments are modifications of standard protocols for the treatment of NHL. Localised therapy such as surgical resection of gastrointestinal lymphomas and radiotherapy may be required for early stage disease, or in debilitated patients with a poor prognosis.

Recently, results have improved with median survivals over 1 year, due to:

- growth factors for therapy induced neutropenia;
- prophylactic use of antimicrobials;
- more effective ART;
- lower dose, less toxic chemotherapy and avoidance of intensive chemotherapy even in high-grade disease.

Treatment is given to maximal response followed by two further cycles with 40% to 60% achieving a complete response. Approximately 10% of these patients achieve disease-free survival beyond two years and some may be cured of their NHL.

SQUAMOUS CELL CARCINOMA (SCC)

Cervix

There is a marked increase in risk of cervical intraepithelial neoplasia (CIN). Over 40% of HIV-infected women may develop CIN. The risk increases with worsening immune function, independent of other known risk factors such as younger age of first sexual contact, increased number of sexual partners and cigarette smoking. Almost all cases are associated with HPV infection, particularly with the oncogenic subtypes 16, 18, 31, 33, 35 and 51. Infection with more than one subtype is also common and further increases risk.

No increase in established cases of squamous cell carcinoma (SCC) of the cervix has yet been detected. While the reasons for this are unclear, cervical cancer is an AIDS-defining diagnosis because of the expected increase in these cancers and their aggressive behaviour.

Anus

Similarly, an HPV-related anal intraepithelial neoplasia (AIN) occurs more commonly in HIV-positive homosexual men who practice ano-receptive intercourse. As for CIN the same serotypes of HPV are implicated and these lesions are more common with severe immunosuppression.

SCC of the anus has an increased incidence in homosexual men but is not greater in HIV-seropositive homosexual men.

Screening Strategies for the Cervix and Anus when HIV Positive

Detectable pre-malignant lesions should allow a surveillance strategy to be developed to contain these potential cancers.

- Regular screening with Papanicolou smears is recommended for all HIV-positive women at least once a year; every 6 months may be indicated for patients who are severely immunosuppressed (CD4 count < 200 cells) with a previously abnormal smear.
- Some recommend colposcopy rather than smears, but an improved outcome for this approach has not been established.
- Surveillance for HIV-positive males at risk of AIN have been proposed using a modified Papanicolou smear technique. Standardisation of this method and outcome data to support its widespread adoption are not yet established.

Conjunctiva

SCC of the conjunctiva has recently been reported with increased incidence in HIV-positive patients in equatorial Africa. Duration of solar exposure also appears an important risk factor.

HODGKIN'S DISEASE AND OTHER LYMPHOPROLIFERATIVE DISEASES

- Hodgkin's disease is not recognised as a AIDS-defining condition.
- Recent epidemiologic studies have demonstrated a 20-fold increased risk for Hodgkin's disease in HIV-seropositive homosexual men and a large number of cases have been reported in the literature.
- Hodgkin's disease has been reported in all risk groups.
- Hodgkin's disease is a more aggressive condition in HIV-seropositives with a poor prognosis compared to HIV-seronegative patients with the disease (30% rather than 90% one-year survival).
- Histology is usually mixed cellularity type.
- Most present with advanced stage disease as for NHL.

- Combination chemotherapy is usually required for effective palliation using modified standard protocols with the same treatment principles relevant as those for NHL.
- Rare cases with limited disease may be treated with radiotherapy.

Other lymphoproliferative disorders, such as low-grade lymphomas, chronic lymphatic leukaemia and multiple myeloma, have been reported but they do not appear to have an increased incidence. Reports of acute lymphoblastic leukaemias likely represent leukaemic presentations of high-grade NHL. These patients generally have a very poor prognosis.

TESTICULAR CANCER AND OTHER SOLID TUMOURS

- Testicular seminoma has been reported to have an increased incidence in some but not all epidemiological studies. The increased risk may be as much as 20-fold.
- An increase in many different tumour types has been reported following long-term iatrogenic immunosuppression after organ transplantation and immunosuppression and cytotoxic therapy following bone marrow transplantation. The same may apply to HIV infection.
- Better anti-HIV therapies may protect against the infective complications of severe immunodeficiency but increase the risk of malignancy if they do not fully correct immunodeficiency and prolong moderate immune dysfunction.
- Generally solid tumours appear to have a poorer prognosis associated with HIV infection. This may be in part due to already debilitated patients having a poorer prognosis.
- Impaired immune function in HIV-seropositives may facilitate more rapid growth and early metastasis of these tumours.
- Patients with preserved or only moderately impaired immune function should be treated with conventional protocols.
- Severely immunosuppressed patients should not be denied appropriate therapy unless debility makes the associated toxicities unacceptable. Treatment guidelines for such patients should be similar to those used for patients with severe intercurrent illness and cancer.

SOFT TISSUE SARCOMAS

Soft tissue sarcomas, usually leiomyoma and leiomyosarcoma, have recently been reported to occur more commonly in HIV-positive children. These tumours predominantly occur in the lungs, spleen or gastrointestinal tract and EBV has been implicated in their development.

REFERENCES

Colematis, B. and DeVita, V. (eds) (1996) *AIDS and Malignancies*. Chichester: John Wiley and Sons.

Crowe, S., Hoy, J., Mills, J. (eds) (1996) *Management of the HIV Infected Patient*. Melbourne: Cambridge University Press.

Krown, S.E. and Von Roehn, J.H. (eds) (1996) *Hematologic and Oncologic Aspects of HIV Infection. Hematology/Oncology*. Philadelphia: W B Saunders.

Stewart, G. (ed) (1997) *Managing HIV*. Sydney: Australian Medical Publishing.

CHAPTER 56

CANCER OF UNKNOWN PRIMARY ORIGIN

John A. Levi

INTRODUCTION

Cancer of unknown primary origin represents a diagnostic and therapeutic challenge as patients present with evidence of malignancy in one or more sites without an obvious primary tumour. Sites of metastatic disease are generally heterogeneous with varying histology and natural histories which often make it difficult to determine a systematic evaluation. Improvements in histopathological techniques and an improved understanding of particular clinical syndromes within this general group of patients has allowed for better determination of relative prognoses and approaches to treatment.

INCIDENCE

- Five to ten percent of patients presenting with metastatic malignancy will have an unknown primary site.
- The mean age of patients is 60 years and with a slight male predominance.
- Identification of the primary site of origin of malignancy is uncommon during the initial and subsequent evaluation with only 10–20% of patients with a primary site defined.
- Post-mortem studies have identified the primary site in up to 60–80% of patients.
- Well-differentiated malignancies have a higher success rate with therapy than undifferentiated carcinoma.

CLASSIFICATION

These patients require an understanding of histological typing, pattern of clinical presentation, sites of disease and overall extent of malignancy to develop a management plan.

Histology

Pathologists require a very generous biopsy specimen to enable them to see the pattern of disease and to undertake all relevant examinations, including special stains, cytogenetic and electron microscopic analyses. Recognised histological categories include the following.

Moderate and Well-differentiated Adenocarcinomas

Moderate and well-differentiated adenocarcinomas comprise 60% of patients and tend to be elderly with multiple metastatic sites, particularly including lymph nodes, liver, lung and bone. Origin of these malignancies is most likely to arise from either gastrointestinal tract or lung, but some arise from breast, prostate or ovary. These sites have varying potential for responsiveness to relevant management, so consideration of the particular clinical features of presentation are important in determining the likelihood of benefit from active therapy.

Poorly Differentiated Carcinomas

Poorly differentiated carcinomas represent 30% of patients with two-thirds of these having poorly differentiated carcinoma without specific histological features, while one-third have poorly differentiated adenocarcinoma. Some of these patients are younger age, predominantly males, with mediastinal masses, retroperitoneal lymph nodes and rapid clinical progression. Such patients are associated with response to aggressive chemotherapy and the potential for prolonged survival. Careful clinical and pathological evaluation is important in these patients.

Squamous Cell Carcinomas

Squamous cell carcinomas comprise 5% of the overall group of patients and the majority of these will have evidence of disease involving cervical and supraclavicular lymph nodes and less commonly inguinal lymph nodes. As effective treatment is regularly possible for these patients, appropriate clinical and radiological work-up is indicated.

Poorly Differentiated Neoplasms

Poorly differentiated neoplasms represent 5% of the total incidence of cancer of unknown primary site and with careful histological evaluation defined pathology is frequently possible. The most common malignancies within this group are non-Hodgkin's lymphomas comprising 35–65% of these patients with the remainder comprising a variable number of patients with melanoma, sarcoma and carcinomas.

Clinical Classification

In addition to the histological classification, the clinical presentation further defines subgroups of these patients and identifies potential benefit from therapeutic interventions.

Cervical and/or Axillary Lymph Node Presentation

- Patients with disease confined to these sites, with squamous cell carcinoma, are most commonly found to have tumours within the head and neck, especially when the upper and middle cervical lymph nodes are involved. Surgical excision and radiotherapy may prolong survival.
- Lower cervical and supraclavicular lymph node presentation with squamous cell carcinoma is more likely to arise from the lung and have poor prognosis.
- Poorly differentiated neoplasms presenting in these sites need to be assessed histologically to exclude lymphomas.

Axillary Lymph Node Involvement in Women

- This presentation should raise the possibility of breast cancer.
- Histology of biopsies should include assessment for oestrogen and progesterone receptors.
- Irrespective of the presence of these receptors, consideration should be given to relevant axillary dissection followed by radiotherapy to the breast and axilla and possible adjuvant chemotherapy.

Inguinal Lymph Nodes

- Presentation with disease confined to inguinal lymph nodes is not common.
- If it is squamous cell carcinoma, the origin of tumour may be from genital or ano-rectal areas.

Mediastinal and/or Retroperitoneal Lymph Nodes

- Presentation in the mediastinal and/or retroperitoneal lymph nodes in younger males, with a short history and histology of poorly differentiated neoplasm or carcinoma may suggest extragonadal germ cell tumours which have a good prognosis with combination chemotherapy.

Peritoneal or Pleural Effusions in Women

Presentation with either or both peritoneal or pleural effusions in women suggest ovarian or primary peritoneal carcinomas.

DIAGNOSTIC WORK-UP

Clinical

- A thorough history and physical examination is required in all patients.
- Assessment should include assessment of performance or activity status, consideration of particular risk factors associated with certain tumour types, including history of tobacco usage, intestinal polyposis, familial carcinomas and reproductive history in women.
- Thorough physical examination should include rectal and pelvic examinations, together with assessment for signs of potential vascular, respiratory, gastrointestinal or urinary obstruction.
- Full blood count and biochemical profiles should be taken which may be of relevance in determining specific organ dysfunction, but are rarely useful to determine the primary site of malignancy.

Pathology

Full pathological evaluation is most important to define possible primary origin of malignancy, particular cell lineage, potential prognosis and relevant therapy. Light microscopy will generally define the four groups described above. Many of these patients will, however, require further histological evaluation including special stains, immunocytochemistry, electron microscopy and, in selected circumstances, cytogenetic analyses.

The use of special stains and immunocytochemistry may allow for differentiation of carcinomas from lymphomas. For example, utilising relevant lymphocyte markers including common leukocyte antigen, neuron-specific enolase, may define endocrine and neuroendocrine tumours including small cell carcinomas; specific immunocytochemical stains including prostate-specific antigen, human chorionic gonadotropin, and alpha feto protein may define prostate cancer, germ cell tumours and hepatomas, oestrogen receptor analysis may define breast cancers.

In selected circumstances electron microscopy may be of value in differentiating malignant melanoma from carcinoma and small cell carcinomas from adenocarcinomas. Cytogenetic analyses may be of value in selected circumstances where specific karyotypic abnormalities may be of value in classifying such malignancies as non-Hodgkin's lymphomas, Ewing's sarcoma and germ cell tumours.

Tumour Markers

Elevation of serum tumour markers is only likely to be present in a minority of patients with cancer of unknown primary site, but are of particular value if present. Alpha feto protein and beta HCG in younger patients, particularly with mediastinal or retroperitoneal lymph node enlargement, is of value. Patients with disease confined to liver should have alpha feto protein analyses to diagnose a possible hepatoma. The presence of pleural and/or peritoneal effusions warrants performing a CA-125 estimation and in older males, particularly with metastatic disease involving bone, PSA estimation for possible prostate origin of tumour is appropriate.

Radiological and Other Investigations

- Extensive investigation using radiology, nuclear medicine and endoscopy is rarely of benefit in the majority of patients with cancer of unknown primary origin. Selective use of these techniques is most appropriate in specific clinical presentations.
- Abdominal CT scan is of relevance in patients with adenocarcinomas or poorly differentiated carcinoma or neoplasm to assess possible involvement of pancreas or intra-abdominal lymph node enlargement.
- Mammographic examination is relevant in women with axillary lymph node presentation or with adenocarcinoma involving selected sites such as lung, bone, mediastinal and above-diaphragmatic lymph nodes.
- Endoscopic examination of lung may be indicated in patients with supraclavicular lymph node presentation, while upper gastrointestinal endoscopy may be indicated in males with peritoneal effusions (ascites).
- Extensive non-directed investigations are not indicated in these patients and any further evaluation should be dependent on specific symptoms and signs demonstrated at presentation.

PROGNOSIS

Several studies have demonstrated that in the heterogeneous population of patients with cancer of unknown primary origin, favourable independent prognostic factors include:

- a good performance or activity status;
- less than two metastatic sites;
- tumour location in lymph nodes, including mediastinum and retroperitoneum but other than supraclavicular lymph nodes;
- female sex;
- a smoking history of less than ten pack years (twenty cigarettes per day for less than ten years); and
- histology other than poorly differentiated adenocarcinoma.

The demonstration of at least two or more of these favourable prognostic factors should encourage more active therapy.

TREATMENT

Selection of appropriate therapy is dependent on determining, as accurately as possible, histology and the number and sites of metastases.

Surgery

Surgical resection is indicated for squamous cell carcinoma or adenocarcinoma histology with limited metastatic sites including cervical, axillary and inguinal lymph nodes and isolated solitary lung or liver lesions. This may be followed with radiotherapy in selected patients.

Radiotherapy

Radiotherapy is indicated for an axillary lymph node mass in women with adenocarcinoma and positive estrogen and/or progesterone receptors.

Patients with squamous cell histology and upper to middle cervical lymph node enlargement are likely to have an occult primary arising from the head and neck. Definitive irradiation to the cervical lymph nodes and upper airway mucosa following radical neck dissection is indicated in such patients.

Chemotherapy

Chemotherapy is indicated in poorly differentiated malignant neoplasm, particularly when immuno-cytochemistry demonstrate a positive common leukocyte antigen suggesting non-Hodgkin's lymphoma. These patients should receive chemotherapy incorporating cyclophosphamide and doxorubicin.

Cisplatin-based combination chemotherapy is indicated in patients with poorly differentiated carcinomas, other than adenocarcinoma. More than 60% of such patients achieve significant tumour regression and 26% complete response for a median duration of 5 years. This group of patients includes those with small cell carcinomas and atypical germ cell carcinomas.

Cisplatin-based combination chemotherapy is also effective in women with predominant perito-neal and/or pleural effusions, particularly associated with an elevated serum CA-125 level indicating likely ovarian and/or primary peritoneal origin.

Chemotherapy for patients with moderate to poorly differentiated adenocarcinoma remains con-troversial. Only a small proportion of patients are likely to benefit. Selection of patients for chemotherapy should be based on younger age, limited number of metastatic sites, good performance or activity status, normal CEA, LDH and alkaline phosphatase. Chemotherapy usually incorporates cisplatin in the combination.

SURVIVAL RATE

Overall, median survival in studies of patients with cancer of unknown primary origin range from 4–5.5 months with approximately 25% surviving one year, 11% at 3 years and 6% at 5 years.

Nevertheless, specific histologies are associated with varying survival rates, including patients with squamous cell carcinoma with median survivals of 9–30.5 months and patients with poorly differen-tiated carcinoma other than adenocarcinoma having a median survival in excess of 12 months. This latter group of patients included those with small cell carcinomas which had a more favourable prognosis, being responsive to both radiotherapy and chemotherapy with response rates of some 60% to combination chemotherapy and 26% of patients achieving complete response with relapse-free survival rate of 26% in 6 years. Also included are a small subgroup of young male patients with disease in mediastinum and retroperitoneum related to atypical germ cell carcinoma when a 50% complete response rate to combination chemotherapy may be obtained and 20% disease-free survival rate beyond 5 years.

Among the patients with a histological classification of poorly differentiated malignant neoplasm, if a common leukocyte antigen on immunocytochemical stain is positive, these patients are also very responsive to chemotherapy, achieving 45% disease-free survival rate at 30 months. These patients are almost certainly an atypical group of non-Hodgkin's lymphoma.

Conversely, patients with a histological diagnosis of adenocarcinoma have a median survival of only 4–6 months.

CONCLUSION

Patients with cancer of unknown primary origin have atypical clinical presentations with sites of metastatic disease often differing from those with an obvious primary. Careful evaluation of these patients is indicated with an emphasis on histological characterisation, including use of special and immunocytochemical stains, electron microscopy and cytogenetics. Appropriate assessment of metastatic sites may define subgroups with potential for significant benefit from active therapy. Clinical investigations should be selective, with an emphasis on defining these specific subgroups of patients with responsive malignancies. An extensive search for the primary site of origin of the malignancy is rarely indicated. Surgery and radiotherapy is indicated for patients with metastatic disease localised to peripheral lymph nodes or with isolated lung and liver lesions. Chemotherapy is indicated for recognised sensitive histologies, including poorly differentiated malignant neoplasm and poorly differentiated carcinoma in selected clinical settings.

REFERENCES

Altman, E. and Cadman, E. (1986) An analysis of 1539 patients with cancer of unknown primary site. *Cancer*, 57, 120–124.

Hainsworth, J.D. and Greco, F.A. (1993) Treatment of patients with cancer of unknown primary site. *New England J. of Med.*, 329, 257–263.

Kirsten, F., Chi, C.H., Leary, J.A., Ng, A.B.P., Hedley, D.W. and Tattersall, M.H.N. (1987) Metastatic adeno or undifferentiated carcinoma from an unknown primary site—natural history and guidelines for identification of treatable subsets. *Quarterly Journal of Med.*, 62, 143–161.

Nystrom, J.S., Wiener, J.M., Wolf, R.M., Bateman, J.R. and Viola M.B. (1979) Identifying the primary site in metastatic cancer of unknown origin: inadequacy of roentgenographic procedures. *JAMA*, 241, 381–383.

Pasterz, R., Savaraj, N. and Burgess, M. (1986) Prognostic factors in metastatic carcinoma of unknown primary. *J. Clin. Oncol.*, 4, 1652–1657.

Van der Gaast, A., Verweij, J., Planting, A.S.T., Hop, W.C.J. and Stoter, G. (1995) Simple prognostic model to predict survival in patients with undifferentiated carcinoma of unknown primary site. *J. Clin. Oncol.*, 13, 1720–1725.

PART XIII

COMPLICATIONS IN
CANCER PATIENTS

CHAPTER 57

ONCOLOGICAL EMERGENCIES

Paul R. Harnett

INTRODUCTION

Patients with malignant disease may develop a variety of problems related to their malignancy and/or its treatment. However, cancer patients may have medical problems unrelated to their malignancy, such as stroke, myocardial infarction or peptic ulcer. Thus, a full range of differential diagnoses should always be considered in every patient, regardless of the stage of their malignancy.

PRESENTATION OF THE UNWELL CANCER PATIENT

The following diagnoses may be present if the patient is non-specifically unwell without obvious localising features.

Differential Diagnosis

- Sepsis: consider recent chemotherapy and the possibility of neutropaenic sepsis.
- Hypercalcaemia: remember the symptoms may be subtle. More likely in bone metastases and some tumours.
- Metabolic disturbances:
  — inappropriate ADH: lung cancer or drugs may be associated.
  — uraemia: possible obstructive uropathy from pelvic/urologic tumours.
- Tumour lysis syndrome: associated with recent treatment in bulky tumours.
- Drug interaction/overdose: consider narcotics and other medications.
- Constipation: consider narcotics, a possible spinal cord obstruction.
- Bedbound: exclude a possible spinal cord lesion.
- Disease relapse/progression: while common is a diagnosis of exclusion.

BONE PAIN

Bone pain in a patient with cancer is an indication for further assessment including a bone scan, followed by plain X-ray of painful 'hot spots', particularly in weight bearing bones. Pain is often a sign of imminent pathological fracture. Following a pathological fracture, major morbidity or mortality may occur. Plain X-rays indicating significant loss of cortical bone, more than one third cortical diameter, requires consideration of prophylactic orthopaedic pinning and/or irradiation.

TUMOUR LYSIS SYNDROME

Tumour lysis syndrome is a result of rapid release of contents of dying tumour cells within hours of therapy. The patient becomes clinically unwell, and biochemically the syndrome is characterised by hyperuricemia, hyperkalaemia, hyperphosphataemia and hypocalcaemia. Lethal cardiac arrythmias, from high serum potassium, and renal failure are the most serious consequences.

The most important management aspect is a high index of suspicion. Patients at risk are those with large tumours likely to be exquisitely sensitive to chemotherapy, such as high-grade lymphomas and leukaemia. Patients can often be recognised before therapy, and at least partially protected by commencement of allopurinol, maintenance of high output of alkaline urine during and after chemotherapy, and appropriate biochemical monitoring. Management of established tumour lysis syndrome is supportive and dictated by the biochemical abnormalities detected.

HYPERCALCAEMIA

Elevated serum calcium is a life-threatening metabolic disorder in cancer patients, usually due to secretion of factors from the tumour which promote bone resorption, and stimulate renal tubular reabsorption of calcium. Hypercalcaemia is typically associated with multiple myeloma, and renal, lung, and breast carcinoma.

Patients can present with polyuria and polydypsia, malaise, lethargy, impaired higher neurological function, nausea, constipation and ileus, or increasing pain despite a previously effective analgesic regimen. The severity of symptoms relates to both the height of the serum calcium and its rate of rise.

Treatment

- The definitive therapy for malignant hypercalcaemia is treatment of the underlying cancer. Unfortunately, hypercalcaemia is most commonly seen as a late manifestation of previously treated malignancy, and in these circumstances specific therapy for the underlying cancer may be limited.
- Correction of dehydration is important, but should not be as aggressive as practised in previous years. The rate of replacement should take into account the degree of dehydration, and any cardiac or renal impairment. With adequate cardiac and renal function, 1–2 litres of saline may be administered over 4 to 6 hours, and more slowly thereafter, with frequent clinical and laboratory reassessment.

Bisphosphonates are chemical analogues of pyrophosphate and include drugs such as pamidronate, clodronate and alendronate. They adsorb to the bone surface and inhibit osteoclast activity, thereby reducing calcium release. These agents are usually administered as a short intravenous infusion, following which the serum calcium will fall towards normal over 48–72 hours.

FEBRILE NEUTROPAENIA

Neutropaenia most commonly occurs following chemotherapy, but may also occur after irradiation of a large amount of marrow bearing bone. It may also be seen as a consequence of marrow infiltration by tumour. In this case, the blood film may show a leukoerythroblastic picture with circulating nucleated red cells and immature white cells.

Neutropaenia predisposes the patient to bacteraemic sepsis. The risk of sepsis depends on the degree of neutropaenia. Patients are at significant risk at and below a neutrophil count of $1 \leftrightarrow 10^9/$ litre. The lower the neutrophil count, and/or the longer the period of neutropaenia, the greater the risk of opportunistic infection. Host and environmental factors also play a role. Any organism may become severely pathogenic if neutropaenia is profound and prolonged.

In cancer patients in the above settings, fever should be assumed to signify sepsis, even in the presence of other potential explanations such as blood transfusion. Careful physical examination with particular attention to potential sites of sepsis is required, together with chest X-ray, blood and urine cultures, and other microbiological samples as indicated.

Untreated neutropaenic sepsis can result in death from septic shock within hours, especially if the responsible organism is a Gram negative bacteria. Therefore, all such patients should be treated immediately after cultures have been taken with broad spectrum antibiotics. A typical regimen is an aminoglycoside and a late generation cephalosporin. Anti-bacterial cover for Staphylococcal species should be considered if potential sources of sepsis include the skin or cannula sites.

NEUROLOGICAL EMERGENCIES

Although many neurologic syndromes arise as a consequence of malignancy, those due to direct compression of nervous tissue are of particular importance because irreversible loss of neuronal function can occur within hours unless the compression can be relieved.

Spinal Cord Compression

Spinal cord compression may arise from expansion or collapse of a vertebra involved by tumour, direct or transforaminal spread, extradural or intramedullary spread. A high index of suspicion should be maintained, as the likelihood of recovery depends upon rapidity of diagnosis and treatment. It is better to overinvestigate some patients, than to wait until neurological signs are pronounced. The more neurologic deficit present, the worse the prognosis for recovery.

Presentation

Particular attention should be paid to the following symptoms:

* localised pain and tenderness in the vertebral column;
* radicular pain, less common, and due to compression of nerve roots;
* minor disturbances of bladder such as unusual urinary hesitancy and changes to bowel function;
* sensory symptoms, which are often vague in the very early stages;
* a report of difficulty with walking or balance, which may not be associated with gross motor weakness in the early stages.

Such findings should prompt urgent investigation to exclude cord compression.

Investigations

Investigations should include:

- urgent plain X-rays if localising features are present.
- urgent specialised imaging, either magnetic resonance scan or myelography.
- high-dose steroids, dexamethasone 4 mg IV then 4 mg orally every 6 hours should be commenced on suspicion of cord compression.

If a localised lesion is detected, urgent irradiation, or possibly neurosurgical decompression, is indicated.

Cerebral Metastases

Cerebral metastases can produce almost any neurological syndrome, and again a high index of suspicion is required. The most common pattern is multiple lesions within the brain parenchyma, although apparently solitary lesions and meningeal disease also occur. Cerebral metastases are most commonly associated with carcinoma of the lung, breast or kidney, melanoma, leukaemia and lymphoma.

On suspicion, high-dose steroids are commenced, and cerebral CT or MRI scans arranged. Further treatment depends upon the specifics of the individual case. Orbital and intraocular metastases are uncommon but important because of the threat posed to vision. Most commonly due to breast and prostate cancer, these lesions should be considered in patients with impaired vision (especially involving one eye), oculomotor palsy or proptosis. Urgent irradiation is indicated.

DYSPNOEA

Although the differential diagnosis of dyspnoea in the cancer patient is identical to that for patients without malignant disease, certain features are more common in cancer. These include:

- pleural effusion
- pulmonary emboli because the presence of cancer produces a 'prothrombotic state'
- lymphangitis carcinomatosa
- pneumonitis, produced by drugs or irradiation

Pericardial Effusion with or without Cardiac Tamponade

Pericardial effusion is most commonly associated with lymphoma, breast or lung cancer. Tamponade is virtually asymptomatic until the onset of symptoms and signs of congestive cardiac failure. In this context, the plain chest radiograph revealing enlargement of the cardiac silhouette may represent the presence of pericardial fluid compressing an otherwise normal heart rather than cardiac enlargement.

The most important physical sign is pulsus paradoxus (a drop of more than 10 mmHg in systolic pressure during inspiration) which distinguishes tamponade from other causes of pump failure. Urgent cardiac echocardiography demonstrates the presence of excess pericardial fluid and allows further assessment of its haemodynamic significance. Initial management involves urgent drainage of the pericardial fluid, with subsequent care being individualised and directed to the underlying cancer.

REFERENCES

Peckham, M., Pinedo, H.M. and Veronesi, U. (1995) Medical and surgical complications of cancer. In *Oxford Textbook of Oncology,* pp. 2193–2369. Oxford University Press.

CHAPTER 58

INFECTIONS IN CANCER PATIENTS

David Mitchell

PREDISPOSING FACTORS

Both the underlying malignancy and its treatment may predispose cancer patients to infection.

- Disruption of normal anatomical barriers
    — Bacteraemia with enteric *Streptococcus* spp. or *Clostridium* spp. may occur in colonic neoplasia.
    — Chemotherapy-induced mucositis predisposes to bloodstream infection with oral/bowel organisms.
    — Intravascular devices predispose to bloodstream infection with skin organisms.

- Obstruction/dysfunction of clearance mechanisms
    — Pneumonia secondary to obstruction from bronchogenic carcinoma.

- Neutropenia
    — occurs following bone marrow infiltration with cancer, or
    — myelosuppressive chemotherapy or radiotherapy. Predisposes to bacteraemia/fungaemia.

- Disordered cell mediated immunity

Lymphoma or immunosuppressive agents, especially steroids, bone marrow transplantation predisposes to infection especially due to intracellular organisms. Organisms commonly identified include:

    — bacteria such as *Listeria monocytogenes*, *Nocardia* spp., *mycobacterium* spp., *Legionella* spp.
    — viruses such as herpes viruses,
    — fungi such as *Aspergillis* spp., *Pneumocystis carinii*, *Cryptococcus neoformans*
    — parasites such as *Toxoplasma gondii*, *Strongyloides stercoralis*.

361

• Deficient immunoglobulin synthesis

Myeloma, chronic lymphocytic leukaemia (CLL) may cause deficient immunoglobulin synthesis which predisposes to infections with encapsulated bacteria such as *Streptococcus pneumoniae, Haemophilus influenzae.*

• Hyposplenism

Myelofibrosis, lymphoma, hairy cell leukaemia or splenectomy may have associated hyposplenism which predisposes to infections with encapsulated bacteria such as *Streptococcus pneumoniae* or haemotropic parasitic infection such as malaria, babesiosis.

INFECTIONS IN NEUTROPENIC CANCER PATIENTS

Neutropenia is the most important risk for life-threatening infection in cancer patients. Whilst mortality has fallen over the past 30 years, approximately 5% of neutropenic patients die from infection, with bacteria and fungi each accounting for about 50% of deaths. The most important causes of infections are as follows.

Gram Negative Bacteria

The relative incidence of Gram negative bacteria has declined in the past 10 years, especially from coliforms (e.g. *E. coli, Klebsiella* spp.) infections. Less virulent but more antibiotic resistant Gram negatives (e.g. *Stenotrophomonas maltiphilia, Acinetobacter* spp., *Flavomonas* spp.) more common and are often central line related. *Pseudomonas aeruginosa* is uncommon in most units but should be covered by empiric antibiotic regimens because of high mortality.

Gram Positive Bacteria

Gram positive bacteria have become relatively more common in the past 10 years. *Staphylococcus* spp., *Corynebacterium* spp. are skin organisms associated with central venous line infection. Viridans group, *Streptococcus* spp. are oral organisms, with infection predisposed by regimens causing severe mucositis or quinolone prophylaxis. They are often penicillin resistant. Bacteraemia with these organisms is associated with septic shock and adult respiratory distress syndrome (ARDS) in approximately 10%. *Enterococcus* spp. Arise from a bowel source, with bacteraemia predisposed to by quinolone prophylaxis and mucositis. They are often multi-resistant (VRE).

Fungi

Fungal infections mainly occur if neutropenia persists for more than 10 days. Yeasts such as *Candida* spp. are usually bowel or central line associated. Chronic disseminated (hepatosplenic) candidiasis is increasingly recognised with a persistent fever after recovery of neutrophils, abnormal liver function tests, characteristic space occupying lesions in liver or spleen on CT scanning. Filamentous fungi such as *Aspergillus* spp., *Scedosporium* spp., *Fusarium* spp. usually arise from a respiratory source. Pulmonary infiltrates, skin lesions, sinus disease are clinical clues. These infections require an aggressive diagnostic and therapeutic approach but are still highly lethal.

Viruses

Viral infections include severe herpes simplex virus (HSV) and varicella zoster virus (VZV) infections. Cytomegalovirus (CMV) is a major problem in bone marrow transplant recipients.

MANAGEMENT OF THE FEBRILE NEUTROPENIC CANCER PATIENT

Febrile neutropenia is defined as a fever $\oplus$ 38.5°C on one recording or a fever $\oplus$ 38°C on two recordings with associated neutrophil count of less than 1 $\leftrightarrow$ 10^6/l. A thorough physical examination must include inspection of the skin and perianal region. Investigations include blood cultures from peripheral vein and each central line lumen, urine cultures, stool examination for *C. difficile* and a CXR. Empiric antimicrobial therapy is commenced after blood cultures are taken. The choice is based on:

- published clinical trials;
- prevalence and resistance patterns of institutional endemic organisms;
- individual patient factors, such as physical examination, whether the patient is on antibiotic prophylaxis, allergies and previous infections.

Regimens used include combination therapy such as anti-pseudomonal penicillin (ticacillin/ clavulanate, piperacillin/tazobactam) with an aminoglycoside. Monotherapy may be used including carbapenem (imipenem, meropenem) or an anti-pseudomonal cephalosporin (ceftazidime, cefipime, cefpirome)

Glycopeptides such as vancomycin, teicoplanin should not be used routinely for empiric therapy because of their toxicity and selection for VRE. They should be considered empirically if there is severe mucositis, obvious line infection, severe hypotension or the patient is on quinolone prophylaxis.

The patient is reviewed daily and therapy altered depending on clinical response and the results of investigations. Microbiological confirmation of infection occurs in only one-third of patients. Antibiotics should usually be continued until the neutrophil count is more than 0.5 x 10^6/l. Amphotericin-B therapy may be indicated if the patient is neutropenic for more than 10 days, with unexplained fever and surface sites have grown fungi and/or if pulmonary infiltrates, skin lesions or sinus disease are present.

CONTROVERSIAL AREAS IN THE MANAGEMENT OF NEUTROPENIC CANCER PATIENTS

Role of Antibacterial Prophylaxis

Most studies have used quinolones (ciprofloxacin, ofloxacin) or co-trimoxazole as antibacterial prophylaxis resulting in a reduction in Gram negative infections, but no reduction in Gram positive infections, overall fever related morbidity or infection related mortality. Selection for resistant organisms is of concern.

Role of Antifungal Prophylaxis

Prophylactic fluconazole or amphotericin B reduces the number of invasive fungal infections but does not reduce the overall infection related mortality. Pre-emptive anti-fungal therapy as indicated above is probably a better strategy.

Role of Colony Stimulating Factors (G-CSF or GM-CSF)

More studies are required, but cytokines are not recommended routinely for therapy of febrile neutropenia. A possible prophylactic role if severe, prolonged neutropenia is expected.

Outpatient Therapy of Febrile Neutropenia

A lower risk patient group with febrile neutropenia has been defined who have solid tumours, the likely period of neutropenia less than 10 days and are clinically stable. In this subset, outpatient management may be appropriate, after initial inpatient assessment.

INFECTIONS IN ASPLENIC/HYPOSPLENIC CANCER PATIENTS

Overall, sepsis rates in asplenic patients are 2–5% and the mortality from sepsis is 1–3%. The risk of sepsis is greater for children, in patients with Hodgkin's disease and in the first 5 years after splenectomy.

Management Strategies

* Comprehensive education of the patient and relatives.
* Immunisation: pneumococcal, meningococcal and H. influenzae B vaccines indicated. Preferably vaccinate > 2 weeks prior to splenectomy.
* Specialist travel medicine advice is indicated prior to travel to malaria endemic area.
* Antibiotic prophylaxis following animal bites because of the risk of disseminated infection with *Capnocytophaga canimorsus.*
* Long-term prophylactic antibiotics are controversial but may be indicated in children less than 5 years of age, in the first 2 years following splenectomy, or following a documented episode of sepsis. Alternatively, patient initiated antibiotics at the first sign of infection may be appropriate.

REFERENCES

Anaissie, E., Vartivarian, S., Bodey, G.P., Legrand, C., Kantarjian, H, Abi-Said, D., Karl, C., Vadhan-Raj, S. (1996) Randomised comparison between antibiotics alone and antibiotics plus GM-CSF in cancer patients with fever and neutropenia. *Am J Med,* **100**, 17–23.

British Committee for Standards in Haematology Clinical Haematology Task Force (1996) Guidelines for the prevention and treatment of infection in patients with an absent or dysfunctional spleen. *Brit Med J,* **312**, 430–434.

Giamarellou, H. (1995) Empiric therapy for infections in the febrile, neutropenic, compromised host. *Med Clin N Am,* **79**, 559–580.

Gotzsche, P. and Johansen, H. (1997) Meta-analysis of prophylactic or empirical antifungal treatment versus placebo or no treatment in patients with cancer complicated by neutropenia. *Brit Med J,* **314**, 1238–1244.

Hughes, W.T., Pizzo, P.A., Wade, J.C., Armstrong, D., Webb, C.D. and Young, L.S. (1992) Evaluation of new anti-infective drugs for the treatment of febrile episodes in neutropenic patients. *Clin Infect Dis,* **15**(Suppl 1), S206–15.

Infectious Diseases Society of America. (1990) Guidelines for the use of antimicrobial agents in neutropenic patients with unexplained fever. *J Infect Dis,* **161**, 381–396.

PART XIV

PSYCHO-SOCIAL ISSUES IN CANCER

CHAPTER 59

BREAKING BAD NEWS

Rhonda F. Brown, Stewart M. Dunn, Afaf Girgis and Robert W. Sanson-Fisher

INTRODUCTION

This chapter provides an overview of the available data on the needs and preferences of patients about breaking bad news, the views and behaviours of health care providers and the evidence of the effects of breaking bad news on patients. A number of general principles relating to breaking bad news are also provided as a guide to clinicians, but should be adjusted according to the individual patient and situation.

PATIENT'S NEEDS AND PREFERENCES

Patients who receive a diagnosis of cancer are in a position of extreme uncertainty and vulnerability. Initially, they may react with significant emotional distress, but in the long term most seem to adjust well.

Uncertainty is a major cause of emotional distress for patients and relief from this uncertainty can, in itself, be therapeutic. Reduced anxiety, peace of mind and better psychological adjustment are just some of the benefits that patients report in relation to having been told their diagnosis of cancer.

However, the way in which bad news is told can significantly impact on the way in which a patient copes. For example, breaking bad news insensitively can increase its negative impact, the use of euphemisms in communicating about cancer may affect patient anxiety, and physician communication which is vague can contribute to psychological morbidity.

There is considerable variability in patients' experiences with and preferences for the communication of bad news. For example, patients may differ in their preference for who should communicate bad news, and whether family members or friends should accompany them to hear the results of diagnostic tests.

However, most cancer patients want to receive all information concerning their health status, whether the news is good or bad. They may regard prognosis and treatment information as being more important than diagnostic disclosure, and often prefer to be actively involved in treatment decision making.

Unfortunately, cancer patients are frequently dissatisfied with the amount of information they receive during medical consultations, as well as the way in which information is provided. It is important to remember that a poorly informed patient is more likely to be unsatisfied with the care provided, to be more anxious, to not cope well with the demands of illness and treatment, and to show lower compliance with recommended treatment.

HEALTH CARE PROVIDER'S VIEWS AND BEHAVIOURS

Physicians face profound problems in breaking bad news. They may feel a sense of failure for not being able to cure the patient or at least improve the situation. They may fear the patient's reaction to this news as well as their own emotional response.

Poor training in communication skills also leaves most doctors unable to give bad news appropriately. For example, most doctors make decisions about when, where and how to communicate with cancer patients based on their early experiences and personal judgements, rather than on the basis of sound empirical data.

As a consequence, doctors often underestimate the amount and sort of information patients require, are not adept at determining how effective they have been in imparting information, and are poor at estimating the extent of psychological distress in cancer patients receiving bad news.

GENERAL GUIDELINES FOR BREAKING BAD NEWS

The following guidelines for breaking bad news were developed by a consensus process by the Professional Education and Training Committee of the New South Wales Cancer Council and the Postgraduate Medical Council of New South Wales, and incorporate much of what is known regarding the needs and preferences of cancer patients, as well as those practices which are likely to reduce distress and psychological morbidity. They also provide a reassuring framework within which the doctor can provide appropriate and empathic care.

Who Should Tell Patients

- One person only should be responsible for breaking bad news. This is the responsibility of the senior clinician involved, and should not be delegated to junior and less experienced staff.
- If you are the person given the responsibility, make sure that the patient knows your name, role and designation.

When to Tell Patients

- The patient should be prepared for the possibility of bad news as early as possible in the diagnostic process, by the doctor of first contact. The possibility of bad news is usually the reason for further tests and referrals, and the patient needs to be made aware of this.
- Tell the patient his/her diagnosis as soon as it is certain. Make every attempt to tell the patient in person, almost never by phone, except in exceptional circumstances. Make sure sufficient time is allocated for this consultation, so that the patient has time to think about what you have said, as well as discuss it with you and ask questions.
- Whenever possible, plan the consultation for when all the test results are available.

Where to Tell Patients

- Make every effort to ensure privacy and make the patient feel comfortable. In a hospital setting, for example:
    - Avoid giving the patient the news during ward rounds or in the recovery room.
    - Find a quiet private room or close the curtains around the patient's bed.
    - Sit at the bedside at eye level with the patient, rather than standing over the patient.
    - Ensure the patient is clothed, not naked.
    - Ensure that interruptions such as beepers and telephone calls do not occur.

What to Tell Patients

- Assess the patient's understanding of the situation. His/her response will provide an appropriate starting point for you.
- Tell the patient the diagnosis and prognosis honestly and in simple language — avoid using technical jargon or euphemisms. Do not provide too much or too detailed information all at once. Give the facts relevant to the diagnosis, reasons for any future investigations, and outline the treatment options and their side effects. These facts may need to be repeated or revised several times and on different occasions, as the patient may remember little of the first consultation. Where relevant, write the information down, use pamphlets and diagrams, and/or provide an audiotape of the consultation.
- Always ask patients how much information they want about their prognosis, and ask this question on more than one occasion. An initial desire not to know, for example, may change during the course of a patient's illness or even during the consultation.
- Avoid giving a prognosis with a definite time scale, but do give the patient a broad, realistic time frame that will allow him/her to sort out personal affairs while still well enough. Avoid conveying the notion that there is no hope. On the other hand, do not pretend that palliative treatment is likely to cure the disease.
- Ask the patient who they would like to tell about the situation and then offer assistance and support in telling these people. If children are involved, recruit the help of a health professional who is used to dealing with children.
- Give the patient information about the availability of various support services, such as chaplains, cancer support groups, palliative care services, bereavement counselling for families and patients, and suggest referral to these, if desired by the patient.

How to Tell Patients

- Use non-verbal cues to convey warmth, empathy, encouragement and reassurance to the patient. For example, face the patient, make eye contact, do not interrupt when the patient is speaking, nod encouragingly, and give your full attention to the patient. It is critical that the patient feels that you have time to talk and listen. Hence, leave enough silence for the patient to express his/her feelings, and avoid writing notes, reading the patient's files, or looking elsewhere when the patient is talking to you. In some cases, touch may be very reassuring for the patient.
- Allow and encourage the patient to express his/her feelings, such as crying, freely. Accept the patient's feelings and concerns by letting him/her know that it is quite normal to feel this way.

This helps the patient feel accepted and makes him/her more likely to discuss concerns. Have tissues available for the patient and relatives.

Involving Others

- Ideally, family and significant others should be present, if the patient so wishes, in order to provide emotional support. They can also help the patient to recall information presented during the consultation.
- Where possible, arrange for another health professional, such as a junior medical officer, nurse or social worker, to be present when breaking bad news. This person should be someone to whom the patient will have access to after you have left and to provide support and supplement information.
- Ensure that the patient's general practitioner and other medical advisers are informed of the patient's level of understanding, so that they can use this as a starting point for giving more information to patients.

Dealing with Language and Cultural Differences

- Employ a trained health interpreter whenever there is a language difference between the doctor and patient. Avoid using untrained people such as family or general hospital staff as they may interpret incorrectly.
- Be sensitive to the person's culture, race, religious beliefs and social background. If appropriate, consult a health professional who has detailed knowledge and experience of that culture.

Documenting Information Given by Patients

- Document what the patient has been told, which family/other members have been told, who is permitted to know about the patient's situation, and the patient's reaction to the news. Be concise and include this on the medical record and discharge summary.

Addressing Your Own Feelings

- The patient may express a number of reactions including anger, denial, depression or acceptance. These reactions may initiate emotions in you that you find hard to handle. Ensure that you acknowledge your own shortcomings and emotional difficulties in breaking bad news, and if appropriate, avail yourself of support services. It is quite normal for the doctor to feel upset and it does no harm if the patient sees this.

REFERENCES

Bennett, M. and Alison, D. (1996) Discussing the diagnosis and prognosis with cancer patients. *Postgraduate Medical Journal*, 72, 25–29.

Butow, P.N., Dunn, S.M. and Tattersall, M.H.N. (1995) Communication with cancer patients: Does it matter? *Journal of Palliative Care*, 11, 34–38.

Butow, P.N., Kazemi, J.N., Beeney, L.J., Griffin, A-M., Dunn, S.M. and Tattersall, M.H.N. (1996) When the diagnosis is cancer: Patient communication experiences and preferences. *Cancer*, 77, 2630–2637.

Fallowfield, L. (1993). Giving sad and bad news. *Lancet*, 341, 476–478.

Girgis, A. and Sanson-Fisher, R.W. (1995) Breaking bad news: Consensus guidelines for medical practitioners. *Journal of Clinical Oncology*, **13**, 2449–2456.

Oken, D. (1961) What to tell cancer patients: A study of medical attitudes. *JAMA*, **175**, 1120–1127.

CHAPTER 60

PATIENTS' EXPECTATIONS OF CANCER

Robert W. Sanson-Fisher

INTRODUCTION

Above all else cancer patients desire a cure. Humans are prepared to endure much in an effort to preserve their lives. Cancer patients reflect this characteristic.

They are prepared to endure physical disfigurement, chemical and radiation assaults upon their bodies in an effort to increase the probability that their disease will be cured, or their life prolonged. People are willing to pay exhorbitant monies in an effort to find a cure, be it within or outside of traditional medicine.

Some individuals who have followed a rational, hard-nosed approach throughout life, will, when faced with a potentially fatal disease, become mystical. They might ascribe to what appears to be fanciful logic in an effort to explain why they may have contracted the disease and what can be done to prevent its spread, and thereby to the termination of their existence.

THE COMMUNITY'S VIEWS ON CANCER

Cancer remains one of the more feared diseases in our society, and is usually equated with pain, disfigurement and a protracted and unpleasant process of dying. These views remain in spite of strenuous efforts to inject a concept of hope and curability into the community's views about cancer.

Increasingly our failure to successfully achieve the goal of a cure for all cancers is being recognised by the community. In the 'war against cancer' it is slowly being acknowledged that there will be no quick 'victories', but rather a protracted, drawn out process with small incremental gains.

There is also a gaining recognition that these gains will require substantive expenditure of health care dollars, and often the active collaboration of the community in screening programs and their acceptance of what are often unpleasant treatments.

PATIENTS' PERCEPTION OF PROVIDERS' TECHNICAL COMPETENCE

Research indicates that patients value the technical skills which the health care profession brings to bear in its attempt to cure cancer. For every case of litigation, there are hundreds of patients who are highly satisfied with the technical care that they receive. This is in spite of its failure to effectively cure their condition.

By ensuring and publicising active quality assurance and strenuous efforts to improve undergraduate and postgraduate training, the health care professions have earned a reputation for pursuing high quality technical care. Patients are also relatively uninformed or not actual approvers about this component of care. This is not surprising given the range of views about what constitutes adequate care for some aspects of cancer treatment.

DESIRE FOR INFORMATION

One area where patients do have strong views about the quality of care relates to the amount of information supplied. It is in this area that there is now substantive data about patients' concerns and our apparent failure to meet their needs.

A growing body of evidence suggests that some patients will actively seek information about their condition. At the extremes, some of these groups indicate an almost insatiable desire for knowledge. They may pursue a wide variety of information gathering strategies in an effort to improve the information and thereby attempt to gain some control over their life. At the other extreme are the so-called 'blunters'. These people are stereotyped as wishing to give all decision making to the health care provider, with them having little desire for data regarding prognosis, treatment options and side effects. As with any population these two groups mark the extremes with a substantive proportion of people falling within the normal curve where individuals wish information on different issues at different times.

What is clear is that there is a need for individually tailored determination of patients' need for involvement and treatment decision making. It is also clear that not all clinicians are effective at determining what an individual patient may desire. That is, a clinician may judge that their patient is a blunter, while in fact their patient may wish to receive substantive amounts of information. The best way of determining what a patient wishes to know, is to simply ask them. While there are potential flaws in this logic, it is preferable to a clinician making judgements on the patient's behalf, given that our perceptions of their needs may be determined by a variety of factors. These include our desire not to have to pass on bad news, or the pressure of work which encourages us to limit the consultation time and our inability to deal with the potential consequences of providing substantive information to cancer patients. Providing choice and hence potential control to patients is likely to make it easier for them to deal with the consequences of the disease. It takes what is vague and unknown and converts it into concrete information from which the patient can then attempt to find some solution.

INFORMATION SUPPLIED IS DIFFICULT FOR A PATIENT TO UNDERSTAND OR RECALL

When one listens to the interactions between clinicians and cancer patients it is clear that a substantive number of clinicians provide information in a way which is difficult for the cancer patient to understand or recall. This view is supported by research exploring patients' recollection of what they have been told.

The most common problems exhibited by clinicians are that they use technical language such as benign, malignant, simple mastectomy and radical mastectomy. These words often have specific and have shared meanings for clinicians, but they may not be understood in the same way by the patient. For example, it is not uncommon to hear a clinician say that the success rate for this particular cancer is very good. Upon questioning, they could indicate that success rate for this cancer means that there is an 80% survival over a five-year period. A patient hearing this information may understandably not accept the value system of the clinician. For the patient a 20% probability that they will be dead in five years may be horrific.

Even when simple language is used it is often presented in a way which is difficult for the patient to recall. For example, to provide information to a patient after you have told them that they have a diagnosis of cancer is likely to be ineffective. Given the high anxiety rates which are associated with the confirmation of cancer as diagnosis, much of what is subsequently told to them will be forgotten. High anxiety is a powerful antidote to recall.

Clinicians often do not use those strategies which have been shown to increase the probability that an individual will be able to recall what they have been told. For example, gathering all the information about one topic, such as prognosis, and saying 'I'm now going to give you a prognosis', providing that information, and then summarising it, are strategies which aid recall.

The repetitious presentation of important units of information and the stressing that it is important, are also strategies which increase the probability of recall. Rather than asking patients whether they have understood what you have told them, a more effective technique is to ask them to repeat the information which you have just transmitted. It is then possible to correct if they have been mistaken about some of the information.

The responsibility for a failure to recall should not rest with the patient but with the clinician. It is the clinician's skill and ability which will largely determine how much an individual patient can recall.

SIDE EFFECTS OF THE DISEASE AND ITS TREATMENT SHOULD BE MINIMISED

Cancer patients are willing to tolerate substantive, unpleasant treatment in an effort to increase the probability that they will live for a longer period. Health care deliverers have a responsibility to minimise these negative side effects of treatment wherever possible. There must be an acknowledgment that the prevalence of side effects associated with some treatment may be high. For example, a recent study of patients under the care of medical oncologists indicate that the prevalence of physical symptoms, anxiety and depression are quite high (see Table 60.1).

Oncologists may not be aware of their patient's physical or psycho-social status in some of these areas. While most care givers believe that their awareness of these physical and psycho-social dimensions of a patient's wellbeing is important, it is clearly difficult for them to cover all issues in a limited time.

To address this, a number of strategies are being introduced by which clinicians can get accurate feedback from their patients concerning these dimensions of clinical care. One mechanism by which this could be achieved is the use of touch screen computers, which have been found to be highly acceptable to cancer patients. For example, in a recent survey patients indicated that a computer

Table 60.1 The prevalence of physical and psychological symptoms in patients with cancer

Measure	%
Physical Symptoms	
Hair loss	32.8
Nausea	40.2
Vomiting	11.5
Fatigue	66.4
Diarrhoea	23.0
Sore mouth	32.0
Constipation	22.0
Appetite loss	30.3
Hot flushes	38.7
Metallic taste in mouth	32.2
Psychological Symptoms	
Anxiety (clinical)	18.8
Depression (clinical)	18.7

survey was easy to complete, enjoyable, not stressful, not too personal, and a good way for their oncologist to get this type of information. Interestingly a majority of the patients (96.1%) also agreed that they would be happy for their doctors to receive a summary of the material which they had entered into the computer to put into their medical records. This mechanism provides a cost-efficient strategy by which a patient's perceptions can be routinely collected and provided to the clinician for future action.

SUMMARY

- Psycho-social issues and needs are an important area for clinicians to consider when providing high quality care.
- There is now an abundance of data suggesting that patients perceive that they are not receiving adequate care in the psycho-social domain.
- Patients are dissatisfied with the amount of information that they receive about their condition and their involvement with clinical decision making.
- Individual patients may vary in the amount of information that they require but a substantive proportion appear to want more information and involvement.
- There are few stringent methodological studies undertaken to examine the feasibility of meeting cancer patient's psycho-social and informational needs. That little evidence exists should not be a reason for not attempting to develop mechanisms by which their needs might be addressed.
- What is required is innovative strategies which could be incorporated into existing care and would allow the rigorous testing of approaches to improving the quality of care in this domain.

Table 60.2 Agreement between medical oncologists' perceptions and patients' reported levels of physical and psychological symptoms

Measure	Sensitivity (%)	Specificity (%)
Physical Symptoms		
Hair loss	80.0	79.3
Nausea	57.1	78.1
Vomiting	57.1	88.0
Fatigue	56.8	56.1
Hot flushes	25.0	100.00
Metallic taste in mouth	20.5	95.1
Skin rash	16.7	90.0
Psychological Symptoms		
Anxiety (clinical)	13.5	93.1
Depression (clinical)	13.5	93.8

CHAPTER 61

WORKING WITH AND MANAGING CANCER PATIENTS

Andrea Szendroe

INTRODUCTION

Working with people who have been diagnosed with cancer is both confronting and rewarding. It is difficult to generalise about cancer patients' experiences. However, there are similarities regarding the patients' approach to their illness.

Today's cancer patients are increasingly informed about their rights, specific diseases, treatments, services and resources. This increase in awareness seems to be the result of two very important developments:

1. a commitment to educating patients with increased awareness of medico-legal issues; and
2. patient access to information via information technology, self-help publications and the media.

Cancer patients are part of the broader community bringing with them a social history. The social statistics regarding violence, drug and alcohol issues, familial dysfunction, childhood trauma, literacy, homelessness, unemployment, etc. are the reality for some cancer patients. It is important to acknowledge the significance of 'social' statistics for cancer patients.

REACTIONS TO DIAGNOSIS AND TREATMENT

When any of us becomes seriously ill, four questions arise[1]:

1. Why me?
2. What caused it?
3. Can it be cured?
4. What now?

To answer the first question, requires the skill and experience of a trained counsellor. 'Why me?' is perhaps the most common reaction to a diagnosis of cancer. Most of us have a need to make sense of our experiences and cancer patients are no exception. Since medicine cannot explain the cause of all cancers, the patient must search for their own meaning. The remaining three questions are best addressed by the medical and nursing staff.

Initially, the newly diagnosed patient experiences a mourning process encapsulated by feelings of loss and grief. There is no psychological equilibrium which assists the patient with a cancer diagnosis. Patients are not given a rule book explaining how to manage a cancer diagnosis instead they rely on previous coping skills, whether they are helpful or not. A range of reactions may be expressed at the time of diagnosis including fear, disbelief, confusion, numbness, anger or withdrawal. People often cry, scream, cease to listen or hear, lose their concentration or stop communicating. Whilst it is difficult to observe raw grief, it is important to accept the patients' reactions as normal.

LISTENING TO AND PROCESSING INFORMATION FOR CANCER PATIENTS

There is an expectation amongst health care professionals that patients hear and understand the information provided. However, patients retain very little content from the initial information about diagnosis or treatment. Many patients have difficulty appreciating the meaning of information imparted by health care professionals. This is not because the information is complex but more commonly because the information is not delivered in plain English.

Establishing how patients learn is important. Health care professionals should be aware of the different learning tools as such, audio, visual and verbal. Where English is not the patient's first language, health care interpreters are an essential ally.

Social work counsellors are able to ascertain the learning needs of patients and guide the treating team as to the best tool for communicating with individual patients. Whilst social work counsellors do not deliver disease information they do assist the patient in understanding the content.

Patients are interested in how information translates to them, their carers and family. Social work counsellors can recognise the uniqueness of the patient's situation by translating both information and disease processes to the individual context.

COMMON ISSUES ARISING FOR CANCER PATIENTS

A range of issues arise for cancer patients during the course of their treatment and can continue to have an impact after treatment is ceased.

Isolation

Isolation is a common concern for cancer patients. After the initial attention from family and friends, cancer patients are often left to manage alone. Health care professionals often assume family will offer support, encouragement, practical and emotional assistance throughout the treatment phase. This is not always the case for cancer patients, some of whom manage the entire experience alone.

Changing Roles

A common issue is the change to roles previously held by the patient. Roles such as parent, partner, friend, employee, sibling and child change at the point of diagnosis. Whether the patient is unwell or not, others will automatically treat them differently. The patient may be forced to relinquish certain roles for practical reasons or because others have decided they are unable to manage. Either way the patient is further compromised by a loss of identity and control.

The reverse can happen in that the patient is expected throughout treatment to continue to perform certain roles as this allows significant others to feel secure. Cancer patients have a vested interest in keeping up appearances in order to reduce the stress experienced by loved ones and will go to enormous lengths to protect their loved ones.

Loss of Sexual Function

Some cancers directly affect patients', sexuality and sexual function. This loss of control for some cancer patients is overwhelming. The patient experiences a mourning for the loss of intimacy which may never return. This may be due to the particular medical intervention, a loss of opportunity to explore options or an inability of the patient and/or their partner in pursuing intimacy. Whatever the reason, many cancer patients cease sexual activity and expression at diagnosis.

Coping Strategies

Coping strategies are often learnt, automatic and often the most public of expressions. Many cancer patients display coping strategies which are confronting to others, such as seeking open discussion regarding their diagnosis and treatment or not communicating at all. Most of us retreat to learnt coping strategies in a time of crisis whether these strategies are helpful or not. Cancer patients are the same, however their crisis does not necessarily go away they simply learn to live with it and in it.

Social work counsellors can assist patients in identifying which coping skills are helpful or unhelpful. Working together, the patient and social work counsellor can explore new and different coping strategies.

FACTORS INFLUENCING PATIENT DECISION MAKING

There are a number of factors which influence the decision making of patients. Whilst these influences are not always well understood by health care professionals they are meaningful to the patient. The following list summarises the most common factors and situations:

- superstitious beliefs about disease, treatment and prognosis
- spiritual beliefs about the purpose of life experiences
- disbelief in medical technology
- commitment and belief in 'alternative' healing
- cultural practices which disallow certain medical practices
- cultural differences with regard to sickness and healing
- impact of previous exposure to cancer treatments as patient, carer or observer
- childhood memories or experience of the death of a loved one to cancer
- lack of understanding of information and/or consent process
- time pressure for decision making with an indecisive character
- emotional reactions to information

Social work counsellors work with patients in an attempt to ascertain the cause of indecision or incongruent decision making in contrast to what has been advised. Assessing the patients understanding of their disease and treatment plan is a fundamental aspect of counselling cancer patients. Skilled explorative questioning will unpack the layers of learnt protection to reveal the patients' belief system.

How the patient makes sense of their diagnosis often indicates how they view the task ahead of them. Similarly, establishing a patients' coping history using previous experiences indicates a potential pattern for future coping strategies and acts as the basis for a therapeutic contract.

GUIDELINES FOR CONSIDERATION WHEN WORKING WITH CANCER PATIENTS

- Reassurance is helpful, assurance can not be guaranteed.
- Information will be processed in the patients' own way and time.
- Patients require information to be given more than once.
- Establish how individual patients best absorb information, whether in verbal, visual, or written form or in a combination of these forms.
- Remember the patient's environment is unique and includes spiritual, psychological, sexual, emotional, social, practical, economic and cultural aspects.
- Remind patients of the side effects of each treatment modality.
- Acknowledge the patients ability to self-monitor especially when at home.
- Explore what is influencing the patient's ability to make decisions.
- Be realistic about the time frame for each treatment modality.
- Remember to include recovery time when completing paperwork for the patient.
- Always offer an interpreter when English is not the patient's first language.
- Acknowledge the patient as a partner in the working relationship.
- Acknowledge the importance of coping mechanisms and work with them.

REFERENCES

1. Bates, E. and Lapsley, H. (1985) *The Health Machine: The Impact of Medical Technology*, p. 22. Ringwood, Australia: Penguin.

CHAPTER 62

MEDICAL STATISTICS
AND CLINICAL TRIALS

Jane P. Matthews

INTRODUCTION

An understanding of basic statistical concepts is essential for the proper design, conduct, analysis and interpretation of clinical trials. This is particularly important in oncology, which requires a rigorous and unbiased evaluation of new cancer therapies to determine 'world's best practice'.

P-VALUES AND STATISTICAL SIGNIFICANCE

Let us suppose we want to determine whether drug A is superior, inferior or equivalent to drug B in treating a particular condition, and we have run a randomised trial with 50 patients receiving drug A and 50 receiving drug B. If 19 patients have responded to drug A and only 11 to drug B, can we confidently conclude that drug A is superior to drug B? If we were a pharmaceutical company, would we abandon production of drug B and gear up to producing drug A instead? Although our best estimate of the response rate for drug A is 38% and that for drug B is 22%, how likely is it that we could have obtained such a big difference, or an even bigger difference, by chance if the true response rates for the two drugs were identical?

Statistical theory enables us to calculate this probability, the p-value[1], as 0.13, or about one chance in eight. All else being equal, a doctor might prefer to prescribe drug A to his or her next patient, but if there were a considerable difference in costs or more side effects with drug A, he or she would be wanting more evidence of a true difference. The pharmaceutical company would certainly be hesitant to commit vast resources to producing drug A on such slender evidence. If the same percentage response rates had been observed in a trial with 100 patients on each drug, the p-value would have been 0.014, about one chance in 72, and would have provided much more compelling evidence of a true difference.

Conventionally, p-values less than 0.05 (one chance in 20) have been labelled as being statistically 'significant' and p-values less than 0.01 (one chance in 100) as 'highly significant'. If the trial had had 10,000 patients on each drug, with 11% of patients on drug A responding and 10% on drug B responding, the difference in response rates would have been statistically 'significant' with a p-value of 0.02. However, the 1% difference in response rates might not be considered to be sufficiently important to outweigh any disadvantages of drug A. A statistically significant difference is not necessarily a clinically important difference, just as a statistically non-significant difference may actually be clinically important, if it can be validated. A p-value on its own does not provide sufficient information for rational decision making.

CONFIDENCE INTERVALS

More information can be obtained from a confidence interval, which in this context is essentially the set of true differences in response rates which are compatible with the data obtained in the trial[2]. A 95% confidence interval (CI) for a particular parameter is one which has a probability of 0.95 of containing the true value of the parameter, or, in other words, one chance in 20 of not including the true value. If we had run our trial comparing drugs A and B on a different set of patients, we would probably have obtained different response rates for A and B and a different confidence interval for the difference in the response rates. If we ran the trial 100 times then we would expect 95% of the 95% confidence intervals to contain the true value of the difference in the response rates.

In many situations the limits of a 95% confidence interval for a parameter can be estimated by taking an estimate of the parameter plus or minus two times (or, more exactly, 1.96 times) the standard error of the estimate, where the standard error is a measure of the variability of the estimate. In our first trial, $^{19}/_{50}$ patients (38%) responded to drug A and $^{11}/_{50}$ (22%) to drug B. Our best estimate of the difference in response rates is 16%, and this estimate has a standard error of approximately 9%. The estimated 95% confidence interval for the true difference is thus –2% to 34%. The width of this confidence interval (approximately four times the standard error of the estimated difference) shows how poorly the difference in response rates has been estimated by this trial. The results are compatible with the response rate on A being 2% lower than that on B right through to it being 34% higher than that on B. Inclusion of the value 0% in the confidence interval reflects the fact that there was no significant difference between the response rates.

In our second trial with 100 patients in each arm, the 95% confidence interval would have been 3% to 29%. Non-inclusion of the value 0% reflects the fact that the difference was statistically significant. Again the confidence interval is wide and the true difference has been poorly estimated. In our trial with 10,000 patients on each drug, the estimated difference in response rates was 1% with an estimated standard error of 0.4% and thus the estimated 95% confidence interval for the true difference in response rates was 0.2% to 1.8%.

As a rule of thumb, to reduce the width w of a confidence interval by a factor f say to w/f, it is necessary to reduce the standard error of the estimate by the factor f^2, which requires the sample size to be increased by a factor f^2; for example, to reduce a confidence interval to half its width, four times as many patients are required, whereas to reduce a confidence interval to one tenth its width, 100 times as many patients are required.

PLANNING A TRIAL

The most important ingredient in planning any trial is to determine clearly what the objectives of the trial are, both in the short and the long term, that is, to determine not only what question the trial is asking, but how the answer to that question will be used in future practice. The trial should be useful no matter what its outcome is.

Two types of errors can be made. The trial might demonstrate a statistically significant benefit when no such benefit exists (false positive or type I error), or the trial might fail to detect a clinically important benefit when such a benefit does exist (false negative or type II error). The probability of the first error is known as the 'significance level' or alpha, and is conventionally taken to be 0.05. The probability of the second error is known as beta; it is more common to refer to (1 − beta) which is known as the 'power' of a study. It represents the probability that the study will be able to detect a pre-specified clinically important benefit if it exists. This probability depends on what is considered to be a clinically important benefit. The smaller the benefit, the larger the trial will need to be to pick it up. Trials are often planned to have a power of 0.8 or 0.9. Although higher powers are desirable, the number of patients required for powerful trials is often prohibitively large. Furthermore there is an ethical requirement to limit the number of patients in a trial to reduce the number of patients treated on a potentially inferior treatment.

PHASE I TRIALS

New drugs or treatments in cancer often go through three phases of testing in humans[3]. Phase I trials are run to determine the 'maximum tolerated dose' (MTD) for a given method of treatment delivery, working on the principle that the higher the dose the more effective the treatment will be in killing the tumour cells. However, the higher the dose the greater the risk of damage to normal cells. Criteria for grading different organ toxicities exist with grades from 0 to 4 corresponding essentially to none, mild, moderate, severe and life-threatening toxicities respectively[4].

A typical phase I trial might treat three patients at each dose level in a series of increasing doses until at least one patient experiences a life-threatening toxicity or two patients experience a severe toxicity. The preceding dose might then be considered the most appropriate dose for future trials, but a further three or so patients may be treated on this dose level before the phase I trial is considered closed.

PHASE II TRIALS

Phase II trials are run to determine how effective the new treatment is likely to be in different types of tumours. Efficacy is usually based on the objective response rate, that is the percentage of patients who achieve a complete response (corresponding to complete disappearance of the disease) or a partial response (corresponding to at least a 50% reduction in the disease present at the time of commencing the treatment)[4].

Separate trials may be run for each tumour type. Each trial may be set up in two stages. In the first stage a fixed number of patients may be treated. If none of these patients respond, the trial will be closed. For example, if a new treatment would only be considered worthy of further study in a particular tumour type if it produced responses in at least 20% of patients with that tumour, the first stage of the trial would include 14 patients. If the true response rate is 20%, the probability that none of the first 14 patients treated will respond is simply $(0.8)^{14}$ or 0.044. Thus the probability of closing the trial after the first stage if the treatment has a response rate > 20% will be < 0.05. If at least one of the first fourteen patients responds, the trial may proceed to accrue a fixed total number of patients to enable the response rate to be estimated with a pre-specified degree of precision. For example, if the true response rate were 25% and 50 patients were entered in the trial, the expected standard error of the estimate of the response rate would be 6%. The maximum standard error for this sample size would be 7%, occurring with a response rate of 50%.

PHASE III TRIALS

A phase III trial is generally run to compare the results of the new treatment with those of the current standard treatment, hoping to show either that the new treatment is more effective than the old or that it is equally effective but less toxic. The study end-points could include survival duration, response rates, time to disease progression, toxicity and quality of life.

Although it is tempting to treat all the patients on the trial with the new treatment and compare their results with the results of past patients on the standard treatment, this could lead to a bias. One could never guarantee that any differences in outcome were due to treatment differences rather than differences in the prognostic characteristics of the groups of patients being treated, or different methods of diagnosing the patients or assessing their outcomes.

The only valid way of comparing the treatments is by randomising patients to one treatment or the other, for example by using a computer-generated randomisation chart. The doctor's decision to enter the patient on the trial must be made before he or she knows which treatment the patient will be allocated, thus eliminating any selection bias. Before randomising the patient, the doctor must confirm that the patient satisfies the eligibility criteria for the trial and has consented to participate regardless of the allocated treatment.

Unfortunately, large numbers of patients are required in a randomised trial to pick up even relatively large treatment effects. For example, a trial comparing two treatments would need to accrue approximately 270 patients to have a probability (power) of 0.9 of detecting a 20% increase in response rates from 50% to 70% with a significance level of 0.05, 480 patients to detect a 15% increase, 1,100 to detect a 10% increase and 4,300 to detect a 5% increase.

META-ANALYSES

Individual trials are unlikely to have the power to detect small but clinically worthwhile differences between treatments, but if several trials have addressed the same issue, for example the role of adjuvant chemotherapy in post-menopausal breast cancer patients, their results can be combined in a meaningful way. A 'meta-analysis' or 'systematic overview' pools the results from individual trials.

To avoid bias, only randomised trials should be included in the meta-analysis and, ideally, the results from all relevant trials (published or unpublished, completed or abandoned) should be included. Similarly, the results from all randomised patients should be included in the analysis, even if some patients did not complete or even commence their allocated treatment ('intention-to-treat' analysis).

It is recognised that treatment effects may differ in the different trials due to different populations studied and different treatment protocols, however it is assumed that the direction of the effect will be the same even if the magnitude is not. Meta-analyses should be carried out according to a well-defined protocol outlining inclusion criteria, methods of identifying eligible trials and methods of analysing and combining the results[5].

REFERENCES

1. Peto, R., Pike, M.C., Armitage, P., Breslow, N.E., Cox, D.R., Howard, S.V., Mantel, N., McPherson, K., Peto, J. and Smith, P.G. Design and analysis of randomized clinical trials requiring prolonged observation of each patient. I. Introduction and design. *Br J Cancer*,1976, **34**, 585–612. II Analysis and examples. *Br J Cancer*, 1977, **35**,1–39.

2. Armitage, P. and Berry, G. (1994) *Statistical Methods in Medical Research* (3rd edn). Oxford, United Kingdom: Blackwell Scientific Publications.

3. Fisher, R.J., Coates, A.S. and Colebatch, J.H. (eds) (1987) *Guidelines for Clinical Trials in Cancer*. Sydney: The Clinical Oncological Society of Australia Inc.

4. Miller, A.B., Hoogstraten, B., Staquet, M. and Winkler, A. (1981) Reporting results of cancer treatment. *Cancer*, **47**, 207–214.

5. Sacks, H.S., Berrier, J., Reitman, D., Ancona-Berk VA and Chalmers TC. (1987) Meta-analyses of randomized controlled trials. *N Engl J Med*, **316**, 450–455.

APPENDIX I

ECOG[a] PERFORMANCE STATUS CRITERIA

Grades	Scale
0	Fully, active, able to carry on all pre-disease performance without restriction (Karnofsky 90–100).
1	Restricted in physically strenuous activity but ambulatory and able to carry out work of a light or sedentary nature, such as light housework, office work (Karnofsky 70–80).
2	Ambulatory and capable of all self-care, confined to bed or chair less than 50% of waking hours (Karnofsky 50–60).
3	Capable of only limited self-care, confined to bed or chair more than 50% of waking hours (Karnofsky 30–40).
4	Completely disable. Cannot carry out any self-care. Totally confined to bed or chair (Karnofsky 10–20).
5	Dead.

[a] Eastern Co-operative Oncology Group

APPENDIX II

COMMONLY USED
CHEMOTHERAPY PROTOCOLS

BREAST CANCER

Adjuvant Therapy

CMF

Cyclophosphamide	100 mg/m^2 po days 1 to14
Methotrexate	40 mg/m^2 IV days 1 and 8
5-Fluorouracil	600 mg/m^2 IV days 1 and 8

Repeat every 28 days for six courses. Radiotherapy may be delivered concurrently or sequentially as appropriate.

AC

Doxorubicin	60 mg/m^2 IV day 1
Cyclophosphamide	600 mg/m^2 IV day 1

Repeat every 21 days for 4 courses. (Epirubicin 90 mg/m^2 may be substituted for doxorubicin (adriamycin). Radiotherapy can not be delivered concurrently with this treatment regimen.

AC/CMF

4 cycles of AC (doses as above) followed by 3 cycles of CMF (doses as above).

Locally Advanced Breast Cancer

AC $\times$ 3 cycles $\rightarrow$ RT and/or Surgery $\rightarrow$ CMF $\times$ 3
(CMF and AC doses are as described above)

Advanced (Metastatic) Breast Cancer

AC

Doxorubicin	50 mg/m^2 IV day 1
Cyclophosphamide	750 mg/m^2 IV day 1

Repeat every 21 days. There is no fixed number of cycles. A total cumulative dose of 450 mg/m^2 of doxorubicin should not be exceeded.

Mitoxantrone

Mitoxantrone	10–14 mg/m^2 IV day 1

Repeat every 21 days.

CMF(P)

Cyclophosphamide	100 mg/m^2 po days 1 to 14
Methotrexate	40 mg/m^2 IV days 1 and 8
5-Fluorouracil	600 mg/m^2 IV days 1 and 8
Prednisolone	40 mg/m^2 po days 1 to 14

Repeat every 28 days.

CARCINOMA OF UNKNOWN PRIMARY SITE

PAC

Cisplatin	60 mg/m^2 IV day 1
Doxorubicin	50 mg/m^2 IV day 1
Cyclophosphamide	500 mg/m^2 IV day 1
Repeat every three weeks.	

Consider when the likely primary site includes ovary, lung or breast.

FAM (Modified)

5-Fluorouracil	600mg/m^2 IV day 1, 22
Doxorubicin	30mg/m^2 IV day 1, 22
Mitomycin C	10mg/m^2 IV day 1 only
Repeat every 6 weeks.	

Consider when the likely primary site includes stomach or pancreas

ECF

Note that this requires a port-a-cath or Hickmans catheter. Unless contraindicated, patients with these indwelling venous access devices on this regimen should receive Warfarin 1 mg daily.

5-Fluorouracil	200 mg/m^2/day by protracted venous infusion
Epirubicin	50 mg/m^2 day 1
Cisplatin	60 mg/m^2 day 1

Cycles of epirubicin and cisplatin repeated every 21 days.

CNS MALIGNANCIES

PCV Regimen

Procarbazine	60 mg/m^2/day po days 8–21
CCNU (Lomustine)	110 mg/m^2 po day 1

Vincristine   1.4 mg/m² (max 2 mg) IV day 8 and 29

Repeat every 8 weeks.

Intensive Course PCV (I-PCV)

Procarbazine   75 mg/m²/day po days 8 to 21
CCNU (Lomustine)   130 mg/m² po day 1
Vincristine   1.4 mg/m² (no max) IV day 8 and 29

Repeat every 6 weeks

This regimen should be used only for selected patients.

ENDOCRINE MALIGNANCIES

Adrenocortical Carcinoma

op-DDD

op-DDD   5–15 mg/kg po daily(in 3 divided doses)

PAC

Cisplatin   60 mg/m² IV day 1
Doxorubicin   50 mg/m² IV day 1
Cyclophosphamide   500 mg/m² IV day 1

Repeat every 21 days.

Malignant Carcinoid

Octreotide   50 g SC bd day 1
                        100 g SC bd day 2
                        150 g SC tds thereafter

For symptom relief.

Streptozotocin   500 mg/m² IV daily for 5 days
Doxorubicin   50 mg/m² IV day 1, 22

Repeat every 6 weeks.

Thyroid Carcinoma

Doxorubicin   60 mg/m² IV day 1

Repeat every 3 weeks.

Doxorubicin   50 mg/ m² IV day 1
Cisplatin   60 mg/ m² IV day 1

Repeat every 3 weeks.

GASTROINTESTINAL MALIGNANCIES

Cisplatin/5-FU
Cisplatin	80 mg/m^2 IV day 1
5-Fluorouracil	800 mg/m^2 continuous IV infusion days 1–4

The usual total dose of RT given concurrently with chemotherapy is 35 Gy although will vary according to indication.

STOMACH

ECF

Epirubicin	50 mg/m^2 day 1
Cisplatin	60 mg/m^2 day 1
5-Fluorouracil	200 mg/m^2/day by protracted venous infusion

Cycles are repeated every 21 days.

Warfarin 1 mg daily is given for prophylaxis of catheter blockage.

COLON

Post-operative adjuvant and chemotherapy for advanced disease

5-Fluorouracil	425 mg/m^2 days 1–5
Leucovorin	20 mg/m^2 days 1–5

Cycles are repeated every 28 days, for 6 cycles.

The initial cycle of 5FU may be at 375 mg/m^2 d 1–5 if impaired 5FU clearance suspected.

Fluorouracil (protracted venous infusion)

5-Fluorouracil 300 mg/m^2/day as a protracted venous infusion (PVI) for 3 month blocks without break (unless toxicity occurs).

ANAL CARCINOMA

5-FU Mitomycin C
5-Fluorouracil	1000 mg/m^2/day as a continuous 4 day IV infusion during the first and last weeks of the RT.
Mitomycin C	10 mg/m^2 IV day 1 of each 5-FU infusion

GERM CELL TUMOURS

First Line Therapy

PEB

Cisplatin	100 mg/m^2 IV day 1 (or 20 mg/m^2 days 1 to 5)
Etoposide	120 mg/m^2 IV days 1 to 3 (or 100 mg/m^2 days 1 to 5)
Bleomycin	30 Units IV or IM days 1, 8, and 15

Give with prophylactic G-CSF, 263 or 300mg sc daily for 7 days, starting one day following initial chemotherapy. Treatment is repeated every 21 days.

Relapsed or Refractory Disease

VIP (Indiana University)

Cisplatin	20 mg/m² IV days 1 to 5
Vinblastine	0.1 mg/kg/day IV days 1,2
Ifosfamide	1.2 g/m²/day IV days 1 to 5, as a 4 hour infusion
Mesna (loading dose)	400 mg IV day 1
Mesna (infusion)	1200 mg/day IV days 1–5

GENITOURINARY MALIGNANCIES

Bladder

M-VAC

Methotrexate	30 mg/m² days 1, 15 and 22
Vinblastine	3 mg/m² days 2, 15 and 22
Doxorubicin	30 mg/m² day 2
Cisplatin	70 mg/m² day 2

Cycles are repeated every 28 days.

CMV

Cisplatin	100 mg/m² day 2
Methotrexate	30 mg/m² days 1 and 8
Vinblastine	4 mg/m² days 1 and 8

Folinic acid 15 mg every 6 hours for 4 doses is given 24 hours after each dose of methotrexate. Cycles are repeated every 21 days

LUNG CANCER

Small Cell Lung Cancer

PE

Cisplatin	25 mg/m² IV, daily for 3 days
Etoposide	120 mg/m² IV, daily for 3 days

Treatment is repeated every 21 days, for 6 cycles

CE

Carboplatin	AUC 5 to 6 (or 100 mg/m² daily for 3 days)
Etoposide	120 mg/m² IV daily for 3 days

Treatment is repeated every 21 to 28 days for 6 cycles.

Non-Small Cell Lung Cancer

CV

Cisplatin   100 mg/m^2 IV on days 1 and 29
Vinorelbine   25–30 mg/m^2 days 1, 8, 15, and 22
(Carboplatin AUC 6 can be used in place of cisplatin)

MELANOMA

Dacarbazine (DTIC)   800 mg/m^2 over 30 mins in 500 ml normal saline.

Cycles are repeated every 21 days

GYNAECOLOGICAL CANCERS

Ovarian Cancer

Cisplatin   75 mg/m^2 IV
Paclitaxel   135–175 mg/m^2 IV over 3 or 24 hours

Carboplatin   AUC 5 or 350 mg/m^2 in 500 ml D5W over one hour.
Cyclophosphamide   500 mg/m^2 in 500 ml N/S over one hour.

Cycles are repeated every 21 days for 6 cycles provided evidence of response.

Mixed Mullerian Carcinomas

Cyclophosphamide 500 mg/m^2
Doxorubicin 50 mg/m^2
Cisplatin 100 mg/m^2

Cycles are repeated every 21/28 days.

Germ Cell Tumours

(Choriocarcinoma, endodermal sinus tumour, embryonal tumour or grade 3 immature teratoma if totally resected)

Cisplatin   100 mg/m^2 IV D1
Etoposide   120 mg/m^2 IV D1–3
Bleomycin   30 units IV D 1 and weekly

Cycles repeated every 3 weeks for 3–4 cycles.

Cisplatin   50 mg/m^2 IV D1
Vinblastine   4 mg/m^2 IV D1
Bleomycin 1   5 mg IV day 1, 8*, 15*

Vulval Carcinoma

Cisplatin   50 mg/m^2 D1 IV (week 1 and 4)
5 Fluorouracil   1,000mg/m^2 IV D1–5 (week 1 and 4)

Gestational Trophoblastic Disease

Low risk

Methotrexate	35 mg/m^2 im D 1, 3, 4, 7
Folinic acid	10–15 mg po/im D 2, 4, 6, 8

Cycles are repeated every 2 weeks 2–3 cycles beyond negative HCG

Medium to high risk

MECCA

D1	Actinomycin D 0.5 mg IV
	Etoposide 100 mg/m^2 IV
	Methotrexate 100 mg IVI stat then 200 mg IV infusion over 12 hours
D2	Actinomycin D 0.5 mg IVI
	Etoposide 100 mg/m^2 IVI
	Folinic acid 15 mg q 6 hourly ↔ 12, starting 24 hours after 1st dose of methotrexate.
D8	Vincristine 1 mg IV
	Cyclophosphamide 600 mg/m^2 IVI

Cycles to be repeated every 2 weeks

LYMPHOMA

Low Grade Non-Hodgkins Lymphoma

Chlorambucil	10 mg daily for 14 days
(± Prednisone 50 mg daily for 14 days)	

Intermediate Grade Non-Hodgkins Lymphoma

CHOP

Cyclophosphamide	750 mg/m^2
Doxorubicin	50 mg/m^2
Vincristine	1.4 mg/m^2 (max. 2 mg)
Prednisone	100 mg po days 1–5
Cycles are repeated every 21 days.	

G-CSF should be used to deliver full dosdes, on schedule.

Hodgkin's Disease

ABVD

Doxorubicin	25 mg/m^2 day 1
Bleomycin	15 mg day 1
Vinblastine	6 mg/m^2 day 1
Dacarbazine	375 mg/m^2 day 1

Cycles are repeated every 2 weeks.

SARCOMA

Soft Tissue Sarcoma (adults)

Doxorubicin	75 mg/m^2 as a single agent, or
Doxorubicin	60 mg/m^2
Dacarbazine	1000 mg/m^2, or
Doxorubicin	60 mg/m^2
Cyclophosphamide	750 mg/m^2

Cycles are repeated every 21 days.

Osteosarcoma

Methotrexate	3 g/m^2
Doxorubicin	60 mg/m^2

Folinic acid rescue (15 mg every 6 hours for 8 doses, starting 24 hours after methotrexate) must be used with this regimen. Patients must have methotrexate levels measured at 36 and 48 hours on at least the first cycle.

Ewing's Sarcoma

OCA/OCA/VIM

OCA

Vincristine	1.5 mg/m^2 (max 2 mg)
Cyclophosphamide	1200 mg/m^2
Doxorubicin	30 mg/m^2 days 1 and 2

VIM

Etoposide	100 mg/m^2 days 1–5
Ifosfamide	1.8 g/m^2 days 1–5
Mesna	1.8 g/m^2 days 1–5, plus 450 mg/m^2 after final ifosfamide dose+

COLOUR PLATES

NON-MELANOMA SKIN CANCERS

(See Chapter 41, page 260.)

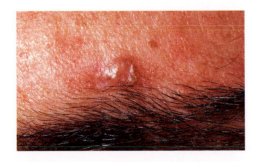

Plate 1A Basal cell carcinoma of the skin (Rodent ulcer). Note classic pearly edge.

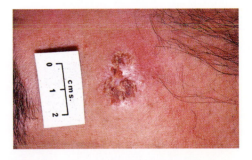

Plate 1B Basal cell carcinoma of the skin (Rodent ulcer)

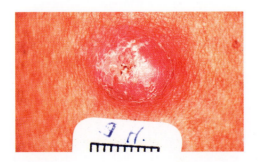

Plate 2A Squamous cell carcinoma of the skin

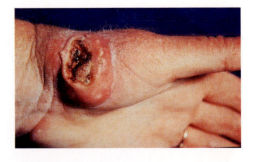

Plate 2B Squamous cell carcinoma of the skin

MALIGNANT MELANOMAS OF THE SKIN

(See Fast Fact Sheet 5, Chapter 41 and 42. For clinical presentation and staging of malignant melanoma, see Chapter 41, page 260.)

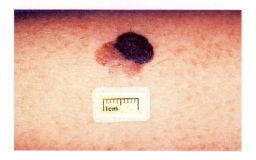

Plate 3A Early malignant melanoma of the skin

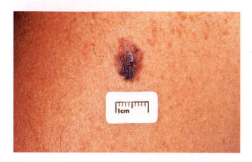

Plate 3B Early malignant melanoma of the skin

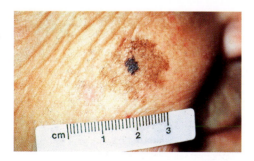

Plate 3C Lentigo malignant melanoma

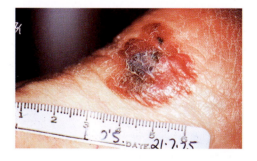

Plate 3D Acral lentiginous malignant melanoma

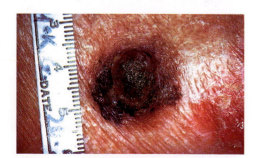

Plate 3E Nodular malignant melanoma

INDEX

Page numbers in bold refer to figures and tables.